T0202449

OXFORD MEDICAL PUBLICATIONS

Drugs in Anaesthesia and Intensive Care

FIFTH EDITION

Drugs in Anaesthesia and Intensive Care

FIFTH EDITION

Edward Scarth
Consultant in Anaesthesia and Intensive Care Medicine,
Torbay Hospital,
Torquay, Devon, UK

Susan Smith
Formerly Consultant in Anaesthesia and Intensive Care,
Cheltenham Hospital, UK, now practising in Pre- and
In-hospital Trauma Care and Event Medicine

OXFORD
UNIVERSITY PRESS

OXFORD
UNIVERSITY PRESS

Great Clarendon Street, Oxford, OX2 6DP,
United Kingdom

Oxford University Press is a department of the University of Oxford.
It furthers the University's objective of excellence in research, scholarship,
and education by publishing worldwide. Oxford is a registered trade mark of
Oxford University Press in the UK and in certain other countries

© Oxford University Press 2016

The moral rights of the authors have been asserted
First edition published in 1990
Second edition published in 1997
Third edition published in 2003
Fourth edition published in 2011

Published in the United States of America by Oxford University Press
198 Madison Avenue, New York, NY 10016, United States of America

British Library Cataloguing in Publication Data
Data available

Library of Congress Control Number: 2015949834

ISBN 978–0–19–876881–4

Printed and bound in Turkey by Promat

Preface to the fifth edition

The aims of this book remain true to those of previous editions. In order to make changes prior to the publication of this edition, a peer review process was undertaken. We have tried to accommodate the changes that were proposed by the reviewers and are grateful for their comments. The book continues in its original structured format, the major changes being the removal of agents no longer in use, the addition of new pharmacological drugs, and the introduction of drug comparison tables and a number of drug structure diagrams. We hope that this new edition will remain popular with critical care professionals, operating department personnel, paramedics, pre-hospital care specialists, and anaesthetists of all grades, in addition to providing sound examination preparation for the FRCA and FFICM. Any comments will be gratefully received via e-mail to edscarth@me.com and susan.smith@glos.nhs.uk.

E.J.S.
S.P.S
Cheltenham, January 2015

Preface to the first edition

The aim of this book is twofold: firstly to summarize concisely the main pharmacodynamic and pharmacokinetic properties of the drugs with which the practising anaesthetist might be expected to be familiar. Secondly, it seeks to introduce the candidate for the FRCAnaes (and, in particular, for the second part of this examination) to an ordered scheme for the presentation of information, which we have found to be of value in both the written and oral sections of the examinations. Examiners are more likely to turn a blind eye to minor errors or omissions of knowledge if they are in the context of a clear and well-ordered presentation. A further advantage of this scheme of presentation is that it allows rapid access to specific information. It is our hope that this compendium will prove to be a useful rapid source of reference for clinical anaesthetists in their day-to-day endeavours, both in the theatre and intensive care unit.

This book is intended to complement, rather than to replace, the standard texts on pharmacology for anaesthetists, since it includes no discussion of the principles of pharmacology, an understanding of which is essential for the clinical use of drugs. We feel that these aspects are very satisfactorily covered elsewhere.

Although our research has been as comprehensive as possible, there will obviously remain some information that will have eluded us, or perhaps remains to be discovered. Many practitioners will disagree with our choice of 172 drugs. Any comments or suggestions will be most gratefully and humbly received in order that further editions of this book may hopefully prove to be more useful.

Finally, we should like to thank the members of the Oxford Regional Drug Information Unit, the many drug company information departments, and all our colleagues for their help and support in this venture. In particular, we should like to thank Professor Roy Spector and Drs John Sear and Tim Peto for their invaluable advice on the manuscript.

M.P.S
S.P.S.
Oxford, 1990

How to use this book

The layout of this book requires some explanation in order for the reader to gain the maximum benefit. The 184 drugs we have included are arranged in alphabetical order to obviate both reference to an index and the artificial categorization of some drugs. Each drug is presented in an identical format and confined to one, two, or three pages under the following headings:

Uses The main clinical uses are listed.

Chemical A brief chemical classification is given.

Presentation The formulations of the commercially available preparations are described.

Main action The fundamental pharmacological properties are briefly indicated.

Mode of action The mode of action at a cellular or molecular level (where known) is described.

Routes of administration/doses The manufacturer's recommended dose ranges are listed in this section; alternative clinical uses are also mentioned.

Effects The pharmacodynamic properties are systematically reviewed. Where a drug has no specific or known action on a particular physiological system, the relevant section has been omitted.

The systems described are:

CVS Cardiovascular system.

RS Respiratory system.

CNS Central nervous system.

AS Alimentary system.

GU Genitourinary system.

Metabolic/other Metabolic, endocrine, and miscellaneous.

Toxicity/side effects The major side effects are listed, with particular reference to the practice of anaesthesia and intensive care.

Kinetics The available pharmacokinetic data are provided. Quantitative data are not available for all drugs, particularly the long established ones. Where information on the absorption, distribution, metabolism, or excretion is unavailable for a particular drug, the relevant section has been omitted.

Absorption Details of the absorption and bioavailability are given.

Distribution This section provides information on the volume of distribution and degree of protein binding of the drug, together with, where appropriate, details of central nervous penetration, transplacental passage, etc.

Metabolism The site and route of metabolic transformation and the nature and activity of metabolites are described.

Excretion The excretory pathways, clearance, and elimination half-life are listed. Although clearances are usually expressed in ml/min/kg, this has not always been possible due to inadequacies in the original source material.

Special points This section describes points of relevance to the practice of anaesthesia and intensive care; in particular, significant drug interactions are reviewed.

This standard format offers great advantages; it enables specific questions to be answered very rapidly. For example, the question 'How is fentanyl metabolized?' may be answered simply by locating the drug alphabetically and then consulting the Metabolism section of the text. This principle holds true for all possible permutations of queries.

Contents

Glossary of terms used in this book

%	percent
<	less than
≤	less than or equal to
>	greater than
≥	greater than or equal to
±	plus or minus
°C	degree Celsius
®	registered
A2RA	angiotensin II receptor antagonist
ACEI	angiotensin-converting enzyme inhibitor
ACT	activated coagulation time
ACTH	adrenocorticotrophic hormone
ADH	antidiuretic hormone
ADHD	attention-deficit/hyperactivity disorder
ADP	adenosine diphosphate
ALT	alanine transaminase
AMP	adenosine monophosphate
ANC	absolute neutrophil count
APTT	activated partial thromboplastin time
ARDS	acute respiratory distress syndrome
AS	abdominal system
AST	aspartate transaminase
ATIII	antithrombin III
ATP	adenosine triphosphate
AUC	area under curve
AV	atrioventricular
BRCP	breast cancer resistance protein
Ca^{2+}	calcium ion
cal	calorie
cAMP	cyclic adenosine monophosphate
cf.	confer (compare with)
cGMP	cyclic guanosine monophosphate
cmH_2O	centimetre of water
CNS	central nervous system
CO_2	carbon dioxide
COX	cyclo-oxygenase

CRP	C-reactive protein
CSF	cerebrospinal fluid
CVS	cardiovascular system
CYP	cytochrome
DIC	disseminated intravascular coagulation
DNA	deoxyribonucleic acid
DVT	deep vein thrombosis
ECG	electrocardiogram
EEG	electroencephalogram
e.g.	*exempli gratia* (for example)
EMLA®	Eutectic Mixture of Local Anaesthetics
ESBL	extended-spectrum beta-lactamase
ESR	erythrocyte sedimentation rate
FEV_1	forced expiratory volume in first second
FiO_2	partial pressure of oxygen in inspired air
FVC	forced vital capacity
g	gram
GABA	gamma-amino-butyric acid
GU	genitourinary
HAFOE	high airflow oxygen enrichment
HAS	human albumin solution
HDL	high-density lipoprotein
HepBsAg	hepatitis B surface antigen
HFIP	hexafluoroisopropanol
HIT	heparin-induced thrombocytopenia
HITT	heparin-induced thrombocytopenia and thrombosis
HIV	human immunodeficiency virus
HMGCoA	3-hydroxy-3-methyl-glutaryl-coenzyme A reductase
5HT	5-hydroxytryptamine
Hz	hertz
i.e.	*id est* (that is)
IgG	immunoglobulin G
IL-1	interleukin-1
IL-6	interleukin-6
IL-8	interleukin-8
INR	international normalized ratio
ITU	intensive treatment unit
IU	international unit
K^+	potassium ion
kcal	kilocalorie

kg	kilogram
KIU	kallikrein inhibitory unit
kPa	kilopascal
l	litre
LMA	laryngeal mask airway
LMWH	low-molecular-weight heparin
MAC	minimal alveolar concentration
MAOI	monoamine oxidase inhibitor
mb	millibar
MDMA	3,4-methylenedioxymethamphetamine
mEq	milliequivalent
mg	milligram
MIC	minimal alveolar concentration
min	minute
ml	millilitre
mmHg	millimetre of mercury
mmol	millimole
MOP	mu-opioid
mOsm	milliosmole
MRI	magnetic resonance imaging
mRNA	messenger ribonucleic acid
MRSA	meticillin-resistant *Staphylococcus aureus*
Na^+	sodium ion
NAC	N-acetylcysteine
NAPQI	N-acetyl-p-benzo-quinoneimine
ng	nanogram
nm	nanometre
NMB	neuromuscular-blocking
NMDA	N-methyl-D-aspartate
NO	nitric oxide
N_2O	nitrous oxide
NSAID	non-steroidal anti-inflammatory drug
$PaCO_2$	partial pressure of carbon dioxide in arterial blood
PaO_2	partial pressure of oxygen in arterial blood
PBP	penicillin-binding protein
PCO_2	partial pressure of carbon dioxide in arterial blood
PEFR	peak expiratory flow rate
PIFE	pentafluoroisopropenyl fluoromethyl ether
PMFE	pentafluoromethoxy isopropyl fluoromethyl ether
PONV	post-operative nausea and vomiting

ppm	part per million
PVR	pulmonary vascular resistance
RDS	respiratory distress syndrome
REM	rapid eye movement
RNA	ribonucleic acid
RS	respiratory system
rtPA	recombinant tissue plasminogen activator
spp.	species
SSRI	selective serotonin reuptake inhibitor
STP	standard temperature and pressure
TCI	target-controlled infusion
TNF	tumour necrosis factor
TPN	total parenteral nutrition
tRNA	transfer ribonucleic acid
UK	United Kingdom
USA	United States of America
V_D	volume of distribution
VD_{ss}	volume of distribution at steady state
VIE	vacuum-insulated evaporator
VMA	vanillylmandelic acid
vpm	volume per million
VRE	vancomycin-resistant *Enterococcus*
vWF	von Willebrand factor
w/v	weight per volume
w/w	weight per weight

Drugs in anaesthesia and intensive care, A–Z

A2RAs

Uses Angiotensin II receptor antagonists (A2RAs) are used in the treatment of:
1. essential and renovascular hypertension
2. diabetic nephropathy
3. congestive cardiac failure, and
4. in patients intolerant of angiotensin-converting enzyme inhibitors (ACEIs).

Chemical A2RAs belong to the tetrazoles group.

Presentation A2RAs are available in tablet, capsule, liquid, and a powder form as an oral suspension. A number of commercially available types are available, including losartan, irbesartan, candesartan, and valsartan. The drug may also be combined with a thiazide diuretic.

Main actions Antihypertensive.

Mode of action A2RAs selectively block the G-protein-coupled angiotensin II receptor AT1, therefore preventing the physiological effects of angiotensin II via the renin–angiotensin–aldosterone system. The drug does not affect bradykinin-induced vasodilatation.

Routes of administration/doses A2RAs are available for oral administration. The specific dose and frequency of an agent administered are dependent on the clinical indication, age of the patient, and particular agent being used.

Effects

CVS A reduction in the systemic vascular resistance occurs, leading to a fall in the systolic and diastolic blood pressures.

GU A2RAs cause a significant increase in the renal blood flow.

Toxicity/side effects A2RAs are generally well tolerated. Dizziness secondary to hypotension may occur. Angio-oedema occurs rarely. The development of a dry cough (cf. ACE inhibitors) is not associated with A2RAs. Hyperkalaemia can occur.

Kinetics Data are incomplete.

Absorption A2RAs are generally well absorbed from the gastrointestinal tract. Bioavailability for some A2RAs are as follows: losartan (33%), irbesartan (60–80%), candesartan (15%), and valsartan (23%).

Distribution The percentage of drug bound to plasma proteins (predominantly albumin) is high: losartan (99.7%), irbesartan (90%), candesartan (>99%), and valsartan (94–97%). The volume of distribution (V_D) of A2RAs is highly variable: losartan (34 l), irbesartan (53–93 l), candesartan (9.1 l), and valsartan (17 l).

Metabolism A2RA metabolism varies widely. Losartan undergoes extensive hepatic metabolism, generating an active metabolite. Irbesartan undergoes hepatic glucuronide conjugation and oxidation to inactive metabolites. Candesartan is a pro-drug presented as candesartan cilexetil, which undergoes rapid ester hydrolysis in the intestinal wall to the active drug candesartan. Valsartan undergoes minimal hepatic metabolism.

Excretion Losartan is excreted 35% in the urine, and 60% in faeces. It has a half-life of 2 hours for the parent drug, and 6–9 hours for its active metabolite. Irbesartan has a half-life of 11–15 hours. Candesartan is excreted 75% unchanged in the urine and faeces, with a half-life of 9 hours. Valsartan is excreted 80% unchanged (83% in faeces and 13% in the urine), with a half-life of 5–9 hours.

ACE inhibitors

Uses ACEIs are used in the treatment of:
1. essential and renovascular hypertension
2. congestive cardiac failure, and
3. diabetic nephropathy.

Chemical ACEIs are derived from peptides originally isolated from the venom of the pit viper *Bothrops jararaca*.

Presentation ACEIs are available in tablet or capsule form, and a number of commercially available types are available, including captopril, enalapril, perindopril, lisinopril, and ramipril.

Main action Antihypertensive.

Mode of action ACEIs inhibit angiotensin-converting enzyme (with an affinity many times greater than that of angiotensin I), so preventing the formation of angiotensin I from angiotensin II. Part of their action may also be exerted through the modulation of sympathetic tone or the kallikrein–kinin–prostaglandin system.

Routes of administration/doses ACEIs are only currently available for oral administration. The specific dose and frequency of an agent administered are dependent on the clinical indication, age of the patient, and particular agent being used.

Effects

CVS The systemic vascular resistance decreases, leading to a decrease in the systolic and diastolic blood pressures; the cardiac output may increase by up to 25%, especially in the presence of cardiac failure.

GU ACEIs cause an increase in the renal blood flow, although the glomerular filtration rate remains unchanged. Natriuresis may ensue, but there is little overall effect on the plasma volume.

Toxicity/side effects ACEIs are generally well tolerated; hypotension, dizziness, fatigue, dry cough (due to an accumulation of bradykinin), gastrointestinal upsets, and rashes may occur. Renal function may deteriorate in patients with renovascular hypertension.

Kinetics Data are incomplete.

Absorption ACEIs are reasonably well absorbed from the gastrointestinal tract. Bioavailability for individual drugs is as follows: captopril (75%), enalapril (40%), perindopril (75%), lisinopril (25%), ramipril (50–60%).

Distribution The percentage of drug bound to plasma proteins is variable: captopril (30%), enalapril (50%), perindopril (76%), ramipril (73%).

Metabolism Captopril undergoes metabolism to a disulfide dimer and cysteine disulfide. Enalapril and perindopril are pro-drugs that are metabolized to their respective active forms. ACEIs undergo minimal metabolism in man.

Excretion ACEIs have markedly variable half-lives and clearance data. The half-life of captopril is 1.9 hours, whereas that of lisinopril is 12 hours, enalapril 35 hours, perindopril 30–120 hours, and ramipril >50 hours. Captopril has a low clearance, compared to enalapril and perindopril which have plasma clearance values of approximately 300 ml/min.

Special points The hypotensive effects of ACEIs are additive with that of anaesthetic agents. However, they do not necessarily protect against the cardiovascular responses to laryngoscopy.

There is an increased risk of renal failure with the co-administration of ACEIs and non-steroidal anti-inflammatory drugs (NSAIDs) in the presence of hypovolaemia.

Acetazolamide

Uses Acetazolamide is used in the treatment of:
1. glaucoma
2. petit mal epilepsy
3. Ménière's disease
4. familial periodic paralysis and
5. the prophylaxis and treatment of altitude sickness.

Chemical A sulfonamide.

Presentation As 250 mg tablets of acetazolamide and in vials containing 500 mg of the sodium salt of acetazolamide for reconstitution with water prior to injection.

Main action Diuresis and a decrease in the intraocular pressure.

Mode of action Acetazolamide is a reversible, non-competitive inhibitor of carbonic anhydrase situated within the cell cytosol and on the brush border of the proximal convoluted tubule. This enzyme catalyses the conversion of bicarbonate and hydrogen ions into carbonic acid and then carbonic acid to carbon dioxide (CO_2) and water. Under normal circumstances, sodium ions (Na^+) are reabsorbed in exchange for hydrogen ions in the proximal and distal renal tubules; acetazolamide decreases the availability of hydrogen ions, and therefore Na^+ and bicarbonate ions remain in the renal tubule, leading to a diuresis.

Routes of administration/doses The adult oral and intravenous dose is 250–1000 mg daily.

Effects

RS Acetazolamide produces a compensatory increase in ventilation in response to the metabolic acidosis and increased tissue CO_2 that the drug causes.

CNS Acetazolamide has demonstrable anticonvulsant properties, possibly related to an elevated CO_2 tension within the central nervous system (CNS). The drug decreases the pressure of both the cerebrospinal fluid (CSF) and the intraocular compartment by decreasing the rate of formation of the CSF and aqueous humour (by 50–60%).

AS The drug inhibits gastric and pancreatic secretion.

GU Acetazolamide produces a mild diuresis, with retention of Na^+ and a subsequent increase in plasma Na^+ concentration. The drug also decreases renal excretion of uric acid.

Metabolic/other The excretion of an alkaline urine results in the development of a hyperchloraemic metabolic acidosis in response to the administration of acetazolamide. The drug also interferes with iodide uptake by the thyroid.

Toxicity/side effects Occur rarely and include gastrointestinal and haemopoietic disturbances, rashes, renal stones, and hypokalaemia.

Kinetics

Absorption Acetazolamide is rapidly and well absorbed when administered orally; the bioavailability by this route is virtually 100%.

Distribution The drug is 70–90% protein-bound in the plasma.

Metabolism Acetazolamide is not metabolized in man.

Excretion The drug is excreted unchanged in the urine; the clearance is 2.7 l/hour, and the elimination-half-life is 1.7–5.8 hours.

Special points The use of acetazolamide is contraindicated in the presence of hepatic or renal failure, as the drug will worsen any metabolic acidosis and may also cause urolithiasis. Pre-treatment with the drug will obtund the increase in intraocular pressure produced by the administration of suxamethonium; however, the use of acetazolamide is of dubious value during eye surgery, as it simultaneously increases the intrachoroidal vascular volume. Acetazolamide has been used effectively for the correction of metabolic alkalosis in the critically ill.

Acetazolamide is removed by haemodialysis.

Aciclovir

Uses Aciclovir is used in the treatment of:
1. Herpes simplex infections of the skin and eye
2. Herpes simplex encephalitis
3. recurrent varicella-zoster virus infections, and
4. for the prophylaxis of herpes simplex infections in immunocompromised patients.

Chemical An analogue of the nucleoside 2'-deoxyguanosine.

Presentation As 200/400/800 mg tablets, a suspension containing 40 mg/ml, a white lyophilized powder in vials containing 250 mg of aciclovir sodium which is reconstituted prior to injection in water, and as a 3% ophthalmic ointment and 5% w/w cream for topical application.

Main action Aciclovir is an antiviral agent, active against herpes simplex (I and II) and varicella-zoster virus.

Mode of action Aciclovir is activated within the viral cell via phosphorylation by a virus-coded thymidine kinase and thus has a low toxicity for normal cells. Aciclovir triphosphate inhibits viral deoxyribonucleic acid (DNA) polymerase by becoming incorporated into the DNA primer template, effectively preventing further elongation of the viral DNA chain.

Routes of administration/doses The adult oral dose is 200–400 mg 2–5 times daily, initially for a period of 5 days. The corresponding intravenous dose is 5–10 mg/kg 8-hourly, infused over a period of 1 hour. A higher dose is used for zoster than for simplex infections. Topical application should be performed 5 times daily, again for an initial period of 5 days.

Effects

Metabolic/other Increases in plasma levels of urea and creatinine may occur if the drug is administered intravenously too rapidly.

Toxicity/side effects Aciclovir is generally well tolerated. CNS disturbances (including tremors, confusion, and seizures) and gastrointestinal upset may occur. Precipitation of the drug in the renal tubules leading to renal impairment may occur if the drug is administered too rapidly or if an adequate state of hydration is not maintained. The drug is an irritant to veins and tissues.

Kinetics

Absorption Oral absorption of the drug is erratic; the bioavailability by this route is 15–30%.

Distribution The drug is 9–33% protein-bound in the plasma; the V_D is 0.32–1.48 l/kg.

Metabolism The major metabolite is 9-carboxymethoxymethyl guanine which is inactive.

Excretion The drug is excreted by active tubular secretion in the urine, 45–80% unchanged. The elimination half-life is 2–3 hours.

Special points A reduced dose should be used in the presence of renal impairment; haemodialysis removes 60% of the drug.

Adenosine

Uses Adenosine is used in the diagnosis and treatment of paroxysmal supraventricular tachycardia.

Chemical A naturally occurring nucleoside that is composed of adenine and d-ribose. Adenosine or adenosine derivatives play many important biological roles, in addition to being components of DNA and ribonucleic acid (RNA).

Presentation As a clear, colourless solution containing 3 mg/ml adenosine in saline.

Main action Depression of sinoatrial and atrioventricular (AV) nodal activity and slowing of conduction. The drug also antagonizes cyclic adenosine monophosphate (cAMP)-mediated catechol stimulation of ventricular muscle. Both actions result in negative chronotropic and inotropic effects.

Mode of action Adenosine acts as a direct agonist at specific cell membrane receptors, classified into A1 and A2 subsets. A1 receptors are coupled to potassium channels by a guanine nucleotide-binding protein in supraventricular tissue.

Routes of administration/doses Adenosine is administered as a rapid intravenous bolus, followed by a saline flush. The initial adult dose is 3 mg, followed, if necessary, by a 6 mg and then a 12 mg bolus at 1- to 2-minute intervals until an effect is observed. The paediatric dose is 0.0375–0.25 mg/kg. The drug acts within 10 seconds and has a duration of action of 10–20 seconds.

Effects

CVS Depression of sinoatrial and AV nodal activity leads to the termination of paroxysmal supraventricular tachycardia. Atrial dysrhythmias are revealed by AV nodal block, leading to a transient slowing of the ventricular response. Adenosine has no clinically important effects on the blood pressure when administered as a bolus. A continuous high-dose infusion may result in a decrease in the systemic vascular resistance and decreased blood pressure. When administered as an infusion, adenosine causes a dose-dependent reflex tachycardia and an increase in the cardiac output. The drug also causes a dose-dependent increase in myocardial blood flow, secondary to coronary vasodilation mediated via endothelial A2 receptors. Adenosine decreases the pulmonary vascular resistance (PVR) in patients with pulmonary hypertension.

RS Bolus administration of adenosine leads to an increase in both the depth and rate of respiration, probably mediated by A2 receptor stimulation in the carotid body. Infusion of the drug results in a fall in $PaCO_2$. Bronchospasm may occur.

CNS Infusion of adenosine results in increased cerebral blood flow. Low-dose adenosine induces neuropathic pain, hyperalgesia, and ischaemic pain. Adenosine itself is a neurotransmitter.

GU Hypotensive doses of adenosine stimulate A2 receptors, resulting in renal and hepatic arterial vasoconstriction, although low doses have no effect on the glomerular filtration rate or sodium excretion.

Metabolic/other Adenosine inhibits lipolysis and stimulates glycolysis.

Toxicity/side effects The commonest side effects are transient facial flushing, dyspnoea, and chest discomfort. Bronchospasm has also been reported. The induced bradycardia predisposes to ventricular excitability and may result in ventricular fibrillation. Profound bradycardia requiring pacing may occur.

Kinetics

Absorption Adenosine is inactive when administered orally.

Metabolism Exogenous adenosine is absorbed from the plasma into red blood cells and the vascular endothelium where it is phosphorylated to adenosine monophosphate (AMP) or deaminated to inosine and hypoxanthine. The plasma half-life is <10 seconds.

Special points No dose adjustment is necessary in the presence of renal or hepatic impairment. Adenosine has been used to induce hypotension perioperatively.

Intraoperative use of adenosine decreases the minimal alveolar concentration (MAC) of isoflurane and decreases post-operative analgesic requirements.

Adrenaline

Uses Adrenaline is used in the treatment of:
1. anaphylactic and anaphylactoid shock
2. asystole
3. low cardiac output states
4. glaucoma and
5. as a local vasoconstrictor, and
6. is added to local anaesthetic solutions to prolong their duration of action.

Chemical A catecholamine.

Presentation As a clear solution for injection containing 0.1/1 mg/ml of adrenaline hydrochloride, a 1% ophthalmic solution, and as an aerosol spray delivering 280 micrograms metered doses of adrenaline acid tartrate.

Main action Sympathomimetic.

Mode of action Adrenaline is a directly acting sympathomimetic amine that is an agonist of alpha- and beta-adrenoreceptors; it has approximately equal activity at both alpha- and beta-receptors.

Routes of administration/doses The drug may be administered intravenously either as an intravenous bolus in doses of 0.1–1 mg for the treatment of asystole or as an infusion at the rate of 0.01–0.1 micrograms/kg/min, titrated according to response; low doses tend to produce predominantly beta-effects, whilst higher doses tend to produce predominantly alpha-effects. The dose by the subcutaneous route is 0.1–0.5 mg. Adrenaline may be administered by inhalation; a maximum daily dose of 10–20 metered doses is recommended.

Effects

CVS Adrenaline is both a positive inotrope and a positive chronotrope, and therefore causes an increase in the cardiac output and myocardial oxygen consumption. The drug causes an increase in the coronary blood flow. When administered as an intravenous bolus, adrenaline markedly increases the peripheral vascular resistance, producing an increase in the systolic blood pressure with a less marked increase in the diastolic blood pressure. When administered as an intravenous infusion, the peripheral vascular resistance (a direct beta-2 effect) and diastolic blood pressure both tend to decrease. The heart rate initially increases and subsequently decreases due to a vagal reflex. The plasma volume decreases as a result of the loss of protein-free fluid into the extracellular fluid. Adrenaline increases platelet adhesiveness and blood coagulability (by increasing the activity of factor V).

RS Adrenaline is a mild respiratory stimulant and causes an increase in both the tidal volume and respiratory rate. The drug is a potent bronchodilator but tends to increase the viscosity of bronchial secretions.

CNS Adrenaline only penetrates the CNS to a limited extent but does have excitatory effects. The drug increases the cutaneous pain threshold and enhances neuromuscular transmission. Adrenaline has little overall effect on the cerebral blood flow. It has weak mydriatic effects when applied topically to the eye.

AS The drug decreases the intestinal tone and secretions; the splanchnic blood flow is increased.

GU Adrenaline decreases the renal blood flow by up to 40%, although the glomerular filtration rate remains little altered. The bladder tone is decreased and the sphincteric tone increased by the drug, which may lead to difficulty with micturition. Adrenaline inhibits the contractions of the pregnant uterus.

Metabolic/other The drug has profound metabolic effects; it decreases insulin secretion whilst increasing both glucagon secretion and the rate of glycogenolysis, resulting in elevation of the blood sugar concentration. The plasma renin activity is increased by the drug (a beta-1 effect), and the plasma concentration of free fatty acids is increased by the activation of triglyceride lipase. The serum potassium concentration transiently rises (due to release from the liver), following the administration of adrenaline; a more prolonged decrease in potassium concentration follows. Adrenaline administration increases the basal metabolic rate by 20–30%; in combination with the cutaneous vasoconstriction that the drug produces, pyrexia may result.

Toxicity/side effects Symptoms of CNS excitation, cerebral haemorrhage, tachycardia, dysrhythmias, and myocardial ischaemia may result from the use of adrenaline.

Kinetics Data are incomplete.

Absorption The drug is inactivated when administered orally. Absorption is slower after subcutaneous than intramuscular administration. The drug is well absorbed from the tracheal mucosa.

Metabolism Exogenous adrenaline is predominantly first metabolized by catechol-O-methyl transferase, predominantly in the liver, to metadrenaline and normetadrenaline (uptake-2); some is metabolized by monoamine oxidase within adrenergic neurones (uptake-1). The final common products of adrenaline metabolism are 3-methoxy 4-hydroxyphenylethylene and 3-methoxy 4-hydroxymandelic acid (which are inactive).

Excretion The inactive products appear predominantly in the urine.

Special points The dose of adrenaline should be limited to 1 microgram/kg/30 min in the presence of halothane and to 3 micrograms/kg/30 min in the presence of enflurane or isoflurane, in an attempt to prevent the appearance of serious ventricular dysrhythmias. Infiltration of adrenaline-containing solutions should be avoided in regions of the body supplied by end arteries.

Alfentanil

Uses Alfentanil is used:
1. to provide the analgesic component in general anaesthesia
2. in sedation regimens for intensive care, and
3. to obtund the cardiovascular responses to laryngoscopy.

Chemical A synthetic phenylpiperidine derivative.

Presentation As a clear, colourless solution for injection containing 0.5/5 mg/ml of alfentanil hydrochloride. The pKa of alfentanil is 6.5; alfentanil is 89% unionized at a pH of 7.4 and has a relatively low lipid solubility. Despite the low lipid solubility of the drug (octanol:water partition coefficient of 128.1), it has a faster onset of action, compared to fentanyl which has a much higher lipid solubility due to its low pKa and consequently large amount of unionized drug available to cross lipid membranes.

Main actions Analgesia and respiratory depression.

Mode of action Alfentanil is a highly selective mu-opioid (MOP) agonist; the MOP receptor appears to be specifically involved in the mediation of analgesia. Opioids appear to exert their effects by interacting with pre-synaptic Gi protein receptors, leading to a hyperpolarization of the cell membrane by increasing potassium conductance. Inhibition of adenylate cyclase, leading to a reduced production of cAMP and closure of voltage-sensitive calcium channels, also occurs. The decrease in membrane excitability that results may decrease both pre- and post-synaptic responses.

Routes of administration/doses Alfentanil is administered intravenously in boluses of 5–50 micrograms/kg. The drug may be administered by intravenous infusion at a rate of 0.5–1 micrograms/kg/min. Alfentanil acts rapidly, with the peak effect occurring within 90 seconds of intravenous administration, and the duration of effect is 5–10 min. Administration of alfentanil reduces the amount of hypnotic/volatile agents required to maintain anaesthesia.

Effects

CVS The most significant cardiovascular effect that alfentanil demonstrates is bradycardia of vagal origin; cardiac output, mean arterial pressure, pulmonary and systemic vascular resistance, and pulmonary capillary wedge pressure are unaffected by the administration of the drug. Doses of 5 micrograms/kg increase left ventricular contractility and cardiac output in animal models. Alfentanil obtunds the cardiovascular responses to laryngoscopy and intubation.

RS Alfentanil is a potent respiratory depressant, causing a decrease in both the respiratory rate and tidal volume; it also diminishes the ventilatory response to hypoxia and hypercarbia. The drug is a potent antitussive agent. Chest wall rigidity (the 'wooden chest' phenomenon) may occur after the administration of alfentanil—this may be an effect of the drug on MOP receptors located on GABA-ergic interneurones. Alfentanil causes minimal histamine release; bronchospasm is thus rarely produced by the drug.

CNS Alfentanil is 10–20 times more potent an analgesic than morphine and has little hypnotic or sedative activity. Miosis is produced as a result of stimulation of the Edinger–Westphal nucleus. Alfentanil reduces the intraocular pressure by approximately 45%. The drug causes an increase in the amplitude of the encephalogram (EEG) and reduces its frequency.

AS The drug decreases gastrointestinal motility and gastric acid secretion; it also doubles the common bile duct pressure by causing spasm of the sphincter of Oddi.

GU Alfentanil increases the tone of the ureters, bladder detrusor muscle, and vesicular sphincter.

Metabolic/other High doses of alfentanil will obtund the metabolic 'stress response' to surgery; the drug appears to be even more effective than fentanyl in this respect. Unlike morphine, alfentanil does not increase the activity of antidiuretic hormone (ADH).

Toxicity/side effects Respiratory depression, bradycardia, nausea, vomiting, and dependence may also complicate the use of the drug.

Kinetics

Distribution Alfentanil is 85–92% bound to plasma proteins, predominantly to alpha-1 acid glycoprotein; the V_D is 0.4–1 l/kg. Alfentanil crosses the placenta.

Metabolism Alfentanil is predominantly metabolized in the liver by N-dealkylation to noralfentanil; the remainder of the drug is metabolized by a variety of pathways, including aromatic hydroxylation, demethylation, and amide hydrolysis followed by acetylation. The major phase II pathway is by conjugation to glucuronide. Cytochrome P450 3A3 and 3A4 play a predominant role in alfentanil metabolism and may be subject to competitive inhibition by the co-administration of midazolam, which may lead to a prolongation of alfentanil and midazolam drug effects. Metabolism of the drug may also be prolonged when other CYP3A4 inhibitors are used concomitantly.

Excretion 90% of an administered dose is excreted in the urine (<1% as unchanged drug). The clearance of alfentanil is 3.3–8.3 ml/kg/min, and the elimination half-life range is 90–111 min. The relatively brief duration of action of a single dose of alfentanil, in comparison to that of fentanyl, is due to the smaller V_D and shorter elimination half-life of the former.

Special points Alfentanil decreases the apparent MAC of co-administered volatile agents. The concomitant use of erythromycin, cimetidine, fluconazole, ketoconazole, ritonavir, and diltiazem may significantly inhibit the clearance of alfentanil.

The half-life of the drug is prolonged in the elderly and debilitated patients and those with significant hepatic and renal impairment.

It is unknown whether alfentanil is removed by haemodialysis.

Allopurinol

Uses Allopurinol is used:
1. in the prophylaxis of gout
2. to prevent renal stone formation in patients with xanthinuria, and
3. in the prophylaxis of the tumour lysis syndrome.

Chemical A hypoxanthine analogue.

Presentation As 100/300 mg tablets of allopurinol.

Main action Xanthine oxidase inhibitor and free-radical scavenger.

Mode of action Allopurinol and its active metabolite oxipurinol inhibit xanthine oxidase, the enzyme responsible for the conversion of hypoxanthine and xanthine to uric acid. Allopurinol also facilitates the incorporation of hypoxanthine and xanthine into DNA and RNA, further reducing serum uric acid concentrations. The drug has no anti-inflammatory, analgesic, or uricosuric actions.

Routes of administration/doses The adult oral dose is 100–900 mg daily, adjusted according to the serum uric acid level. The serum urate levels begin to decrease 24–48 hours after the initiation of treatment; the maximum effect is observed after 1–3 weeks.

Toxicity/side effects A skin rash may be followed by more severe hypersensitivity reactions such as exfoliative, urticarial, and purpuric lesions, as well as Stevens–Johnson syndrome, and/or generalized vasculitis, irreversible hepatotoxicity, and rarely death.

Kinetics

Absorption Allopurinol is well absorbed when administered orally; the bioavailability by this route is 80–90%.

Distribution The drug is not protein-bound in the plasma; the V_D is 0.6 l/kg.

Metabolism Allopurinol is rapidly converted to an active metabolite oxipurinol.

Excretion Occurs predominantly in the urine for both allopurinol and oxipurinol; some 20% is excreted in faeces. The clearance of allopurinol is 680 ml/min/kg, and the elimination half-life is 1–3 hours.

Special points An adequate urine output should be ensured during treatment with the drug; the dose of allopurinol should be reduced in the presence of severe renal impairment.

Allopurinol may protect against stress-induced gastric mucosal injury by scavenging oxygen-derived free radicals.

The drug and its metabolites are removed by haemodialysis.

Amiloride

Uses Amiloride is used in the treatment of:
1. oedema of cardiac, renal, or hepatic origin
2. hypertension, and
3. in combination with loop or thiazide diuretics to conserve potassium.

Chemical A pyrazinoylguanidine.

Presentation As 5 mg tablets of amiloride hydrochloride and in various fixed-dose combinations with thiazide or loop diuretics.

Main action Diuretic.

Mode of action Amiloride selectively blocks sodium reabsorption in the distal convoluted tubule. As a result of the inhibition of Na^+ transport, the electrical potential across the tubular epithelium decreases, and potassium ion (K^+) excretion is inhibited. The net result is a slight increase in renal Na^+ excretion and a decrease in excessive K^+ excretion. Amiloride has been shown to decrease the enhanced urinary excretion of magnesium which occurs when a thiazide or loop diuretic is used alone.

Routes of administration/doses The adult oral dose is 10–20 mg daily. The diuretic effect commences within 2 hours and lasts 24 hours.

Effects

CVS With chronic use, amiloride causes a slight decrease in the systolic and diastolic blood pressures, probably due to a reduction in the Na^+ content of arteriolar smooth muscle, producing a decrease in the systemic vascular resistance.

GU The principal effect is diuresis, with an increased rate of Na^+ and bicarbonate ion excretion and a decreased rate of K^+, calcium (Ca^{2+}), and ammonium and hydrogen ion excretion. The drug has no effect on free water clearance.

Metabolic/other The inhibition of hydrogen ion excretion leads to a slight alkalinization of the urine; serum uric acid concentrations are also increased, following the administration of amiloride. A metabolic acidosis may occur.

Toxicity/side effects The most significant side effect of the drug is hyperkalaemia; other reported side effects, although rare, occur infrequently. These include nausea and vomiting, abdominal pain, diarrhoea, rashes, cramps, CNS and haemopoietic disturbances, impotence, and interstitial nephritis.

Kinetics

Absorption Amiloride is incompletely absorbed when administered orally; the bioavailability by this route is 50%.

Distribution The drug is 5% protein-bound in the plasma; the V_D is 5 l/kg.

Metabolism No metabolism of the drug occurs in man.

Excretion 50% of the dose is excreted unchanged in the urine, the remainder in faeces. The clearance is 264–372 ml/min, and the elimination half-life is 18–24 hours (this is prolonged to 140 hours in the presence of renal failure).

Special points Amiloride inhibits the excretion of co-administered digoxin; concurrent NSAID therapy tends to obtund the diuretic and anti-hypertensive effects of the drug.

Aminoglycosides

Uses Aminoglycosides are used in the treatment of:
1. respiratory tract infections
2. urinary tract infections
3. skin and soft tissue infections
4. ocular infections
5. intra-abdominal sepsis
6. septicaemia
7. neutropenic sepsis
8. severe neonatal infections
9. CNS sepsis, and
10. as surgical prophylaxis.

Chemical Aminocyclitol ring derivatives bound to amino sugars.

Presentation Aminoglycosides in clinical use include gentamicin, amikacin, streptomycin, and neomycin. Gentamicin is available in a liquid form for topical use (ear/eye drops), in an intravenous form, and in a form suitable for intrathecal or intraventricular administration. Amikacin is available for intravenous use only. Neomycin is available in topical formulations combined with steroid (eye/ear/nasal drops; creams/ointments) or in tablet form. Streptomycin is available for intramuscular injection.

Main action Aminoglycosides are active against:
1. Gram-positive bacteria (limited activity against streptococci spp.)
2. Gram-negative bacteria.

These agents are not active against anaerobic bacteria. Acquired resistance is common due to plasmid translocation. Streptomycin is active against *Mycobacterium tuberculosis*. Neomycin is a bowel-sterilizing agent when administered orally.

Mode of action Aminoglycosides bind irreversibly to specific bacterial ribosomal proteins (30S subunit) and inhibit protein synthesis by interfering with the initiation of the polypeptide chain and by inducing misreading of messenger RNA (mRNA).

Routes of administration/doses Aminoglycosides may be administered topically as eye, ear, or nasal drops, as creams or ointments, orally (neomycin), intravenously, or via the intrathecal/intraventricular route. The specific dose, route, and frequency of an agent administered is dependent on the clinical indication, age of the patient, and particular agent being used. Doses should be reduced in patients with renal impairment. Drug doses should be modified using drug level monitoring and trends in renal function.

Toxicity/side effects Ototoxicity (with vestibular and auditory components) and nephrotoxicity (a form of acute tubular necrosis occurring 5–7 days after exposure) are the most serious side effects of the drug, and both are correlated with high trough concentrations of aminoglycosides. Headaches, nausea and vomiting, rashes, and abnormalities of liver function tests have also been reported in association with the use of these agents.

Kinetics

Absorption Aminoglycosides are not significantly absorbed when administered orally due to their low lipid solubility; approximately 3% of neomycin is absorbed. The drugs are not inactivated within the gastrointestinal tract.

Distribution The V_D for gentamicin is 0.14–0.7 l/kg, and that for amikacin is 0.34 l/kg. The percentage of drug bound to plasma proteins is 70–85% for gentamicin and <20% for amikacin. High concentrations are found within the renal cortex. The CSF is poorly penetrated by these agents. Streptomycin penetrates tuberculous cavities well.

Metabolism Aminoglycosides undergo minimal metabolism in man.

Excretion Aminoglycosides are excreted unchanged almost completely by glomerular filtration. The clearance of gentamicin is 1.18–1.32 ml/kg/min, and that of amikacin is 1.42 ml/kg/min. The half-life of gentamicin and amikacin is 2–3 hours (which markedly increases as the renal function deteriorates).

Special points Monitoring of drug levels of gentamicin and amikacin should follow local guidelines. Trough samples are taken immediately before a dose, and peak levels an hour after drug administration. Gentamicin and amikacin are removed by haemofiltration and dialysis.

Direct administration of gentamicin into the CSF via an indwelling extraventricular drain can be undertaken in the treatment of ventriculitis.

Neomycin has been used in the treatment of hepatic coma.

Aminoglycosides prolong the action of non-depolarizing muscle relaxants by inhibiting pre-synaptic acetylcholine release and stabilizing the post-synaptic membrane at the neuromuscular junction. This effect may be reversed by the administration of intravenous calcium. These agents should be used with caution in patients with myasthenia gravis.

Antimicrobial agents should always be administered, following consideration of local pharmacy and microbiological policies.

Aminoglycosides exhibit synergy with other antibiotics, e.g. in the treatment of pneumonia and subacute bacterial endocarditis.

Aminophylline

Uses Aminophylline is used in the treatment of:
1. asthma
2. chronic obstructive airways disease, and
3. heart failure.

Chemical The ethylenediamine salt of theophylline (a methylated xanthine derivative).

Presentation As tablets containing 100/225/350 mg of aminophylline, as 180/360 mg suppositories, and as a clear solution for injection containing 25 mg/ml of aminophylline.

Main action Bronchodilatation associated with an increased ventilatory response to hypoxia and hypercapnia. It has been shown to improve diaphragmatic contractility.

Mode of action Aminophylline acts by inhibiting a magnesium-dependent phosphodiesterase, the enzyme responsible for the degradation of cAMP. The drug has a synergistic effect with those catecholamines which directly activate adenylate cyclase and lead to an increase in the intracellular concentration of cAMP. In addition, aminophylline interferes with the influx of Ca^{2+} into smooth muscle cells and stabilizes mast cells by antagonizing the action of adenosine.

Routes of administration/doses The adult daily oral dose is 900 mg, administered in 2–3 divided doses, and the rectal dose 360 mg daily, titrated according to response. The loading dose by the intravenous route is 5 mg/kg over 10–15 minutes; this may be followed by a maintenance infusion of 0.5 mg/kg/hour. An intravenous loading dose should be administered with extreme caution to patients already receiving oral or rectal aminophylline. The therapeutic range is narrow (10–20 micrograms/ml), and estimations of the plasma concentration of aminophylline are valuable during chronic therapy.

Effects

CVS The drug has mild positive inotropic and chronotropic effects, producing an increase in the cardiac output and a decrease in the systemic vascular resistance, thus leading to a decrease in the arterial blood pressure. The left ventricular end-diastolic pressure and pulmonary capillary wedge pressure tend to decrease with the use of the drug. Aminophylline is arrhythmogenic at the upper extremes of its therapeutic range; it is synergistic with halothane in this respect.

RS Aminophylline causes bronchodilatation, leading to an increase in the vital capacity. It also increases the sensitivity of the respiratory centre to CO_2 and increases diaphragmatic contractility. Intravenous administration of the drug inhibits hypoxic pulmonary vasoconstriction and necessitates the administration of oxygen during therapy.

GU Aminophylline increases the renal blood flow and glomerular filtration rate and decreases renal tubular sodium absorption, leading to a diuretic effect.

Metabolic/other Hypokalaemia may occur, secondary to the diuretic effect and also to increased cellular uptake of potassium. Abnormalities of liver function tests and inappropriate ADH secretion are also recognized effects of the drug.

Toxicity/side effects Gastrointestinal and CNS disturbances (including convulsions after rapid intravenous administration) and cardiac dysrhythmias (including ventricular fibrillation) may occur, especially with plasma concentrations in excess of 20 micrograms/ml.

Kinetics

Absorption Aminophylline is rapidly absorbed when administered orally and has a bioavailability by this route of 88–96%. Rectal absorption is slow and erratic.

Distribution The drug is 50–60% protein-bound in the plasma; the V_D is 0.4–0.5 l/kg.

Metabolism Occurs in the liver by demethylation and oxidation; a 3-methyl xanthine derivative is active.

Excretion Demethylated metabolites are excreted in the urine; 10–13% of the dose is excreted unchanged. The clearance is 0.83–1.16 ml/min/kg; this is decreased in the presence of heart failure, liver disease, and in the elderly. Saturation of the metabolic pathways occurs near the therapeutic range; whilst obeying zero-order kinetics, the elimination half-life varies with the dose. Under conditions of first-order kinetics, the elimination half-life is 8 hours.

Special points Co-administration of cimetidine, propranolol, or erythromycin will elevate plasma concentrations of aminophylline; conversely, co-administration of barbiturates, alcohol, or phenytoin will decrease plasma concentrations of aminophylline. The site of these interactions is at cytochrome P450. In high concentrations, the drug will antagonize nondepolarizing neuromuscular blockade.

Aminophylline infusion shortens the recovery time from enflurane–nitrous oxide (N_2O) anaesthesia.

Amiodarone

Uses Amiodarone is used in the treatment of:
1. tachydysrhythmias inappropriate for, or resistant to, other drugs and
2. those associated with the Wolff–Parkinson–White syndrome.

Chemical An iodinated benzofuran derivative.

Presentation As 100/200 mg tablets of amiodarone hydrochloride and in ampoules and prefilled syringes containing 30/50 mg/ml of amiodarone hydrochloride for injection.

Main action A class III antiarrhythmic agent.

Mode of action Amiodarone acts by partial antagonism of alpha- and beta-agonists by reducing the number of receptors or by inhibiting the coupling of receptors to the regulatory subunit of the adenylate cyclase system. In addition, the drug has a direct action in isolated myocardial preparations to decrease the delayed slow outward potassium current and, in higher doses, additionally depresses the fast and slow inward currents which are due to sodium and calcium, respectively.

Routes of administration/doses The initial intravenous dose is 5 mg/kg, administered by infusion diluted in 250 ml of 5% glucose over 20–120 minutes via a central vein (the drug carrier is highly irritant). Most patients respond to an intravenous loading dose within 1 hour. Subsequently, 15 mg/kg/day may be administered intravenously if oral administration is not desirable or feasible. The adult oral dose is initially 200 mg 8-hourly, reducing to 100–200 mg daily after 1 week. The therapeutic level is 0.1 micrograms/ml.

Effects

CVS Sinus rhythm is slowed by 15%, secondary to a reduction in the slow diastolic depolarization in nodal cells after the administration of amiodarone. AV nodal automaticity is depressed, and AV nodal conduction is slowed by 25% in the face of atrial tachycardia due to a decreased speed of depolarization of cells and an increase in the duration of the action potential. Amiodarone has no effect on conduction in the His bundle or ventricular myocardium. After oral administration, little effect is seen on the blood pressure or left ventricular contractility; the systemic vascular resistance decreases, and coronary sinus blood flow increases. After intravenous administration, left ventricular contractility may decrease; the effects are otherwise similar to those observed after oral administration.

Metabolic/other Abnormalities of liver function tests occur in up to 50% of patients; abnormalities of thyroid function tests may also occur due to inhibition of triiodothyronine and enhancement of reverse triiodothyronine production.

Toxicity/side effects Almost all patients receiving amiodarone develop corneal microdeposits, and one-third develop signs of CNS toxicity. Pneumonitis, cirrhosis, peripheral neuropathy, photosensitivity, and gastrointestinal upsets are well-recognized complications. Hypotension, cardiovascular collapse, and AV block have been reported after intravenous injection. Other dysrhythmias may arise, especially in the presence of hypokalaemia.

Kinetics

Absorption The drug is incompletely absorbed after oral administration and has a bioavailability of 22–86%.

Distribution Amiodarone is 96–98% protein-bound in the plasma; the V_D is 1.3–65.8 l/kg, according to the dose.

Metabolism The metabolic pathways of amiodarone have not been fully elucidated; it appears to be extensively metabolized in the liver, the major metabolite being desethyl-amiodarone which has antiarrhythmic properties and is cumulative.

Excretion 1–5% of the dose appears in the urine; the drug appears to be extensively excreted in the bile and faeces. The clearance is 0.14–0.6 l/min, and the elimination half-life has been estimated at 4 hours to 52 days, depending on the dose and route of administration.

Special points Modification of the dose is not required in the presence of renal impairment; amiodarone is not removed by haemodialysis. The actions of digoxin, calcium antagonists, oral anticoagulants, and beta-adrenergic antagonists may be potentiated by amiodarone due to displacement from plasma proteins. Bradycardia, and complete and AV heart block resistant to atropine, adrenaline, and noradrenaline have been reported in patients receiving amiodarone undergoing general anaesthesia; it has been suggested that such patients may require temporary pacing in the perioperative period.

The drug is contraindicated in porphyria.

Amitriptyline

Uses Amitriptyline is used for the treatment of:
1. depression
2. nocturnal enuresis, and
3. can be used as an adjunct in the treatment of chronic pain syndromes, including chronic tension headache, post-herpetic neuralgia, painful neuropathies, and chronic spinal syndromes.

Chemical A dibenzocycloheptadiene derivative.

Presentation As tablets containing 10/25/50 mg and a clear, colourless solution for injection containing 10 mg/ml of amitriptyline hydrochloride. A syrup containing 2 mg/ml of amitriptyline embonate is also available.

Main actions Antidepressant, sedative, and analgesic.

Mode of action Tricyclic antidepressants potentiate the action of biogenic amines within the CNS by inhibiting the pre-synaptic reuptake of noradrenaline and serotonin. They also antagonize muscarinic cholinergic, alpha-1 adrenergic, and H1 and H2 histaminergic receptors.

Routes of administration/doses The adult oral dose is initially 75–150 mg/day, decreasing to 50–100 mg/day for maintenance. The corresponding parenteral dose is 10–20 mg 6-hourly. The drug takes from 3 to 30 days to become fully effective.

Effects

CVS In high doses, amitriptyline may cause postural hypotension, tachycardia, dysrhythmias, and an increase in the conduction time through the AV node.

RS The drug may cause respiratory depression when administered in toxic doses.

CNS The predominant effect of the drug is an antidepressant action which may take several weeks to develop; sedation, weakness, and fatigue are also commonly produced.

Toxicity/side effects A wide spectrum of cardiovascular, CNS, gastrointestinal, and haematological disturbances may complicate the use of amitriptyline. Anticholinergic side effects (blurred vision, dryness of the mouth, constipation, and urinary retention) tend to predominate.

Kinetics

Absorption The drug is rapidly absorbed when administered orally; the bioavailability is 45% by this route.

Distribution Amitriptyline is 95% protein-bound in the plasma; the V_D is 18–22 l/kg.

Metabolism Occurs by N-demethylation and hydroxylation, with subsequent conjugation to glucuronide and sulfate. Nortriptyline is an intermediate active metabolite.

Excretion The conjugates are excreted in the urine. The clearance is 9.7–15.3 ml/min/kg, and the elimination half-life is 12.9–36.1 hours.

Special points Hyoscine and the phenothiazines displace tricyclic antidepressants from their binding sites on plasma proteins and thus increase the activity of the latter; barbiturates increase the rate of hepatic metabolism of tricyclic antidepressants and decrease their activity. Amitriptyline accentuates the cardiovascular effects of adrenaline; care should be exercised when local anaesthetic agents containing adrenaline are used in patients receiving the drug. Amitriptyline also increases the likelihood of dysrhythmias and hypotension occurring during general anaesthesia.

Amoxicillin

Uses Amoxicillin is used in the treatment of:
1. ear, nose, and throat, and respiratory tract infections
2. urinary tract infections, including gonorrhoea
3. septicaemia
4. gastroenteritis
5. endocarditis, and
6. meningitis.

Chemical An aminopenicillin derivative of ampicillin.

Presentation Amoxicillin is available in the following formulations:
1. in vials containing 250/500/1000 mg of amoxicillin sodium
2. in sachets containing 3 g of amoxicillin trihydrate for reconstitution
3. in capsules containing 250/500 mg of amoxicillin trihydrate
4. as a suspension containing 125 mg of amoxicillin trihydrate per 1.25 ml
5. as a syrup containing 125 mg/5 ml and 250 mg/5 ml of amoxicillin trihydrate.

The drug is also available in a variety of formulations in combination with the beta-lactamase inhibitor clavulanic acid as co-amoxiclav.

Main actions Amoxicillin is bactericidal against a wide range of organisms, including some strains of the Gram-negative *Haemophilus influenzae* and *Escherichia coli* (benzylpenicillin showing lower activity against these species), *Proteus mirabilis, Bordetella pertussis*, and *Neisseria, Salmonella,* and *Shigella* spp. The drug is nearly always effective against the Gram-positive *Streptococcus* and *Clostridium* spp. (not *Clostridium difficile*). Ninety percent of staphylococci are resistant. It is ineffective against *Pseudomonas* and *Klebsiella* spp. and penicillinase-producing organisms. The addition of clavulanic acid reduces the minimum inhibitory concentration (MIC) against the following organisms: *Staphylococcus aureus, Escherichia coli, Haemophilus influenzae*, and *Klebsiella* spp.

Mode of action Amoxicillin acts in the manner typical of penicillins; it binds to penicillin-binding proteins (PBPs) in the bacterial cell wall and inhibits pentapeptide cross-linking during its formation, resulting in cell wall disruption.

Route of administration/doses The adult oral dose is 250–500 mg 8-hourly, and the corresponding parenteral dose is 500 mg 8-hourly, increased to 1 g 6-hourly in severe infections. Drug dosage and frequency may be modified on an individual patient basis in the treatment of severe infections.

Toxicity/side effects Allergic phenomena, gastrointestinal upsets, interstitial nephritis, and haemopoietic disturbances may complicate the use of the drug. Amoxicillin and clavulanic acid use are associated with the late development of cholestatic jaundice.

Kinetics

Absorption The drug is rapidly absorbed when administered orally; the bioavailability by this route is 72–94%. The bioavailability of clavulanic acid is approximately 60%, although it exhibits marked variability between individuals.

Distribution Amoxicillin is 17–20% protein-bound in the plasma, predominantly to albumin; the V_D is 0.3–0.4 l/kg. Clavulanic acid is 22% protein-bound; the V_D is 0.2 l/kg.

Metabolism 30% is metabolized in the liver. Clavulanic acid undergoes 50–70% hepatic metabolism.

Excretion The clearance of amoxicillin is 250–370 ml/min, and the elimination half-life is 61.3 min. Forty percent of clavulanic acid undergoes renal elimination (18–35% as unchanged drug). It has a clearance of 260 ml/min and an elimination half-life of approximately 1 hour.

Special points A reduced dosing frequency should be considered in patients with severe renal impairment. Both amoxicillin and clavulanic acid are removed by haemodialysis.

Amphotericin

Uses Amphotericin is used in the treatment of life-threatening systemic fungal infections, especially disseminated candidosis, coccidiomycosis, histoplasmosis, aspergillosis, and cryptococcosis. Amphotericin may also be administered orally for selective decontamination of the gut.

Chemical Amphotericin is a mixture of two polyene macrolides (amphotericin A and B) produced by *Streptomyces nodosus*.

Presentation As 100 mg tablets and a yellow powder in vials containing 50 000 units of amphotericin (with sodium deoxycholate which solubilizes amphotericin); the mixture forms a colloidal suspension in water; as a yellow opaque suspension of 5 mg/ml of amphotericin B complexed with two phospholipids in a 1:1 drug-to-lipid molar ratio with a ribbon-like structure, pH 5–7; as liposomal amphotericin, a lyophilized 50 mg product presentation where the 100-nm liposomes are created, so that the amphotericin is intercalated within the unilamellar bilayer structure; as an elongated disc structure, 100 nm in diameter, in a 1:1 molar ratio of amphotericin B and cholesteryl sulfate in 50 and 100 mg vials, presented in lyophilized powder for reconstitution to form a colloidal dispersion.

Main actions Amphotericin is a fungistatic antibiotic which is active against a wide range of yeasts and yeast-like fungi, including *Candida albicans*.

Mode of action The drug binds to cell membrane sterols, leading to altered membrane permeability to univalent ions, water, and small non-electrolyte molecules. Leakage of intracellular components occurs; cell growth is inhibited, and cell death may result. Amphotericin binds preferentially to sterols (especially ergosterol) in fungal cell membranes, although it does bind to sterols (especially cholesterol) in animal cell membranes where it exerts similar effects.

Routes of administration/doses Amphotericin is administered by slow intravenous infusion (via a dedicated vein), diluted in 5% glucose, over 6 hours; the daily dose is 0.25–1.5 mg/kg, and treatment will usually be required for a period of several weeks. Intrathecal, topical, and nebulized administrations of the drug have also been described.

Effects

GU Deterioration of renal function leading to hypokalaemia, renal tubular acidosis, or nephrocalcinosis occurs in >80% of patients who receive the drug; this is usually reversible but may need renal replacement therapy.

Metabolic/other The drug may decrease serum magnesium levels. Amphotericin may alter immune function (especially that of T cells and monocytes) and thereby potentiate host defences.

Toxicity/side effects The list of side effects reported with the use of amphotericin is lengthy. Gastrointestinal upsets (anorexia, nausea and vomiting, loss of weight), haematological impairment (anaemia, thrombocytopenia, leucopenia), and disturbances of the CNS (headache, muscle pains, vision disturbances, hearing loss, convulsions, peripheral neuropathy) may occur. The drug may also cause fever and phlebitis; acute dysrhythmias have also been reported.

Kinetics The assay only distinguishes amphotericin B.

Absorption The drug is poorly absorbed when administered orally.

Distribution Amphotericin is 90–95% bound in the plasma to lipoproteins; the V_D is 3.6–4.4 l/kg.

Metabolism The metabolic pathway of amphotericin has not been established; the liver appears to be the principal site of metabolism.

Excretion The drug is predominantly excreted in the urine, 2–5% unchanged. The dose should be reduced in the presence of renal impairment, as continued use of the drug may lead to further renal impairment. The clearance is 0.35–0.51 ml/min/kg, and the elimination half-life is 15 days. The high clearance and large V_D indicate tissue uptake, and the long half-life indicates slow redistribution from tissues. Non-linear behaviour occurs with increasing dosage.

Special points Liposomal encapsulation or incorporation into a lipid complex can substantially affect the action of amphotericin, compared to the free drug. There is a theoretical risk of amphotericin enhancing the effect of non-depolarizing relaxants and digoxin, secondary to the hypokalaemia that the former produces. Liposomal amphotericin (amphotericin incorporated into unilamellar liposomes) is safe, effective, and better tolerated, but may cause disordered liver function tests. The drug is poorly dialysable.

Aspirin

Uses Aspirin is used:
1. for the treatment of pain of mild to moderate severity and severe bone pain
2. as an anti-inflammatory agent, e.g. in rheumatoid arthritis and osteoarthritis
3. as an antipyretic
4. for the prevention of recurrence after myocardial infarction
5. for the prevention of graft occlusion after coronary artery surgery
6. in the treatment of pre-eclampsia
7. for the prevention of transient ischaemic attacks, and
8. deep vein thrombosis (DVT) prophylaxis post-fractured neck of femur.

Chemical An aromatic ester of acetic acid.

Presentation As 75/100/300/600 mg tablets of aspirin and in a variety of fixed-dose combinations.

Main actions Antipyretic, analgesic, and anti-inflammatory.

Mode of action Aspirin acetylates, and thereby inhibits, the enzyme cyclo-oxygenase (COX) which converts arachidonic acid to cyclic endoperoxides, thus preventing the formation of prostaglandins and thromboxanes. Prostaglandins are involved in the sensitization of peripheral pain receptors to noxious stimuli. It may also inhibit the lipo-oxygenase pathway by an action on hydroperoxy fatty acid peroxidase. The drug inhibits cyclooxygenase irreversibly in platelets, but not in the endothelium.

Routes of administration/doses The adult oral dose is 300–900 mg, 6- to 8-hourly; aspirin is not recommended for use in children under 12 years of age.

Effects

CVS Aspirin has minimal haemodynamic effects at normal doses; however, platelet aggregation is inhibited, and bleeding time is increased by a decrease in thromboxane A2 production (with large doses, the concentration of prothrombin is decreased).

RS Therapeutic doses of aspirin increase oxygen consumption and CO_2 production by uncoupling oxidative phosphorylation. Overdosage may lead to hyperventilation (by a direct action of the drug on the respiratory centre), pulmonary oedema, and respiratory failure.

CNS The analgesic effect of the drug appears to be exerted by both central and peripheral mechanisms; the antipyretic effect may be a manifestation of inhibition of prostaglandin synthesis at the hypothalamic level.

AS Aspirin increases gastric acid production.

GU The drug may cause proteinuria and an increase in the number of renal tubular casts appearing in the urine. Aspirin is uricosuric in high doses but paradoxically decreases urate excretion at low doses.

Metabolic/other Blood sugar tends to decrease with low doses and increase with high doses of aspirin. Transient elevation of serum urea concentrations and elevation of liver enzymes may occur. Lipogenesis is decreased; very large doses of aspirin stimulate steroid secretion.

Toxicity/side effects Gastrointestinal upsets occur in 2–6%; haemorrhage and gastric ulceration occur in about 1 in 10 000 of habitual users of aspirin. Large doses of the drug taken over a prolonged period may cause hepatic impairment and renal papillary necrosis, leading to chronic renal failure. Allergic response (including bronchospasm), CNS disturbances, and aplastic anaemia may also occur. The use of aspirin is associated with the development of Reye's syndrome in children.

Kinetics

Absorption Aspirin is rapidly and completely absorbed from the upper gastrointestinal tract and has a bioavailability of 70% due to an extensive first-pass metabolism.

Distribution Aspirin is rapidly hydrolysed to salicylic acid; the pharmacokinetics are of this compound. Salicylic acid is 80–90% protein-bound in the plasma, primarily to albumin. The V_D is 9.6–12.71. The drug has only a limited ability to cross the blood–brain barrier.

Metabolism/excretion At therapeutic doses, 50% of salicylic acid is metabolized to salicylurate in the liver via a saturable enzyme pathway. A further 20% is metabolized to salicylphenolic glucuronide which is also a saturable pathway. First-order kinetics occurs with the metabolic pathways of salicylacyl glucuronide (10%) and gentisic acid (5%) production and with the urinary excretion of salicylic acid (15%). Due to the two saturable metabolic pathways, the elimination of salicylic acid obeys non-linear kinetics, i.e. the half-life varies with the dose administered.

Special points Salicylates may increase the effect of co-administered oral anticoagulants and sulfonylureas due to displacement from plasma proteins.

Overdosage with aspirin has a mortality of 1–2% and may result in respiratory alkalosis or metabolic acidosis, according to the age of the patient and the time of ingestion. Alkalization of the urine increases the excretion of free salicylic acid; the fraction of free drug may increase from 5 to 85%. This principle is used in forced alkaline diuresis, and aspirin is removed by haemodialysis. A normal bleeding time should be demonstrated before embarking upon spinal or epidural anaesthesia in patients receiving aspirin.

Preoperative ingestion of aspirin is associated with increased blood loss during open heart surgery and prostatectomy.

Atenolol

Uses Atenolol is used in the treatment of:
1. hypertension
2. angina
3. tachydysrhythmias, and
4. in the acute phase of myocardial infarction and prevention of reinfarction.

Chemical A phenoxypropanolamine.

Presentation As 25/50/100 mg tablets (and in fixed-dose combinations with nifedipine, amiloride, and chlortalidone), a 0.5% syrup, and as a clear, colourless solution for injection containing 0.5 mg/ml of atenolol.

Main action Atenolol is negatively inotropic and chronotropic, leading to a fall in myocardial oxygen consumption; it also has antihypertensive and antiarrhythmic properties.

Mode of action Atenolol acts by reversible, competitive blockade of cardiac beta-1 receptors and also has some action at beta-2 receptors.

Routes of administration/doses The adult oral dose is 50–100 mg daily. Intravenously, 2.5–10 mg may be administered at a rate of 1 mg/min until the desired effect is achieved.

Effects

CVS Sinus node automaticity and AV nodal conduction are decreased. The effective refractory periods of the atrial and AV nodes are all increased by the administration of atenolol. No effect is seen on conduction in the His–Purkinje system or the effective refractory period of the ventricles. The ensuing negative inotropic and chronotropic effects lead to a decrease in myocardial oxygen consumption. Atenolol has no intrinsic sympathomimetic activity. The drug has a prolonged antihypertensive effect and can lead to regression of left ventricular hypertrophy in hypertensive patients.

RS Little effect is seen on lung function due to the cardioselectivity of atenolol.

CNS Poor CNS penetration means that little effect is seen; however, sleep disturbances and vivid dreams have been reported.

GU A clinically insignificant elevation in serum urea or creatinine may be produced by the drug.

Metabolic/other The plasma triglyceride levels may increase, and high-density lipoprotein (HDL) cholesterol levels may decrease, following the use of atenolol.

Toxicity/side effects The side effects are predictable manifestations of the pharmacological effects of the drug: exacerbation of peripheral vascular disease, bronchospasm, masking of the signs of hypoglycaemia, depression, impotence, and altered bowel habit. The precipitation of heart failure by atenolol is rare.

Kinetics

Absorption The oral bioavailability is 50%.

Distribution Atenolol is 3% protein-bound in the plasma; the V_D is 0.7 l/kg.

Metabolism <10% is metabolized in the liver.

Excretion The drug is excreted largely unchanged in the urine. The clearance is 77 ml/min/kg (which is decreased in the presence of renal failure), and the elimination half-life is 6–9 hours.

Special points The dosage should be reduced in renal failure if the glomerular filtration is <35 ml/min; the drug is readily dialysable.

Beta-blockade should be continued throughout the perioperative period; a single preoperative dose of atenolol may be as valuable as chronic treatment in the anaesthetic management of patients with borderline hypertension and in decreasing the hypertensive response to intubation and subsequent dysrhythmias. Beta-blockade may improve perioperative mortality from cardiovascular events.

Atracurium

Uses Atracurium is used to facilitate intubation and controlled ventilation.

Chemical A benzyl isoquinolinium ester which is a mixture of ten stereo-oisomers due to the presence of four chiral centres.

Presentation As a clear, colourless or pale yellow solution for injection available in 2.5 ml, 5 ml, and 25 ml vials, containing 10 mg/ml of atracurium besilate (equivalent to atracurium 7.5 mg/ml), needing to be stored at 2–8°C. It has a pH of between 3.25 and 3.65.

Main action Competitive, non-depolarizing neuromuscular blockade.

Mode of action Atracurium acts by competitive antagonism of acetylcholine at nicotinic (N2) receptors in the post-synaptic membrane of the neuromuscular junction.

Routes of administration/doses The drug is administered intravenously. The ED95 of atracurium is estimated to be 0.23 mg/kg. An initial dose of 0.3–0.6 mg/kg is recommended, providing muscle relaxation for between 15 and 35 minutes. Endotracheal intubation can be achieved within 90–120 seconds of an intravenous dose of 0.5–0.6 mg/kg, with maximal resultant neuromuscular blockade achieved within 3–5 minutes following administration. Ninety-five percent recovery of the twitch height occurs within approximately 35 minutes. Maintenance of neuromuscular blockade may be achieved with bolus doses of 0.1–0.2 mg/kg. Atracurium may be administered by intravenous infusion at a rate of 0.3–0.6 mg/kg/hour, although there is wide inter-patient variability in dosage requirements, particularly in patients on ventilation in intensive care. Induced hypothermia to a temperature of approximately 25°C reduces the rate of metabolism of atracurium. Consequently, neuromuscular block can be maintained with approximately half the original infusion rate. The drug is non-cumulative with repeated or continuous administration. Ninety-five percent recovery of twitch height, following a single dose of atracurium, occurs within 35 minutes.

Effects

CVS Atracurium has minimal cardiovascular effects; there is a change of <5% in the heart rate, mean arterial pressure, systemic vascular resistance, central venous pressure, and pulmonary capillary wedge pressure, following administration of the drug. The incidence of transient hypotension ranges from 1% to 14% in clinical trial data using doses of 0.3–0.6 mg/kg or greater.

RS Bronchospasm may occasionally occur, secondary to histamine release, in approximately 0.2% of patients.

CNS The drug has no effect on the intracranial or intraocular pressure.

AS Lower oesophageal sphincter pressure is unaffected by administration of atracurium.

Toxicity/side effects Histamine release may occur (by up to 92%) if doses >0.6 mg/kg are used, leading to cutaneous flushing (2–3%), hypotension, and bronchospasm. Bradycardia has been reported, following the administration of atracurium. There have been rare reports of fatal anaphylactoid reactions with the administration of atracurium. Cross-sensitivity may exist with vecuronium, rocuronium, and pancuronium. Administration of atracurium by intravenous infusion to critically ill patients on intensive care has been associated with the development of a critical illness neuropathy/myopathy.

Kinetics

Distribution Atracurium is 82% protein-bound in the plasma; the V_D is 0.16–0.18 l/kg. The drug does not cross the blood–brain barrier. Atracurium does cross the placenta, but not in clinically significant amounts.

Metabolism Occurs by two pathways. The major pathway is via Hofmann degradation (cleavage of the link between the quaternary nitrogen ion and the central chain) to laudanosine and a quaternary monoacrylate. Laudanosine is cleared primarily by the liver. The minor degradative pathway is via hydrolysis by non-specific esterases in the blood to a quaternary alcohol and a quaternary acid. The metabolites have insignificant neuromuscular-blocking (NMB) activity.

Excretion The clearance is 5.1–6.1 ml/kg/min, and the elimination half-life is 17–21 minutes; these parameters are little altered by renal or hepatic impairment, and no alteration in dose is necessary in these patients.

Special points

The duration of action of atracurium, in common with other non-depolarizing relaxants, is prolonged by hypokalaemia, hypocalcaemia, hypermagnesaemia, hypoproteinaemia, dehydration, acidosis, and hypercapnia. The following drugs, when co-administered with atracurium, increase the effect of the latter: volatile anaesthetic agents (isoflurane increases the activity by up to 35%), induction agents (including ketamine), fentanyl, suxamethonium, diuretics, calcium channel blockers, alpha- and beta-adrenergic antagonists, protamine, lidocaine, metronidazole, and the aminoglycoside antibiotics. Patients with burns may develop resistance to the effect of atracurium. The onset of neuromuscular blockade is likely to be lengthened and the duration of action shortened in patients receiving chronic anticonvulsant therapy. The use of atracurium appears to be safe in patients susceptible to malignant hyperpyrexia.

Laudanosine (in concentrations >17 micrograms/ml) has been shown to cause seizures in animal models and becomes measurable in patients who have received atracurium by infusion for 6 days; the clinical significance of this is unclear. Haemofiltration has a minimal effect on plasma levels of atracurium or laudanosine. The stereoisomer cisatracurium causes less histamine release and is available commercially. Atracurium, due to its acidic pH, should not be mixed with alkaline solutions (e.g. barbiturates).

Atropine

Uses Atropine is used:
1. traditionally to dry secretions prior to ether or chloroform anaesthesia (nowadays when a dry airway is desirable, especially in children under 1 year of age)
2. to counter bradycardia due to increased vagal tone
3. to counter the muscarinic effects of anticholinergic agents
4. during cardiopulmonary resuscitation
5. as a cycloplegic
6. as a constituent of cold cures, and
7. in the treatment of organophosphorus poisoning and
8. tetanus.

Chemical An alkaloid from *Atropa belladona*; atropine is a tertiary amine which is the ester of tropic acid and tropine. Commercial atropine is the racemic mixture of D- and l-hyoscyamine (l-form is active).

Presentation As a clear, colourless solution for injection containing 0.5/0.6 mg/ml and 3 mg in 10 ml of atropine sulfate; it is also available as 0.6 mg tablets.

Main action Anticholinergic.

Mode of action Atropine exerts its effects by competitive antagonism of acetylcholine at muscarinic receptors (having little effect at nicotinic receptors, except at high doses).

Routes of administration/doses Atropine may be administered intramuscularly or intravenously in a dose of 0.015–0.02 mg/kg. The adult oral dose is 0.2–0.6 mg. A total of 3 mg is needed for complete vagal blockade in adults.

Effects

CVS In low doses, atropine may produce an initial bradycardia (Bezold–Jarisch reflex), followed by tachycardia (the usual effect). The cardiac output is increased, but there is little effect on the blood pressure. Atropine decreases the AV conduction time and may produce dysrhythmias. Dilatation of facial capillaries may occur with the use of high doses.

RS Atropine produces bronchodilation with an increase in the physiological dead space. Bronchial secretions are reduced by the drug. The respiratory rate is increased, and a decreased incidence of laryngospasm has been reported following the administration of the drug.

CNS Central excitation or depression may occur (central anticholinergic syndrome). The syndrome is characterized by somnolence, confusion, amnesia, agitation, hallucinations, dysarthria, ataxia, or delirium. Atropine also has antiemetic and anti-parkinsonian actions.

AS The drug reduces salivation, the volume of gastric secretions, and tone and peristalsis throughout the gut. Atropine has a mild antispasmodic action on the biliary tree. The lower oesophageal tone is reduced by the drug.

GU Tone and peristalsis in the urinary tract are decreased.

Metabolic/other Cycloplegia, mydriasis, and an increase in intraocular pressure may be produced by the drug. Sweating is inhibited, and the basal metabolic rate is increased. The drug suppresses ADH secretion. Atropine has local anaesthetic properties.

Toxicity/side effects Atropine is painful when injected intramuscularly, and the sensation of a dry mouth is unpleasant. The central anticholinergic syndrome may occur in the elderly, and inhibition of sweating may lead to hyperpyrexia in children. Urinary retention may be precipitated by the drug. Glaucoma may result from ocular (but not intravenous or intramuscular) administration.

Kinetics

Absorption Atropine is rapidly absorbed from the gut; the bioavailability by oral route is 10–25%.

Distribution Atropine is 50% protein-bound in the plasma, the V_D is 2.0–4.0 l/kg. The drug crosses the placenta and blood–brain barrier.

Metabolism Atropine is hydrolysed in the liver and tissues to tropine and tropic acid.

Excretion 94% of the dose is excreted in the urine in 24 hours, some unchanged. The clearance is 70 l/hour, and the elimination half-life is 2.5 hours.

Special points Atropine reduces the incidence and morbidity of oculocardiac crises.

Bendroflumethiazide

Uses Bendroflumethiazide is used in the treatment of:
1. hypertension
2. oedema due to heart failure or the nephrotic syndrome
3. diabetes insipidus
4. renal tubular acidosis
5. hypercalciuria, and
6. for the inhibition of lactation.

Chemical A thiazide.

Presentation As 2.5/5 mg tablets of bendroflumethiazide and in a variety of fixed-dose combinations with beta-adrenergic antagonists.

Main actions Diuretic and antihypertensive.

Mode of action Thiazide diuretics inhibit sodium chloride co-transport in the distal convoluted tubule. They inhibit Na^+ reabsorption, which results in an increased urinary excretion of sodium, potassium, and water.

Routes of administration/doses The adult oral dose is 2.5–10 mg daily. Bendroflumethiazide has a duration of action of 12–18 hours.

Effects
CVS Bendroflumethiazide exerts its antihypertensive effect by decreasing the plasma volume and as a vasodilator. It also causes a slight decrease in the cardiac output.

CNS In toxic doses, the drug causes depression of the CNS.

GU Bendroflumethiazide decreases the renal blood flow and may also cause a reduction in the glomerular filtration rate. The drug decreases the urinary excretion of calcium and increases that of sodium, potassium, and magnesium.

Metabolic/other Thiazide diuretics may increase the blood sugar concentration by enhancing glycogenolysis and decreasing the rate of glycogenesis and insulin secretion. They may also increase serum urate, triglyceride, and cholesterol concentrations and give rise to a hypochloraemic acidosis.

Toxicity/side effects CNS and haemopoietic disturbances, rashes, impotence, and acute pancreatitis may complicate the use of the drug. Bendroflumethiazide may interfere with diabetic control and produce hypercholesterolaemia and gout, and it may aggravate renal or hepatic insufficiency.

Kinetics
Absorption Bendroflumethiazide is completely absorbed when administered orally.

Distribution Bendroflumethiazide is completely absorbed when administered orally.

Metabolism The drug is 94% protein-bound in the plasma; the V_D is 1.18 l/kg.

Excretion Occurs predominantly in the urine, 30% unchanged. The clearance is 3.68 ml/min/kg, and the elimination half-life is 2.7–4.1 hours.

Special points The drug may cause hypokalaemia and hypercalcaemia, which may precipitate digoxin toxicity, potentiate the effect of non-depolarizing muscle relaxants, and increase the likelihood of dysrhythmias occurring during general anaesthesia.

The hypotension occurring secondary to the administration of opioids, barbiturates, and halothane is reportedly exaggerated in patients receiving thiazide diuretics.

Bupivacaine

Uses Bupivacaine is used as a local anaesthetic.

Chemical An amide which is a structural homologue of mepivacaine.

Presentation As a clear, colourless solution containing racemic bupivacaine (S- and R-enantiomers) in concentrations of 0.25% (2.64 mg/ml equivalent to bupivacaine hydrochloride anhydrous 2.5 mg/ml) and 0.5% (5.28 mg/ml equivalent to bupivacaine hydrochloride anhydrous 5.0 mg/ml). The 0.25/0.5% solutions are available combined with 1:200 000 adrenaline, which contain the preservative sodium metabisulfite. A 0.5% ('hyperbaric' or 'heavy') solution containing 80 mg/ml of glucose (with a specific gravity of 1.026) is also available. Bupivacaine 0.1% is available as a mixture with 2 micrograms/ml of fentanyl for epidural use. The S-enantiomer is available as levobupivacaine hydrochloride in the following concentrations: 2.5 mg/ml, 5 mg/ml, and 7.5 mg/ml. Levobupivacaine is also available for epidural use in the following concentrations: 0.625 mg/ml and 1.25 mg/ml. The pKa of bupivacaine is 8.1, and it is 15% unionized at a pH of 7.4. The heptane:buffer partition coefficient is 27.5.

Main action Local anaesthetic.

Mode of action Local anaesthetics diffuse in their uncharged base form through neural sheaths and the axonal membrane to the internal surface of cell membrane Na^+ channels; here they combine with hydrogen ions to form a cationic species which enters the internal opening of the Na^+ channel and combines with a receptor. This produces blockade of the Na^+ channels, thereby decreasing Na^+ conductance and preventing the depolarization of the cell membrane.

Routes of administration/doses Bupivacaine may be administered topically, by infiltration, intrathecally, or epidurally; the toxic dose of bupivacaine is 2 mg/kg (with or without adrenaline). The maximum dose is 150 mg. The drug acts within 10–20 minutes and has a duration of action of 5–16 hours.

Effects

CVS Bupivacaine is markedly cardiotoxic; it binds specifically to myocardial proteins, in addition to blocking cardiac sodium channels and decreasing the rate of increase of phase 0 during the cardiac action potential. In toxic concentrations, the drug decreases the peripheral vascular resistance and myocardial contractility, producing hypotension and possibly cardiovascular collapse. K^+ and Ca^{2+} channels may also be affected at toxic doses. Levobupivacaine-induced cardiotoxicity requires a greater dose to be administered, compared with racemic bupivacaine.

CNS The principal effect of bupivacaine is reversible neural blockade; this leads to a characteristically biphasic effect in the CNS. Initially, excitation (light-headedness, dizziness, visual and auditory disturbances, and seizure activity) occurs due to inhibition of inhibitory interneurone pathways in the cortex. With increasing doses, depression of both facilitatory and inhibitory pathways occurs, leading to CNS depression (drowsiness, disorientation, and coma). Local anaesthetic agents block neuromuscular transmission when administered intraneurally; it is thought that a complex of neurotransmitter, receptor, and local anaesthetic is formed, which has negligible conductance. Levobupivacaine produces less motor blockade, but longer sensory blockade, following epidural administration.

Toxicity/side effects Allergic reactions to the amide-type local anaesthetic agents are extremely rare. The side effects are predominantly correlated with excessive plasma concentrations of the drug, as described above. The use of the drug for intravenous regional blockade is no longer recommended, as refractory cardiac depression, leading to death, has been reported when it is used for this purpose.

Kinetics

Absorption The absorption of local anaesthetic agents is related to:
1. the site of injection (intercostal > caudal > epidural > brachial plexus > subcutaneous)
2. the dose—a linear relationship exists between the total dose and the peak blood concentrations achieved, and
3. the presence of vasoconstrictors which delay absorption.

The addition of adrenaline to bupivacaine solutions does not influence the rate of systemic absorption, as:
1. the drug is highly lipid-soluble, and therefore its uptake into fat is rapid, and
2. the drug has a direct vasodilatory effect.

Distribution Bupivacaine is 95% protein-bound in the plasma to albumin and alpha-1 acid glycoprotein; the V_D is 21–103 l. An *in vitro* study of levobupivacaine protein binding in man demonstrated plasma protein binding to be >97% at concentrations between 0.1 and 1.0 micrograms/ml.

Metabolism Occurs in the liver by N-dealkylation, primarily to pipecoloxylidide. N-desbutyl bupivacaine and 4-hydroxy bupivacaine are also formed. There is no evidence of *in vivo* racemization of levobupivacaine. *In vitro* studies of levobupivacaine demonstrate that CYP3A4 and CYP1A2 are responsible for its metabolism to desbutyl levobupivacaine and 3-hydroxy levobupivacaine, respectively.

Excretion 5% of the dose is excreted in the urine as pipecoloxylidide; 16% is excreted unchanged. The clearance is 0.47 l/min, and the elimination half-life (after intravenous administration) is 0.31–0.61 hours.

Special points The onset and duration of conduction blockade are related to the pKa, lipid solubility, and the extent of protein binding. A low pKa and high lipid solubility are associated with a rapid onset time; a high degree of protein binding is associated with a long duration of action. In infants under 6 months of age, the low level of albumin and alpha-1 acid glycoprotein results in an increase in the free fraction of bupivacaine. Local anaesthetic agents significantly increase the duration of action of both depolarizing and non-depolarizing relaxants. Levobupivacaine may precipitate if diluted in alkaline solutions. Clonidine (8.4 micrograms/ml), morphine (0.05 mg/ml), and fentanyl (4 micrograms/ml) have been shown to be compatible with levobupivacaine.

Buprenorphine

Uses Buprenorphine is used:
1. in the treatment of moderate to severe pain and has been used
2. in sequential analgesia.

Chemical A synthetic derivative of the alkaloid thebaine.

Presentation As a clear, colourless solution containing 300 micrograms/ml of buprenorphine hydrochloride, 200/400 micrograms tablets, and various strengths of transdermal patches.

Main actions Analgesia.

Mode of action The mode of action of buprenorphine remains to be fully elucidated. The drug acts as a partial agonist at MOP receptors but dissociates slowly from the latter, leading to prolonged analgesia. Buprenorphine appears also to have a high affinity for (but a low intrinsic activity at) kappa-opioid receptors. One unusual property of buprenorphine hydrochloride observed *in vitro* is its very slow rate of dissociation from its receptor. This may explain its longer duration of action than morphine, the unpredictability of its reversal by opioid antagonists, and its low level of manifest physical dependence.

Routes of administration/doses The adult intramuscular and intravenous dose is 0.3–0.6 mg 6- to 8-hourly; the corresponding sublingual dose is 0.2–0.4 mg 6- to 8-hourly. The drug is also effective when administered by the epidural route; a dose of 0.3 mg has been recommended. The dose for transdermal delivery should be evaluated after 24–72 hours and adjusted according to instructions, due to the slow rise in plasma levels. Buprenorphine has a significantly longer latency period and duration of action than morphine.

Effects

CVS Buprenorphine has minimal cardiovascular effects; the heart rate may decrease (by up to 25%) and the systolic blood pressure may fall by 10%, following administration of the drug.

RS The drug produces respiratory depression and an antitussive effect, similar to that produced by morphine. Buprenorphine may cause histamine and tryptase release from lung parenchymal mast cells and may increase the PVR.

CNS The drug is 25 times as potent an analgesic as morphine. In common with other opioids, buprenorphine produces miosis. The drug decreases cerebral glucose metabolism by up to 30%.

GU The drug has been shown to reduce the rate of urine output in animals.

Metabolic/other Buprenorphine decreases the release of luteinizing hormone and increases the release of prolactin.

Toxicity/side effects Side effects are similar in nature and incidence to those produced by morphine. Drowsiness, dizziness, headache, confusion, dysphoria, and nausea and vomiting may be produced by the drug. Buprenorphine appears to be less liable to produce dependence than pure mu-agonists.

Kinetics

Absorption The drug is absorbed when administered orally but undergoes a significant first-pass metabolism, and the sublingual route is therefore preferred. The bioavailability is 40–90% when administered intramuscularly and 44–94% when administered sublingually.

Distribution Only unchanged buprenorphine appears to reach the CNS. The drug is 96% protein-bound *in vitro*; the V_D is 3.2 l/kg.

Metabolism Occurs in the liver by dealkylation with subsequent conjugation to glucuronide; the polar conjugates then appear to be excreted in the bile and hydrolysed by bacteria in the gastrointestinal tract.

Excretion Occurs predominantly via the faeces as unchanged buprenorphine; the remainder is excreted in the urine as conjugated buprenorphine and dealkylated derivatives. The clearance is 934 ml/min (this is decreased by 30% under general anaesthesia), and the elimination half-life is 5 hours.

Special points Being a partial agonist, buprenorphine antagonizes the effects of morphine and other opioid agonists and may precipitate abstinence syndromes in opiate-dependent subjects. The respiratory depressant effects of the drug are not completely reversed by even large doses of naloxone; doxapram, however, will do so. Severe respiratory depression has occurred when benzodiazepines have been co-administered with buprenorphine.

Buprenorphine is not removed by haemodialysis.

The addition of buprenorphine to local anaesthesia for brachial plexus blockade triples the length of post-operative analgesia, compared to local anaesthesia alone.

Carbamazepine

Uses Carbamazepine is used in the treatment of:
1. epilepsy, especially temporal lobe and tonic–clonic seizures
2. trigeminal neuralgia, and
3. prophylaxis of bipolar disorder.

Chemical An iminostilbene derivative structurally related to the tricyclic antidepressants.

Presentation As 100/200/400 mg tablets, 125/250 mg suppositories, and as a white syrup containing 20 mg/ml of carbamazepine.

Main actions Anticonvulsant and analgesic.

Mode of action The mode of action of carbamazepine is unknown; it may act via alterations in adenosine disposition within the CNS. It does not appear to act in the same manner as tricyclic antidepressants.

Routes of administration/doses The adult oral dose is 100–1600 mg daily in divided doses.

Effects

CVS Carbamazepine has antiarrhythmic properties and depresses AV conduction.

CNS The drug is more effective than phenytoin in raising the threshold for minimal electroshock seizures. Carbamazepine also has analeptic properties.

GU Carbamazepine has an antidiuretic effect that may lead to water intoxication.

Toxicity/side effects Diplopia, nausea and vomiting, drowsiness, and ataxia are relatively common side effects of the drug. Rashes occur in 3% of patients. Carbamazepine may also cause renal and liver damage. Mild neutropenia occurs commonly; fatal aplastic anaemia is extremely rare.

Kinetics

Absorption The drug is well absorbed when administered orally; the bioavailability by this route is nearly 100%.

Distribution Carbamazepine is 75% protein-bound in the plasma; the V_D is 1 l/kg.

Metabolism Occurs via oxidation in the liver to an epoxide which is active. With chronic use, the drug induces its own metabolism.

Excretion The drug is predominantly excreted in the urine as unconjugated metabolites; the clearance is 20 ml/kg/hour, and the elimination half-life is 16–36 hours.

Special points Sodium valproate and calcium antagonists may increase the plasma concentrations of free carbamazepine if administered concurrently. The efficacy of both pancuronium and vecuronium is reportedly decreased in patients receiving carbamazepine. Regular liver function tests and estimation of white cell counts need to be performed during chronic carbamazepine therapy.

The drug is not removed by haemodialysis.

Carbapenems

Uses Carbapenems are used in the treatment of:
1. respiratory tract infections
2. urinary tract infections
3. infections of bone, joint, skin, and soft tissues
4. intra-abdominal sepsis
5. gynaecological sepsis
6. meningitis
7. septicaemia
8. neutropenic sepsis, and
9. as surgical prophylaxis.

Chemical Beta-lactam derivatives.

Presentation Imipenem, meropenem, and ertapenem are presented as a dry powder. Imipenem is presented in an ampoule containing 500 mg of imipenem monohydrate and 500 mg of cilastatin sodium, which blocks renal imipenem metabolism. Meropenem is presented in ampoules containing 500 mg and 1 g as meropenem trihydrate. Ertapenem is presented in vials containing 1 g of ertapenem (as ertapenem sodium). Each 1 g dose of ertapenem contains approximately 137 mg of sodium.

Main action Carbapenems are broad-spectrum antibiotics with activity against:
1. Gram-positive bacteria (not meticillin-resistant *Staphylococcus aureus* (MRSA) or *Enterococcus faecalis*)
2. Gram-negative bacteria (not *Stenotrophomonas maltophilia*)
3. Anaerobic bacteria
4. Extended-spectrum beta-lactamase (ESBL)-producing organisms.

Mode of action Carbapenems act by binding to PBPs on the bacterial cytoplasmic membrane, thereby blocking peptidoglycan synthesis and thus cell wall formation. Cilastatin sodium, presented with imipenem, is a competitive, reversible inhibitor of dehydropeptidase-1, which mediates the renal metabolism of imipenem. The drug itself has no intrinsic antibacterial activity.

Routes of administration/doses Carbapenems are administered intravenously. The specific dose and frequency of an agent administered are dependent on the clinical indication, age of the patient, and particular agent being used. Doses should be reduced in patients with renal impairment.

Toxicity/side effects Hypersensitivity reactions, diarrhoea, vomiting, a positive Coombs' test, and pseudomembranous colitis have been reported, following the administration of carbapenems. Patients with underlying CNS disorders and/or renal impairment may develop CNS side effects.

Kinetics

Distribution The V_D for imipenem is 16 l, for meropenem 12.5–20 l, and for ertapenem 8 l. The percentage of drug bound to plasma proteins is 20% for imipenem, 2% for meropenem, and 85–95% for ertapenem.

Metabolism Imipenem is combined with cilastatin, which prevents renal hydrolysis of the beta-lactam ring. However, 20–25% of an administered dose undergoes non-renal systemic metabolism that remains to be fully elucidated. Meropenem is metabolized to an inactive metabolite. Ertapenem is metabolized to a ring-open derivative, following hydrolysis mediated by dehydropeptidase-1.

Excretion The clearance of imipenem is 225 ml/min (reduced to 194 ml/min when administered with cilastatin), and it has a half-life of 62 minutes. The clearance of meropenem is equivalent to the creatinine clearance, and it has a half-life of 60 minutes. Seventy percent of an administered dose of meropenem is excreted unchanged in the urine. The clearance of ertapenem is 207 ml/min, and it has a half-life of 4 hours. Eighty percent of an administered dose is excreted in the urine (38% unchanged, 37% as the inactive metabolite) and 10% in faeces.

Special points Imipenem is cleared by dialysis, and the dose should be halved and the dose interval doubled. Meropenem and ertapenem are unaffected by hepatic dysfunction. No data are available regarding the use of imipenem in patients with hepatic dysfunction.

Co-administration of imipenem and ganciclovir may lead to focal seizures. Carbapenems may reduce sodium valproate levels, leading to seizure activity.

Carbapenemase-producing organisms, such as *Klebsiella pneumoniae*, have been isolated.

Antimicrobial agents should always be administered, following consideration of local pharmacy and microbiological policies.

Carbon dioxide

Uses CO_2 is used:
1. to reverse apnoea due to passive hyperventilation
2. to facilitate the inhalational induction of anaesthesia and blind nasal intubation
3. to speed the onset of action of local anaesthetics
4. to increase cerebral blood flow during carotid artery surgery
5. for the insufflation of body cavities during endoscopy
6. for cryotherapy, and
7. in the treatment of hiccups.

Chemical An organic gas.

Presentation As a liquid in cylinders at a pressure of 50 bar at 15°C; the cylinders are grey and are available in three sizes (C–E, containing 450–1800 l, respectively). CO_2 is a colourless gas with a pungent smell in high concentrations; it is non-flammable and does not support combustion. The specific gravity of the gas is 1.98, the critical temperature 31°C, and the critical pressure 73.8 atmospheres.

Main action Respiratory and sympathetic stimulation.

Routes of administration/doses The gas is generally administered by inhalation but may be insufflated into, for example, the peritoneal cavity. Any concentration that is desired may be employed; concentrations of up to 5% are generally administered by inhalation.

Effects

CVS In vitro, the gas has negative inotropic and chronotropic effects; in vivo, these effects are offset by sympathetic stimulation. The overall effect of the administration of 5% CO_2 is to increase the heart rate, systolic and diastolic blood pressures, and cardiac output. Dysrhythmias may occur in vivo, although, in vitro, the gas increases the threshold for catecholamine-induced dysrhythmias. The peripheral vascular resistance is decreased in vivo; CO_2 is a potent coronary arterial vasodilator.

RS CO_2 (in a concentration of 5%) stimulates respiration by an action on the respiratory centre and peripheral chemoreceptors, leading to an increase in the tidal volume and respiratory rate; bronchodilatation is also produced. At high concentrations, respiratory depression occurs. The presence of an increased partial pressure of CO_2 in the blood shifts the oxygen dissociation curve to the right (the Bohr effect).

CNS A $PaCO_2$ of 8–11 kPa will increase the cerebral blood flow by 100% and lead to an increase in the intracranial pressure and progressive narcosis. A $PaCO_2$ of 3.5 kPa will reduce the cerebral blood flow by 30%.

Metabolic/other The administration of exogenous CO_2 causes a respiratory acidosis which may, in turn, lead to hyperkalaemia. The plasma concentrations of adrenaline, noradrenaline, angiotensin, and 15-hydroxycorticosteroid are increased by the administration of CO_2.

Toxicity/side effects When administered in concentrations of 10%, the gas may cause dyspnoea, headache, dizziness, restlessness, paraesthesiae, diaphoresis, and dysrhythmias.

Kinetics

Absorption The gas is freely permeable through normal alveolar tissue.

Distribution CO_2 is transported in the blood in solution, in the form of bicarbonate ions, and in combination with plasma proteins and haemoglobin.

Metabolism The gas is transformed in the blood to the forms described above.

Excretion Predominantly by exhalation and some as renally excreted bicarbonate.

Special points A respiratory acidosis may alter drug action by altering both the degree of ionization and protein binding of drugs; an increased dose of thiopental and a decreased dose of tubocurarine are required in the face of an uncompensated respiratory acidosis.

Caspofungin

Uses Caspofungin is used for:
1. treatment of invasive candidiasis
2. treatment of invasive aspergillosis, and
3. empirical therapy for presumed fungal infections (such as *Candida* or *Aspergillus*) in febrile, neutropenic patients.

Chemical Semi-synthetic lipopeptide (echinocandin) compound synthesized from a fermentation product of *Glarea lozoyensis*.

Presentation As off-white powder in 50 mg and 70 mg vials containing 35.7 mg and 50 mg of sucrose, respectively—store in a refrigerator at 2–8°C. It is reconstituted with 10.5 ml of water to make a clear solution and should be used immediately. Stability data show the concentrate solution for infusion can be stored for up to 24 hours when the vial is stored at 25°C. It contains no preservatives. Diluted patient infusion solution should be used immediately, diluted with 100 ml or 250 ml of 0.9/0.45% sodium chloride solution or lactated Ringer's solution. Stability data have shown that this can be used within 24 hours when stored at 25°C or less, or within 48 hours when the intravenous infusion bag is stored refrigerated at 2–8°C.

Main actions Fungicidal activity with lysis and death of hyphal apical tips and branch points where cell growth and division occur. Caspofungin is active against *Aspergillus fumigatus/flavus/niger/terreus/candidus* and *Candida* spp. (*Candida albicans/dubliniensis/glabrata/guilliermondii, kefyr, krusei, lipolytica, lusitaniae, parapsilosis, rugosa*, and *tropicalis*), including isolates with multiple resistance transport mutations and those with acquired or intrinsic resistance to fluconazole, amphotericin B, and 5-flucytosine.

Mode of action Caspofungin acetate inhibits the synthesis of beta (1,3)-D-glucan, an essential component of the cell wall of many filamentous fungi and yeast. Beta (1,3)-D-glucan is not present in mammalian cells.

Route of administration/doses A single 70 mg intravenous loading dose is given on day 1, followed by 50 mg daily thereafter. In patients weighing >80 kg, after the initial 70 mg loading dose, caspofungin 70 mg daily is recommended. After reconstitution and dilution, the solution should be administered by slow intravenous infusion over approximately 1 hour. The duration of treatment is unknown and should be based on the patient (duration of clinical response to empirical therapy), up to 72 hours after the resolution of neutropenia (absolute neutrophil count, ANC ≥500): fungal infections for a minimum of 14 days, and continue for at least 7 days after both neutropenia and clinical symptoms are resolved; invasive candidiasis after symptoms have resolved, and antifungal therapy should continue for at least 14 days after the last positive culture; invasive aspergillosis is based upon the severity of the patient's underlying disease, recovery from immunosuppression, and clinical response. In general, treatment should continue for at least 7 days after the resolution of symptoms.

Effects

GU Caspofungin is not an inhibitor of cytochrome P450 (CYP).

Metabolic/other Hypokalaemia, decreased haemoglobin level, decreased haematocrit, and decreased white blood cell count.

Toxicity/side effects
Anaphylaxis, histamine-mediated adverse reactions, including rash, facial swelling, angio-oedema, pruritus, sensation of warmth, or bronchospasm have been reported.

Kinetics

Absorption Poor oral bioavailability.

Distribution Caspofungin is 97% protein-bound to albumin. Peak concentrations occur in tissues at 1.5–2 days where 92% of the dose is distributed. Only a small fraction of caspofungin taken up into tissues returns to the plasma, so a true estimate of the V_D of caspofungin is impossible to calculate.

Metabolism It undergoes spontaneous degradation to an open ring compound, with further peptide hydrolysis and N-acetylation. Two intermediate products form covalent adducts to plasma proteins, resulting in a low-level, irreversible binding.

Excretion Elimination from the plasma is slow, with a clearance of 10–12 ml/min. Plasma concentrations of caspofungin decline in a polyphasic manner, following single 1-hour intravenous infusions. A short alpha-phase occurs immediately post-infusion, followed by a beta-phase with a half-life of 9–11 hours. An additional gamma-phase also occurs with a half-life of 45 hours. Distribution is the dominant mechanism influencing the plasma clearance. Approximately 41% of the dose is excreted in the urine, and 34% in faeces. Caspofungin displays moderate non-linear pharmacokinetics.

Special points
No dosage adjustment is needed for renal or liver impairment; there is little knowledge about severe liver impairment. Weight was found to influence caspofungin pharmacokinetics; the plasma concentrations decrease with increasing weight with 23% AUC, hence a higher dose for patients weighing >80 kg. Less common non-*Candida* yeasts and non-*Aspergillus* moulds may not be covered by caspofungin. Close monitoring of liver enzymes should be considered if caspofungin and ciclosporin are used concomitantly due to elevation of aspartate transaminase (AST) and alanine transaminase (ALT). This product contains sucrose, so patients with rare hereditary problems of fructose intolerance or sucrase–isomaltase insufficiency should not have caspofungin.

Cephalosporins

Uses Cephalosporins are used in the treatment of:
1. respiratory tract infections
2. urinary tract infections
3. infections of bone, joint, and soft tissues
4. intra-abdominal, gynaecological, and obstetric sepsis
5. meningitis
6. septicaemia, and
7. as surgical prophylaxis.

Chemical Derivatives of penicillin containing a beta-lactam and a hydro-thiazine ring.

Presentation Cephalosporins are divided into first (cefradine), second (cefuroxime), and third (cefotaxime, ceftazidime, ceftriaxone) generations.

Main action Cephalosporins are broad-spectrum bactericidal antibiotics that are variably resistant to hydrolysis by beta-lactamase. The drugs are effective against Gram-positive organisms. Gram-negative cover improves with each subsequent generation of cephalosporin (cefradine < cefuroxime < cefotaxime/ceftazidime/ceftriaxone), although this is at the expense of reduced activity against Gram-positive bacteria. Ceftazidime is active against the following organisms: *Pseudomonas, Klebsiella, Proteus, Salmonella, Shigella, Neisseria* spp., *Haemophilus influenzae*, and *Escherichia coli*.

Mode of action Cephalosporins act by binding to PBPs on the bacterial cytoplasmic membrane, thereby blocking peptidoglycan synthesis and thus cell wall synthesis.

Routes of administration/doses Cefradine is available in capsule form, as a syrup, or as a powder for dissolving in solution for intravenous use. Cefuroxime is available as a tablet, as granules for use as an oral suspension, or as a powder for dissolving in solution for intravenous administration. Third-generation cephalosporins are presented for intravenous use only. The specific dose and frequency of an agent administered are dependent on the clinical indication, age of the patient, and particular agent being used.

Toxicity/side effects Cephalosporins are generally well tolerated. Rashes, hypersensitivity reactions, fever, diarrhoea, transient haematological disturbances (including a positive Coombs' text), and abnormalities of liver function tests may occur with the use of these drugs. If administered in high doses to patients concurrently receiving other nephrotoxic drugs, further deterioration in renal function may result. *Clostridium difficile* infection may complicate the administration of these agents. The development of a 'Jarisch–Herxheimer' reaction may complicate the use of cephalosporins in the treatment of Lyme disease.

Kinetics

Absorption Cefradine is well absorbed from the gastrointestinal tract. The bioavailability of cefuroxime is 36–52%.

Distribution Cephalosporins exhibit variable degrees of protein binding: cefradine 8–17%, cefuroxime and cefotaxime 35–50%, ceftazidime <10%, ceftriaxone 95%. The drugs are widely distributed, and third-generation agents penetrate inflamed tissues well.

Metabolism Most cephalosporins are not metabolized, apart from cefotaxime which is partially metabolized to the active metabolite desacetyl-cefotaxime. The half-life for these agents are short (1–2 hours), compared with ceftriaxone which has a half-life of 8 hours.

Excretion Cephalosporins are predominantly renally excreted unchanged in the urine. Forty percent of ceftriaxone is excreted in the bile and faeces, 60% in the urine.

Special points Cephalosporins are removed by haemodialysis.

Cephalosporins are associated with an increased potential for *Clostridium difficile* infection.

Antimicrobial agents should always be administered, following consideration of local pharmacy and microbiological policies.

Chloroprocaine

Uses Chloroprocaine is used for spinal anaesthesia for surgical procedures lasting no longer than 40 minutes.

Chemical An ester of aminobenzoic acid.

Presentation As a clear, colourless solution containing 5 ml of chloroprocaine hydrochloride in a glass ampoule at a concentration of 10 mg/ml. The pH of the solution is 3–4. The pKa is 8.96.

Main actions Local anaesthetic.

Mode of action Local anaesthetics diffuse in their uncharged base form through neural sheaths and the axonal membrane to the internal surface of cell membrane Na^+ channels; here they combine with hydrogen ions to form a cationic species which enters the internal opening of the Na^+ channel and combines with a receptor. This produces blockade of the Na^+ channel, thereby decreasing Na^+ conductance and preventing depolarization of the cell membrane.

Route of administration/doses Chloroprocaine is licensed for intrathecal administration. The duration of action of the drug is dose-dependent. For example, a sensory block to T10 can be achieved with 40 mg of the drug lasting 80 minutes, or 50 mg of the drug lasting 100 minutes.

Effects

CVS Chloroprocaine is cardiotoxic; it binds specifically to myocardial proteins, in addition to blocking cardiac sodium channels and decreasing the rate of increase of phase 0 during the cardiac action potential. In toxic concentrations, the drug decreases the peripheral vascular resistance and myocardial contractility, producing hypotension and possibly cardiovascular collapse. K^+ and Ca^{2+} channels may also be affected at toxic doses.

CNS The principal effect of chloroprocaine is reversible neural blockade; this leads to a characteristically biphasic effect in the CNS. Initially, excitation (lightheadedness, dizziness, visual and auditory disturbances, and seizure activity) occurs due to inhibition of inhibitory interneurone pathways in the cortex. With increasing doses, depression of both facilitatory and inhibitory pathways occurs, leading to CNS depression (drowsiness, disorientation, and coma). Local anaesthetic agents block neuromuscular transmission when administered intraneurally; it is thought that a complex of neurotransmitter, receptor, and local anaesthetic is formed which has negligible conductance.

Toxicity/side effects The side effects are predominantly correlated with excessive plasma concentrations of the drug, as described above.

Kinetics Limited data are available.

Metabolism Chloroprocaine is rapidly metabolized by plasma pseudocholinesterase, producing the metabolites beta-diethylaminoethanol and 2-chloro-4-aminobenzoic acid.

Excretion The metabolites of chloroprocaine are excreted in the urine.

Chlorphenamine

Uses Chlorphenamine is used in the treatment of:
1. allergic rhinitis
2. urticaria
3. pruritus, and
4. anaphylactic and anaphylactoid reactions.

Chemical An alkylamine.

Presentation As 4 mg tablets, a syrup containing 0.4 mg/ml, and a clear, colourless solution for injection containing 10 mg/ml of chlorphenamine maleate.

Main action Antihistaminergic (H1 receptors) and anticholinergic.

Mode of action Chlorphenamine acts by reversible competitive antagonism of histamine H1 receptors.

Routes of administration/doses The adult oral dose is 4 mg 6- to 8-hourly. The drug may also be administered intravenously (over a period of 1 min), intramuscularly, or subcutaneously as a stat dose of 10 mg.

Effects

CVS The drug inhibits histamine-induced vasodilation and increased capillary permeability.

RS Chlorphenamine decreases bronchial secretions; it does not completely reverse anaphylactic bronchospasm in man, since leukotrienes are involved in the mediation of allergic bronchoconstriction.

CNS The drug has a sedative effect and local anaesthetic properties.

Metabolic/other Chlorphenamine has anticholinergic properties.

Toxicity/side effects The predominant side effect of the drug is drowsiness, but it may also produce gastrointestinal disturbances (including nausea and vomiting) and anticholinergic side effects.

Kinetics

Absorption The drug is slowly absorbed when administered orally; the bioavailability by this route is 25–50% due to an extensive first-pass metabolism in the gut wall and liver.

Distribution The drug is 70% protein-bound in the plasma; the V_D is 7.51–7.65 l/kg.

Metabolism Occurs via demethylation and oxidative deamination in the liver.

Excretion The mono- and di-desmethyl derivatives are excreted predominantly in the urine; 1–27% (dependent upon the urinary pH) of an administered dose is excreted unchanged in the urine. The clearance is 4.4–7.92 ml/min/kg, and the elimination half-life is 2–43 hours.

Special points The sedative effect of the drug is additive with that produced by anaesthetic agents.

The drug is not removed by dialysis.

Chlorpromazine

Uses Chlorpromazine is used in the treatment of:
1. schizophrenia and related psychoses
2. nausea and vomiting associated with terminal illness, and
3. intractable hiccup.

Chemical A phenothiazine (with an aliphatic side chain).

Presentation As 10/25/50/100 mg tablets, a syrup containing 5 mg/ml, 100 mg suppositories, and as a straw-coloured solution for injection containing 25 mg/ml of chlorpromazine hydrochloride.

Main action Antipsychotic, antiemetic, and sedative.

Mode of action The antiemetic and neuroleptic effects of the drug appear to be mediated by central dopaminergic (D2) blockade, leading to an increased threshold for vomiting at the chemoreceptor trigger zone. The other pharmacological effects are mediated by antagonism of serotonergic, histaminergic, muscarinic cholinergic, and alpha-adrenergic receptors.

Routes of administration/doses The adult oral dose is 10–50 mg 6- to 8-hourly; the corresponding dose by the intramuscular route is 25–50 mg 6- to 8-hourly.

Effects

CVS Chlorpromazine is negatively inotropic; in combination with the decrease in the systemic vascular resistance mediated by alpha-adrenergic blockade that it produces, postural hypotension with a reflex tachycardia are the main effects observed. The drug increases the coronary blood flow and has a mild quinidine-like action on the heart. Chlorpromazine may produce electrocardiographic (ECG) changes, including prolongation of the PR and QT intervals, T-wave flattening, and ST-segment depression.

RS The drug is a respiratory depressant; it also diminishes bronchial secretions.

CNS The main central effect of the drug is neurolepsis, but sedation and anxiolysis are also produced. Chlorpromazine enhances the effect of co-administered analgesics and lowers the seizure threshold; it also has local anaesthetic properties. The drug causes skeletal muscle relaxation via a central effect. Miosis occurs due to alpha-adrenergic blockade. It increases sleep time but decreases the time spent in the rapid eye movement (REM) phase. The characteristic EEG changes associated with the use of chlorpromazine are slowing with an increase in theta- and delta-wave activity and a decrease in alpha- and beta-wave activity, associated with some increase in burst activity.

AS Chlorpromazine increases appetite and may cause weight gain; it tends to decrease salivation, gastric secretion, and gastrointestinal motility.

GU The drug increases renal blood flow and has a weak diuretic action. Ejaculation and micturition may be inhibited, secondary to the anticholinergic effect of the drug.

Metabolic/other Chlorpromazine impairs temperature regulation by both central and peripheral mechanisms; anaesthetized subjects receiving the drug show a tendency to become poikilothermic. The phenothiazines increase prolactin secretion and tend to decrease adrenocorticotrophic and ADH release. Insulin release, and thus glucose tolerance, may also be impaired by the drug.

Toxicity/side effects Chlorpromazine is generally a well-tolerated and safe drug, despite its panoply of effects. The drug may produce a variety of extrapyramidal syndromes, including the rare neuroleptic malignant syndrome (a complex of symptoms that include catatonia, cardiovascular lability, hyperthermia, and myoglobinaemia) which has a mortality in excess of 10%. A variety of anticholinergic effects, jaundice, blood dyscrasias, and allergic phenomena may also complicate the use of the drug.

Kinetics

Absorption Chlorpromazine is well absorbed when administered orally but has a bioavailability by this route of 30% due to an extensive first-pass metabolism in the liver and gut wall.

Distribution The drug is 95–98% protein-bound in the plasma; the V_D is 12–30 l/kg.

Metabolism Chlorpromazine is extensively metabolized in the liver by oxidation, dealkylation, demethylation, and hydroxylation, with subsequent conjugation to glucuronide; at least 168 metabolites have been described, many of which are active.

Excretion Occurs in equal quantities in the urine and faeces; <1% is excreted unchanged. The clearance is 5.7–11.5 ml/min/kg, and the elimination half-life is 30 hours.

Special points The depressant effects of chlorpromazine are additive with those produced by general anaesthetic agents.

The drug is not removed by haemodialysis.

Cisatracurium

Uses Cisatracurium is used to facilitate intubation and controlled ventilation.

Chemical A benzyl isoquinolinium ester which is one of ten stereoisomers of atracurium due to the presence of four chiral centres.

Presentation As a clear, colourless or pale yellow solution for injection available in 5, 10, and 20 ml vials containing 6.7 mg/ml of cisatracurium besilate (equivalent to cisatracurium 5 mg/ml), needing to be stored at 2–8°C. It contains no antimicrobial preservative. It has a pH of between 3.25 and 3.65.

Main action Competitive, non-depolarizing neuromuscular blockade.

Mode of action Cisatracurium acts by competitive antagonism of acetylcholine at nicotinic (N2) receptors at the post-synaptic membrane of the neuromuscular junction.

Routes of administration/doses The drug is administered intravenously. The ED95 of cisatracurium is estimated to be 0.05 mg/kg during opioid anaesthesia. An initial dose of 0.15 mg/kg is recommended, providing good to excellent intubating conditions in 120 seconds. The time to 90% T1 suppression following this dose is 2.6 minutes; the time to maximal T1 suppression is 3.5 minutes, and the time to 25% spontaneous T1 recovery is 55 minutes. Maintenance of neuromuscular blockade may be achieved with bolus doses of 0.03 mg/kg (0.02 mg/kg in paediatric patients) which will provide approximately 20 minutes of additional neuromuscular blockade (approximately 9 minutes in paediatric patients). Once recovery from neuromuscular blockade has started, the rate of recovery is independent of the dose of cisatracurium administered. Cisatracurium may be administered by intravenous infusion at an initial rate of 3 micrograms/kg/min (0.18 mg/kg/hour), although there is wide inter-patient variability in dosage requirements, particularly in patients ventilated on intensive care. This infusion rate should result in T1 suppression of between 89 and 99%. After an initial period of stabilization of neuromuscular block, a rate of 1–2 micrograms/kg/min (0.06–0.12 mg/kg/min) is recommended to maintain adequate blockade (0.03–0.06 mg/kg/min in patients ventilated on intensive care). Following long-term continuous infusion of cisatracurium (<6 days), the median time to full spontaneous recovery was approximately 50 minutes. When used in conjunction with isoflurane maintenance, the infusion rate may be reduced by up to 40%. The use of cisatracurium in patients undergoing induced hypothermia (25–28°C) has not been studied.

Effects

CVS Cisatracurium has fewer cardiovascular effects than atracurium. There is no change in the mean arterial pressure or heart rate following rapid bolus doses of 0.1–0.4 mg/kg in healthy adults and patients with severe cardiovascular disease. Bradycardia (0.4%), hypotension (0.2%), and cutaneous flushing (0.2%) have all been reported.

RS Bronchospasm following the administration of cisatracurium has been occasionally reported (approximately 0.2%).

CNS The drug has no effect on the intracranial or intraocular pressure.

AS Lower oesophageal sphincter pressure is unaffected by administration of cisatracurium.

Toxicity/side effects There is no dose-dependent increase in histamine release following the administration of cisatracurium at doses of 0.1–0.4 mg/kg. There have been rare reports of fatal anaphylactoid reactions with the administration of atracurium. The administration of cisatracurium by intravenous infusion to critically ill patients on intensive care has been associated with the development of a critical illness neuropathy/myopathy.

Kinetics

Distribution The binding of cisatracurium has not been determined due to its rapid degradation at physiological pH. The V_D at steady state is 0.12–0.16 l/kg.

Metabolism Occurs by two pathways; the major pathway is via Hofmann degradation (cleavage of the link between the quaternary nitrogen ion and the central chain) to laudanosine and a quaternary monacrylate. Laudanosine is cleared primarily by the liver. The minor degradative pathway is via hydrolysis by non-specific esterases in the blood to a quaternary alcohol and a quaternary acid. The metabolites have insignificant NMB activity.

Excretion The clearance is 4.7–5.7 ml/kg/min, and the elimination half-life is 22–29 minutes; these parameters are little altered by renal or hepatic impairment, and no alteration in dose is necessary in these patients. A study in healthy adults demonstrated that 95% of the dose of cisatracurium is excreted in the urine (mostly as conjugated metabolites) and 4% in the faeces. Between 10% and 15% of an administered dose is excreted unchanged in the urine.

Special points The duration of action of cisatracurium, in common with other non-depolarizing relaxants, is prolonged by hypokalaemia, hypocalcaemia, hypermagnesaemia, hypoproteinaemia, dehydration, acidosis, and hypercapnia. The following drugs, when co-administered with atracurium, increase the effect of the latter: volatile anaesthetic agents, ketamine, other non-depolarizing NMB agents, diuretics (furosemide, mannitol, acetazolamide), calcium channel blockers, propranolol, lidocaine, aminoglycoside antibiotics, and magnesium and lithium salts. A decreased effect may be seen in patients receiving chronic anticonvulsant therapy.

The C_{max} values of laudanosine are lower in patients receiving intravenous infusions of cisatracurium, compared with those receiving a continuous atracurium infusion. No dose alteration is required in patients with renal or hepatic impairment, although the half-life values of metabolites are prolonged in patients with renal impairment.

Cisatracurium, due to its acidic pH, should not be mixed with alkaline solutions (e.g. barbiturates). It is not compatible with propofol or ketorolac. The drug is compatible with the following agents: alfentanil, fentanyl, sufentanil, and midazolam.

Porcine studies indicate that cisatracurium does not trigger malignant hyperthermia, although the drug has not been studied in susceptible humans.

Clomethiazole

Uses Clomethiazole is used:
1. in the management of alcohol withdrawal states
2. as an anticonvulsant (emergency use only)
3. as a hypnotic for the elderly
4. in the treatment of eclampsia and pre-eclampsia, and
5. for sedation in patients undergoing surgery under regional blockade or intensive care.

Chemical A thiamine derivative.

Presentation As a clear, aqueous solution containing 8 mg/ml of clomethiazole edisylate, and in 192 mg capsule and 50 mg/ml syrup form.

Main action Anticonvulsant, sedative, and anxiolytic.

Mode of action The anticonvulsant and sedative actions are due to enhancement of central GABA-ergic transmission and possibly inhibition of central dopaminergic transmission.

Routes of administration/doses For the control of convulsions in adults, 40–100 ml of the 0.8% solution are infused intravenously over 5–10 minutes; subsequently, the infusion rate is tailored to the response. For sedation, 25 ml/min are administered intravenously for 1–2 minutes, followed by a maintenance infusion of 1–4 ml/min. As a hypnotic, 1–2 capsules or 5–10 ml of the syrup are administered orally.

Effects

CVS Tachycardia and hypotension are the only clinically significant effects of the drug. It is also powerfully amnesic.

RS No effects are seen with the use of clomethiazole, but, at high doses, airway obstruction may occur.

CNS Clomethiazole has anticonvulsant, sedative, and hypnotic properties.

Toxicity/side effects Nasal and conjunctival irritation, headache, and increased bronchial secretions may occur. Prolonged intravenous infusion of clomethiazole may lead to volume overload and electrolyte abnormalities due to the water load involved. Renal failure has been reported after prolonged use associated with hypotension. Physical dependence and withdrawal states have been reported, following chronic use of the drug.

Kinetics

Absorption Clomethiazole is well absorbed when administered orally; the bioavailability by this route is 25–34% due to a high hepatic clearance.

Distribution The drug is 65–70% protein-bound in the plasma, predominantly to albumin; the V_D is 3–5 l/kg.

Metabolism Occurs predominantly by oxidation in the liver; there is an extensive first-pass effect. Ten to 20% is metabolized in the lung; there may also be some renal extraction of the drug.

Excretion 0.1% is excreted unchanged in the urine. The clearance is 2.1 l/min, and the elimination half-life is 1–6 hours.

Special points Clomethiazole is absorbed by plastic giving-sets.

It is removed by haemodialysis, but this may not significantly affect the degree of sedation.

Clonidine

Uses Clonidine is used in the treatment of:
1. all grades of essential and secondary hypertension
2. hypertensive crises and in the management of
3. migraine
4. menopausal flushing and may be of use in
5. chronic pain
6. during opiate and alcohol withdrawal, and
7. for intravenous regional analgesia for chronic regional pain syndromes.

Chemical An aniline derivative.

Presentation As 0.1/0.25/0.3 mg tablets and as a clear, colourless solution for injection containing 0.15 mg/ml of clonidine hydrochloride.

Main action Antihypertensive, analgesic, sedative, and anxiolytic.

Mode of action Clonidine acts acutely by stimulating alpha-2 (pre-synaptic) adrenoceptors, thereby decreasing noradrenaline release from sympathetic nerve terminals and consequently decreasing sympathetic tone; it also increases vagal tone. The drug acts chronically by reducing the responsiveness of peripheral vessels to vasoactive substances and to sympathetic stimulation. The analgesic effects are also mediated by activation of alpha-2 adrenoceptors in the dorsal horn of the spinal cord.

Routes of administration/doses The adult oral dose is 0.05–0.6 mg 8-hourly; the corresponding intravenous dose is 0.15–0.3 mg. When administered by the epidural route, a dose of 0.15 mg has been used. The drug acts within 10 minutes and lasts for 3–7 hours when administered intravenously.

Effects

CVS When administered intravenously, clonidine causes a transient increase in the blood pressure (due to the stimulation of vascular alpha-1 receptors), followed by a sustained decrease. The heart rate and venous return may decrease slightly; the drug has no effect on cardiac contractility, and the cardiac output is well maintained. The coronary vascular resistance is decreased by clonidine; the systemic vascular resistance is decreased with long-term treatment.

CNS Clonidine decreases the cerebral blood flow and intraocular pressure. It exerts a depressant effect on both spontaneous sympathetic outflow and afferent A delta- and C-fibre-mediated somatosympathetic reflexes.

AS Clonidine decreases gastric and small bowel motility and is an antisialogogue.

GU Clonidine reduces renovascular resistance; however, little alteration in the glomerular filtration rate occurs.

Metabolic/other The drug causes a decrease in plasma catecholamine concentrations and plasma renin activity. Blood sugar concentration may increase, secondary to alpha-adrenergic stimulation.

Toxicity/side effects Drowsiness and a dry mouth may occur in up to 50% of patients who receive the drug. CNS disturbances, fluid retention, impotence, and constipation have also been reported. Rapid withdrawal of the drug may lead to life-threatening rebound hypertension and tachycardia.

Kinetics

Absorption The drug is rapidly well absorbed when administered orally; the oral bioavailability is 100%.

Distribution Clonidine is very lipid-soluble and penetrates the CNS. The drug is 20% protein-bound in the plasma; the V_D is 1.7–2.5 l/kg.

Metabolism Less than half of an administered dose is metabolized in the liver to inactive metabolites.

Excretion 65% of the dose of clonidine is excreted unchanged in the urine; some 20% is excreted in the faeces. The clearance is 1.9–4.3 ml/min/kg, and the elimination half-life is 6–23 hours. The latter is markedly increased in the presence of renal impairment; the dose of clonidine should be reduced if the glomerular filtration rate is 10 ml/min.

Special points Clonidine decreases the MAC of co-administered volatile agents. It decreases the incidence of post-anaesthetic shivering and post-operative nausea and vomiting (PONV).

Clonidine decreases the propofol dose needed for laryngeal mask airway (LMA) insertion.

It obtunds tourniquet-induced hypertension.

Clonidine decreases post-operative agitation in children undergoing sevoflurane anaesthesia.

It prolongs the duration of local anaesthesia when co-administered for neural and retrobulbar blockade.

The drug is not removed by haemodialysis.

Clopidogrel

Uses Clopidogrel is used in the treatment of:
1. acute coronary syndrome
2. recent myocardial infarction
3. recent stroke and transient ischaemic attacks
4. established peripheral vascular disease, and
5. as part of revascularization procedures to reduce the incidence of thrombotic events.

Chemical Clopidogrel is a thienopyridine.

Presentation As 75/300 mg tablets.

Main actions Inhibitor of platelet activation and aggregation; prolongation of bleeding time.

Mode of action Clopidogrel is a pro-drug and a class inhibitor of P2Y12 adenosine diphosphate (ADP) platelet receptors. The active metabolite of clopidogrel selectively and irreversibly inhibits the binding of ADP to its platelet P2Y12 receptor and the subsequent ADP-mediated activation of the glycoprotein GPIIb/IIIa complex, thereby inhibiting platelet aggregation. It acts by irreversibly modifying the platelet ADP receptor. Platelets exposed to clopidogrel are affected for their lifespan. Dose-dependent inhibition of platelet aggregation can be seen 2 hours after a single oral dose.

Route of administration/doses Orally 75 mg once daily in combination with aspirin, with or without thrombolytic agents. For acute coronary syndromes and prevascularization procedures, use a 300 mg loading dose orally, then continue at 75 mg once daily.

Effects

CVS No effect is seen with normal clinical dosages.

RS The drug has no effect on respiratory parameters.

AS No effect is seen with normal clinical dosages.

Metabolic/other Interaction with other drugs affecting platelet function, thus enhancing the potential for bleeding.

Toxicity/side effects Minor bleeding (5%); major bleeding, including intracranial, gastrointestinal, and retroperitoneal, 4%; life-threatening bleeding, 2%; agranulocytosis, aplastic anaemia/pancytopenia, thrombotic thrombocytopenic purpura, usually in the first 2 weeks of treatment.

If undergoing routine surgery and antiplatelet effect is not desired, discontinue clopidogrel 5 days prior. If an emergency surgery is needed or trauma has been sustained with the attendant risk of bleeding, platelet transfusion may be used.

Kinetics

Absorption Clopidogrel is rapidly absorbed. Bioavailability is 50%.

Distribution The drug and the main circulating metabolite bind reversibly *in vitro* to human plasma proteins (98% and 94%, respectively). The data for V_D are incomplete.

Metabolism Clopidogrel is a pro-drug and is extensively metabolized in the liver, undergoing rapid hydrolysis to carboxylic acid derivative (active). The metabolic pathway is the cytochrome P450 (CYP) system.

Excretion 50% is excreted in the urine, and approximately 46% in faeces, over the 5 days post-dosing. After a single oral dose of 75 mg, clopidogrel has a half-life of approximately 6 hours. The half-life of the active metabolite is about 8 hours.

Kinetics Clopidogrel at recommended doses in patients who are CYP2C19-poor metabolizers forms less of the active metabolite and so has a smaller effect on platelet function. Poor metabolizers with acute coronary syndrome or undergoing percutaneous coronary intervention treated with clopidogrel at recommended doses exhibit higher cardiovascular morbidity. It is possible to identify the CYP2C19 genotype.

The risk of bleeding may be increased with aspirin. NSAIDs, anticoagulants, and proton pump inhibitors decrease its efficacy. Bleeding during surgery is increased.

Cocaine

Uses Cocaine is used as a topical vasoconstrictor.

Chemical An ester of benzoic acid (a naturally occurring alkaloid derived from the leaves of *Erythroxylon coca*).

Presentation As 1–4% solutions and as a non-proprietary paste of varying concentration.

Main action Local anaesthesia, vasoconstriction, and euphoria.

Mode of action Local anaesthetics diffuse in their uncharged base form through neural sheaths and the axonal membrane to the internal surface of cell membrane Na^+ channels; here they combine with hydrogen ions to form a cationic species which enters the internal opening of the Na^+ channel and combines with a receptor. This produces blockade of the Na^+ channel, thereby decreasing Na^+ conductance and preventing depolarization of the cell membrane. Cocaine also produces blockade of the uptake-1 pathway of noradrenaline and dopamine, leading to vasoconstriction and CNS excitation.

Routes of administration/doses Cocaine is administered topically; the toxic dose is 3 mg/kg. The drug has a duration of action of 20–30 minutes.

Effects

CVS The usual effect of cocaine is to produce hypertension and tachycardia due to a combination of central sympathetic stimulation and the blockade of noradrenaline reuptake at peripheral adrenergic nerve terminals, leading to intense peripheral vasoconstriction. Large doses produce myocardial depression and may precipitate ventricular fibrillation.

RS Therapeutic concentrations of the drug cause stimulation of the respiratory centre and an increase in ventilation.

CNS The principal effect of cocaine is reversible neural blockade; this leads to a characteristically biphasic effect in the CNS. Initially, excitation (euphoria, light-headedness, dizziness, visual and auditory disturbances, and fitting) occurs due to the blockade of inhibitory pathways in the cortex; with increasing doses, depression of both facilitatory and inhibitory pathways occurs, leading to CNS depression (drowsiness, disorientation, and coma). Cocaine may also cause hyperreflexia, mydriasis, and an increase in the intraocular pressure.

AS The drug produces hyperdynamic bowel sounds and marked nausea and vomiting (a central effect).

Metabolic/other Cocaine causes a marked increase in body temperature due to increased motor activity combined with cutaneous vasoconstriction and a direct effect of the drug on the hypothalamus.

Toxicity/side effects Allergic phenomena occur occasionally with the use of cocaine. The side effects are predominantly correlated with excessive plasma concentrations of the drug. These include confusion, hallucinations, seizures, cerebral haemorrhage and infarction, and medullary depression leading to respiratory arrest. Chest pain is common; myocardial infarction, pulmonary oedema, gut infarction, rhabdomyolysis, and disseminated intravascular coagulation (DIC) may also occur. Cocaine is a drug of dependence; maternal use may result in neonatal dependence. Nasal septum necrosis is reported.

Kinetics

Absorption The drug is well absorbed from mucosae, including that of the gut. The bioavailability when administered intranasally is 0.5%.

Distribution Cocaine is 98% protein-bound in the plasma; the V_D is 0.9–3.3 l/kg.

Metabolism In common with the other ester-type local anaesthetic agents, cocaine is predominantly degraded by plasma esterases, predominantly to benzoylecgonine.

Excretion The metabolites are excreted in the urine, 10% unchanged. The clearance is 26–44 ml/min/kg, and the elimination half-life is 25–60 minutes.

Codeine

Uses Codeine is used for the treatment of:
1. pain of mild to moderate severity
2. diarrhoea and excessive ileostomy output and
3. as an antitussive agent and
4. traditionally to provide analgesia for head-injured patients.

Chemical A naturally occurring phenanthrene alkaloid which is a methylated morphine derivative.

Presentation As 15/30/60 mg tablets, a syrup containing 5 mg/ml, and as a clear, colourless solution for injection containing 60 mg/ml of codeine phosphate. A number of fixed-dose preparations containing paracetamol, ibuprofen, or aspirin in combination with codeine phosphate are also available.

Main action Analgesic, antitussive, and a decrease in gastrointestinal motility.

Mode of action Codeine has a very low affinity for opioid receptors; 10% of the drug is metabolized to morphine, and the analgesic and constipating effects are due to the morphine metabolite. The antitussive effects of codeine appear to be mediated by specific high-affinity codeine receptors.

Routes of administration/doses The adult oral and intramuscular dose is 30–60 mg 4- to 6-hourly. Rectal administration in a dose of 1 mg/kg can be used in paediatrics. It should not be given intravenously due to hypotension probably due to histamine release.

Effects

RS The principal effect of the drug is an antitussive effect; it also produces some respiratory depression with a decreased ventilatory response to hypoxia and hypercapnia.

CNS Codeine is ten times less potent an analgesic, compared to morphine, and produces few of the central effects associated with opioids.

AS The drug markedly inhibits gastrointestinal motility, leading to constipation.

Toxicity/side effects Nausea and vomiting, dizziness, and excitatory phenomena may complicate the use of the drug; cardiovascular collapse may occur when codeine is taken in overdose or administered intravenously. Bowel perforation, secondary to decreased gastrointestinal transit, has been reported. Codeine has a low propensity to cause dependence.

Kinetics

Absorption Codeine phosphate is well absorbed when administered orally and rectally; the bioavailability by these routes is 60–70%, as little first-pass metabolism of the drug occurs. Absorption is faster after intramuscular absorption (0.5 hours). Peak concentration occurs at 1 hour.

Distribution Codeine is 7% protein-bound in the plasma; the V_D is 5.4 l/kg.

Metabolism Codeine is extensively metabolized in the liver by three methods: principally (10–20%) by glucuronidation to codeine-6-glucuronide, by N-demethylation (10–20%) to norcodeine, and by O-demethylation to morphine (5–15%).

Other minor metabolites (normorphine and norcodeine-6-glucuronide) have been found.

Genetic variability occurs with the cytochrome P450 enzyme CYP2D6 which causes conversion to morphine, so 'fast' metabolizers produce more morphine.

Excretion Occurs predominantly in the urine as free and conjugated codeine, norcodeine, and morphine; 17% of the dose is excreted unchanged. The clearance is 98 l/hour after oral administration, and the elimination half-life is 2.8 hours. The dose should be reduced in the presence of renal failure.

Special points There are no published data to support the use of codeine in the management of head-injured patients. The drug has traditionally been used in these circumstances due to its low potency and consequent relative lack of respiratory and neurological depressant effects.

Co-trimoxazole

Uses Co-trimoxazole should be used in the treatment of:
1. Pneumocystis carinii infections
2. toxoplasmosis, and
3. nocardiasis.

Chemical (trimethoprim + sulfamethoxazole) Trimethoprim is a diaminopyrimidine, and sulfamethoxazole is a sulfonamide.

Presentation All preparations contain trimethoprim and sulfamethoxazole in the ratio of 1:5. The tablets contain 20/80/160 mg of trimethoprim in a fixed-dose combination with 100/400/800 mg of sulfamethoxazole, respectively. A suspension for oral administration is also available. A pale yellow preparation of co-trimoxazole is available for intravenous use and contains 16 mg of trimethoprim and 80 mg of sulfamethoxazole per ml. The intramuscular preparation contains 160 mg of trimethoprim and 800 mg of sulfamethoxazole in 3 ml.

Main action Co-trimoxazole is bactericidal against a broad spectrum of Gram-positive and Gram-negative aerobic bacteria, including the Gram-positive *Staphylococcus* and *Streptococcus* spp., the Gram-negative *Proteus*, *Salmonella*, *Shigella*, and *Klebsiella* spp., and *Escherichia coli*. It is also effective against some protozoa, *Chlamydia* spp., and some anaerobic species. Bacterial resistance to the drug is widespread.

Mode of action Co-trimoxazole inhibits the synthesis of tetrahydrofolic acid which is needed for the synthesis of nucleic acids and amino acids. The two components of the drug act at separate stages in the biosynthetic pathway of tetrahydrofolic acid; sulfamethoxazole inhibits the synthesis of dihydrofolic acid, and trimethoprim is a competitive inhibitor of dihydrofolate reductase. Mammalian dihydrofolate reductase is minimally affected by co-trimoxazole; in any case, mammalian cells utilize preformed folate derived from the diet.

Routes of administration/doses The adult oral dose is 2–3 of the 80/400 mg tablets 12-hourly. The corresponding dose by the intravenous or intramuscular route is 160/800 to 240/1200 mg 12-hourly. The intravenous preparation should be diluted in a crystalloid prior to use and infused over a period of 90 minutes.

Effects

Metabolic/other Serum creatinine concentrations may increase with the use of the drug, due to competition for tubular secretory mechanisms and an effect on the assay of creatinine. The plasma concentration of thyroid hormone may also decrease.

Toxicity/side effects The use of co-trimoxazole may be complicated by allergic phenomena, and gastrointestinal and haematological disturbances, especially neutropenia. Patients known to be deficient in vitamin B12 or folate are at increased risk for the latter complication.

Kinetics

Absorption Both components of the drug are well absorbed; the bioavailability of both sulfamethoxazole and trimethoprim is 100%.

Distribution The plasma ratio of trimethoprim:sulfamethoxazole is 1:20, which appears to be optimal for synergistic activity. Trimethoprim is 45% protein-bound in the plasma; its V_D is 1.6–2.0 l/kg. Sulfamethoxazole is 66% protein-bound in the plasma; its V_D is 0.19–0.23 l/kg.

Metabolism 5–15% of the dose of trimethoprim is metabolized to inactive products; sulfamethoxazole is extensively metabolized, the major metabolite being an acetyl derivative.

Excretion Both components are excreted predominantly in the urine; 80% of the dose of trimethoprim is excreted unchanged, whereas sulfamethoxazole is excreted predominantly as inactive metabolites. The clearance of trimethoprim is 1.6–2.8 ml/min/kg, and the elimination half-life is 11 hours. The clearance of sulfamethoxazole is 0.28–0.36 ml/min/kg, and the elimination half-life is 9 hours. The dose of co-trimoxazole should be reduced if the creatinine clearance is 30 ml/min; hepatic impairment has no effect on the kinetics of the drug.

Special points Co-trimoxazole potentiates the anticoagulant effect of co-administered warfarin and the hypoglycaemic effect of co-administered sulfonylureas. The drug has a theoretically synergistic action with N_2O on folic acid metabolism. Both components of the drug are haemodialysable.

Cyclizine

Uses Cyclizine is used in the treatment of nausea and vomiting due to:
1. opioid or general anaesthetic agents
2. motion sickness
3. radiation sickness, and
4. Ménière's disease.

Chemical A piperazine derivative.

Presentation As tablets containing 50 mg of cyclizine hydrochloride and as a clear, colourless solution for injection containing 50 mg/ml of cyclizine lactate which should be protected from light. Fixed-dose combinations with morphine, caffeine, ergotamine, and dipipanone are available. It has a pH of 3.2.

Main action Antiemetic.

Mode of action Cyclizine is a competitive antagonist of histamine at H1 receptors and has anticholinergic activity at the muscarinic M1, M2, and M3 receptors. The antiemetic effect is mediated via blockade of central histamine and muscarinic receptors within the vomiting area of the chemoreceptor trigger zone. Cyclizine produces its antiemetic effect within 2 hours and lasts approximately 4 hours.

Route of administration/doses Cyclizine may be given orally or by intramuscular or intravenous injection. Given the low pH of the parenteral preparation, injection by either route may be painful. The maximum daily dose is 150 mg. The paediatric dose is 1 mg/kg.

Effects

CVS The drug has mild anticholinergic action and can produce tachycardia and hypotension due to alpha-blockade.

RS Cyclizine, although it has antihistaminergic properties, does not completely reverse anaphylactic bronchospasm, as leukotrienes are involved in the mediation of allergic bronchoconstriction.

CNS The principal effect of the drug is antiemetic, with a slight degree of sedation. Cyclizine reduces the sensitivity of the labyrinthine apparatus and depresses vestibular stimulation.

AS Cyclizine increases the tone of the lower oesophageal sphincter.

Toxicity/side effects The predominant side effects are anticholinergic, including drowsiness, dryness of the mouth, and blurred vision. Restlessness, nervousness, insomnia, and auditory and visual hallucinations have been reported. Confusion in the elderly is common.

Kinetics Data are incomplete.

Absorption The drug is well absorbed when administered orally; the bioavailability by this route is 80%. Following oral administration of 50 mg of cyclizine, peak plasma concentrations of 70 ng/ml occur at approximately 2 hours.

Metabolism Cyclizine is metabolized in the liver by N-demethylation to nor-cyclizine. Norcyclizine has little antihistamine activity.

Excretion The elimination half-life is 10–20 hours. Limited data suggest that only 1% of the total administered dose is excreted unchanged in the urine.

Special points Cyclizine appears to be as effective as perphenazine in counteracting the nausea and vomiting associated with the use of opioids. The sedative effect of the drug is additive with that produced by anaesthetic agents.

The drug should be used with caution in patients with severe heart failure, as a fall in cardiac output may occur following the administration of cyclizine, secondary to increases in the heart rate, mean arterial pressure, and pulmonary capillary wedge pressure.

The drug should be avoided in patients with porphyria.

Dabigatran

Uses Dabigatran is used for the primary prevention of:
1. venous thromboembolic events post-elective total hip replacement and
2. venous thromboembolic events post-elective total knee replacement surgery.

Chemical A benzamidine-based thrombin inhibitor.

Presentation As 75/110 mg capsules containing dabigatran etexilate.

Main actions Competitive, reversible direct thrombin inhibitor.

Mode of action Dabigatran etexilate is a pro-drug. Following oral administration, it undergoes plasma and hepatic esterase-catalysed hydrolysis to dabigatran which acts as a direct thrombin inhibitor. Inhibition of thrombin prevents cleavage of fibrinogen to fibrin. The drug also inhibits:
1. free thrombin
2. fibrin-bound thrombin, and
3. thrombin-induced platelet aggregation.

Routes of administration/doses Dabigatran is available in 75 and 110 mg capsules as dabigatran mesilate. The recommended dose for prevention of venous thromboembolism following elective knee replacement surgery is 110 mg, taken 1–4 hours after surgery, followed by 220 mg once daily for 10 days. The recommended dose following elective hip replacement surgery is the same, but treatment is continued for 28–35 days. The dose should be reduced in the elderly and in patients with moderate renal impairment to 75 mg, taken 1–4 hours after surgery, followed by 150 mg once daily.

Effects

Metabolic/other In addition to its anticoagulant effects, dabigatran inhibits platelet aggregation.

Toxicity/side effects Excessive bleeding is the most common reported side effect (14% of patients). The colourant 'sunset yellow' is present within capsules of dabigatran, which has been associated with allergic reactions. The use of neuroaxial blocks in patients receiving the drug must be carefully considered, and the timing of lock/catheter insertion/removal and commencement/withholding/discontinuation of dabigatran must be appropriately timed to minimize the risk of spinal/epidural haematoma formation.

Kinetics

Absorption Dabigatran is rapidly converted from its etexilate form to the active drug via esterase hydrolysis. The bioavailability of the drug is 6.5%. Following oral administration, C_{max} is reached within 0.5–2 hours.

Distribution The drug is 35% protein-bound in the plasma; the V_D is 60–70 l.

Metabolism Dabigatran is metabolized by conjugation to active acylglucuronides. Four isomers may exist: 1-O-, 2-O-, 3-O-, and 4-O-acylglucuronide, accounting for <10% of total drug in the plasma.

Excretion The drug is excreted predominantly unchanged in the urine at a rate proportional to the glomerular filtration rate. Plasma levels of the drug demonstrate a bi-exponential decline, with a terminal elimination half-life of 12–14 hours. Six percent of an administered dose is excreted in faeces. Renal impairment increases the time of drug exposure. Consequently, the dose should be reduced in moderate renal impairment, and the drug should be avoided in patients with severe renal impairment. Limited data from patients with hepatic impairment did not demonstrate increased time of drug exposure following the administration of dabigatran.

Special points The use of unfractionated heparin, low-molecular-weight heparins (LMWHs), fondaparinux, desirudin, thrombolytic agents, glycoprotein IIb/IIIa receptor antagonists, clopidogrel, ticlopidine, dextran, sulfinpyrazone, and vitamin K antagonists is not recommended in patients concurrently receiving dabigatran.

The time of drug exposure is increased when dabigatran is administered to patients concurrently receiving amiodarone, and the daily dose should be reduced to 150 mg of dabigatran daily. The mechanism of this interaction has not been fully elucidated. However, amiodarone is an inhibitor of the efflux transporter P-glycoprotein of which dabigatran is a substrate. Strong inhibitors of P-glycoprotein include verapamil and clarithromycin. The drug should be used with caution in patients receiving these drugs. Dabigatran should not be administered to patients also receiving the P-glycoprotein inhibitor quinidine.

The time of drug exposure may be reduced when dabigatran is administered to patients concurrently receiving P-glycoprotein inducers such as rifampicin and *Hypericum perforatum* (St John's wort).

There is no antidote currently available for dabigatran.

The drug may be removed by haemodialysis.

Dantrolene

Uses Dantrolene is used in the treatment of:
1. malignant hyperthermia and the neuroleptic malignant syndrome
2. heat stroke, and
3. muscle spasticity and may be of use
4. as an adjunct in the treatment of tetanus.

Chemical A phenyl hydantoin derivative.

Presentation As 25 or 100 mg capsules of dantrolene sodium, as a lyo-philized orange powder which contains 20 mg of dantrolene sodium and 3 g of mannitol (to improve the solubility), together with sodium hydroxide in each vial; this is reconstituted prior to use with 60 ml of water. A solution of pH 9.5 is produced.

Main action Muscular relaxation.

Mode of action Dantrolene acts within skeletal muscle fibres to inhibit Ca^{2+} release through the inhibition of ryanodine receptors in the sarcoplasmic reticulum to cause a reduction in muscular contraction to a given electrical stimulus. Part of its action may be due to a marked GABA-ergic effect.

Routes of administration/doses For the treatment of acute hyper-thermia, 1–10 mg/kg administered intravenously (either via a central vein or into a fast-running infusion), as required—an average of 2.5 mg/kg is required. For the prophylaxis of malignant hyperthermia, 4–8 mg/kg/day are given for 1–2 days prior to surgery in 3–4 divided doses; the role of this regime is controversial. The oral adult dose used for the prevention of spasticity is 25–100 mg 6-hourly. Therapeutic effects are observed within 15 minutes; the mean duration of action is 4–6 hours.

Effects

CVS No consistent effects have been reported from animal studies. Dantrolene may have antiarrhythmic effects in man. Dantrolene improves beta-adrenergic responsiveness in the failing human myocardium.

RS Negligible effects are produced by the drug in man.

CNS Dantrolene has marked central GABA-ergic effects; sedation may occur.

GU Dantrolene increases the effectiveness of voiding in many patients with neuromuscular disorders.

Metabolic/other Dantrolene diminishes the force of electrically induced muscle twitches, whilst having no effect on action potentials in skeletal muscle.

Toxicity/side effects The drug is highly irritant if extravasated. With chronic use, muscular weakness, drowsiness, and gastrointestinal distur-bances may occur. Hepatic dysfunction occurs in up to 2% of patients which is reversible.

Kinetics

Absorption 20–70% of an oral dose is absorbed.

Distribution Dantrolene is 80–90% protein-bound to albumin. The V_D is 0.6 l/kg.

Metabolism Predominantly in the liver by hydroxylation (to an active metabolite) and by reduction and acetylation.

Excretion 15–25% is excreted in the urine, predominantly as the hydroxy metabolite. The clearance is 2.3 ml/kg/min, and the elimination half-life is 3–12 hours.

Special points There are no controlled trials of the effectiveness of dantrolene in the treatment of malignant hyperthermia or the malignant neuroleptic syndrome in man; however, >80% of patients with prodromal signs of the syndromes improve after receiving dantrolene. It has also been used successfully in the management of 'Ecstasy' toxicity.

Verapamil and dantrolene administered concurrently in animals may cause hyperkalaemia, leading to ventricular fibrillation; these drugs are not recommended for use together in man.

Desflurane

Uses Desflurane is used for the induction and maintenance of general anaesthesia.

Chemical A fluorinated methylethyl ether.

Presentation As a clear, colourless liquid that should be protected from light. The commercial preparation contains no additives and is flammable at a concentration of 17%. The molecular weight of desflurane is 168; the boiling point is 22.8°C, and the saturated vapour pressure is 88.5 kPa at 20°C. The MAC of desflurane is age-dependent and ranges from 5.17 ± 0.65% to 10.65% (1.67 ± 0.4% to 7.75% in the presence of 60% N_2O); the blood:gas partition coefficient is 0.45, and the fat:blood partition coefficient is 29. Desflurane is stable in the presence of moist soda lime.

Main action General anaesthesia (reversible loss of both awareness and recall of noxious stimuli).

Mode of action The mechanism of general anaesthesia remains to be fully elucidated. General anaesthetics appear to disrupt synaptic transmission (especially in the area of the ventrobasal thalamus). This mechanism may include potentiation of the gamma-amino-butyric acid (GABA) type A ($GABA_A$) and glycine receptors and antagonism at N-methyl-D-aspartate (NMDA) receptors. Their mode of action at the molecular level appears to involve expansion of hydrophobic regions in the neuronal membrane, either within the lipid phase or within hydrophobic sites in cell membranes.

Routes of administration/dose Desflurane is administered by inhalation. Because of the high saturated vapour pressure, desflurane must be administered by a specific pressurized and heated vaporizer. The concentration used for induction of anaesthesia is quoted as 4–11%, although induction is usually achieved using a different agent. Maintenance of anaesthesia is usually achieved by using between 2% and 6%.

Effects

CVS Desflurane causes a decrease in myocardial contractility, but the sympathetic tone is relatively well preserved. The cardiac index and left ventricular ejection fraction are well preserved in man. Desflurane causes a dose-dependent decrease in the systemic vascular resistance and mean arterial pressure; the heart rate may increase via an indirect autonomic effect, particularly at inspired concentrations of 9% or greater. The drug does not appear to cause the 'coronary steal' phenomenon in man. Desflurane does not sensitize the myocardium to the effects of catecholamines.

RS Desflurane is a respiratory depressant, causing dose-dependent decreases in the tidal volume and an increase in the respiratory rate. The drug depresses the ventilatory response to CO_2. Desflurane is markedly irritant to the respiratory tract in concentrations >6%.

CNS The principal effect of desflurane is general anaesthesia. The drug causes cerebral vasodilation, leading to an increase in the cerebral blood flow; the effects on the intracranial pressure are unclear. As with other volatile anaesthetic agents, desflurane may increase the intracranial pressure in patients with space-occupying lesions. Desflurane decreases cerebral oxygen consumption and is not associated with epileptiform activity. A centrally mediated decrease in the skeletal muscle tone results from the use of desflurane.

AS Desflurane does not decrease the hepatic blood flow.

GU Desflurane does not decrease the renal cortical blood flow.

Metabolic/other Rapid alterations in desflurane concentrations cause transient increases in catecholamine levels.

Toxicity/side effects There is a high incidence of airway irritation and reactivity during the use of high concentrations of desflurane, making it unsuitable for use during gaseous induction. It is not recommended for induction in children, as airway irritation may be severe. Desflurane is a trigger agent for the development of malignant hyperthermia. Desflurane may cause PONV.

Kinetics

Absorption The major factors affecting the uptake of volatile anaesthetic agents are solubility, cardiac output, and the concentration gradient between the alveoli and venous blood. Due to the low blood:gas partition coefficient of desflurane, it is exceptionally insoluble in blood; the alveolar concentration therefore reaches inspired concentration very rapidly (fast wash-in rate), resulting in a rapid induction of anaesthesia. An increase in the cardiac output increases the rate of alveolar uptake and slows the induction of anaesthesia. The concentration gradient between the alveoli and venous blood approaches zero at equilibrium; a large concentration gradient favours the onset of anaesthesia.

Distribution The drug is initially distributed to organs with a high blood flow (brain, heart, liver, kidney) and later to less well-perfused organs (muscle, fat, bone).

Metabolism 0.02% of an administered dose is metabolized, predominantly to trifluoroacetic acid.

Excretion Excretion is via the lungs, predominantly unchanged; trace quantities of trifluoroacetic acid are excreted in the urine. Elimination of desflurane is rapid due to its low solubility, resulting in a fast washout rate. Rapid washout occurs, even after prolonged administration of desflurane.

Special points Desflurane potentiates the action of co-administered depolarizing and non-depolarizing muscle relaxants.

Due to the physical characteristics of desflurane, a specific vaporizer is used to administer the drug. The vaporizer comprises an electrically heated vaporization chamber in which desfludrane is heated to 39°C at a pressure of 1550 mmHg. A percentage control dial controls the flow of desflurane vapour into the fresh gas flow (1% graduations from 0% to 10%;

2% graduations from 10% to 18%). A fixed restriction in the fresh gas flow path and the use of a differential pressure transducer allow the vaporizer to match the pressure of desflurane vapour upstream of the control valve, with the pressure of the fresh gas flow at the fixed restriction.

As with other volatile anaesthetic agents, the co-administration of N_2O, benzodiazepines, or opioids lowers the MAC of desflurane.

Desflurane may be used safely in patients breathing spontaneously via a laryngeal mask.

Drug structure For the drug structure, please see Fig. 1.

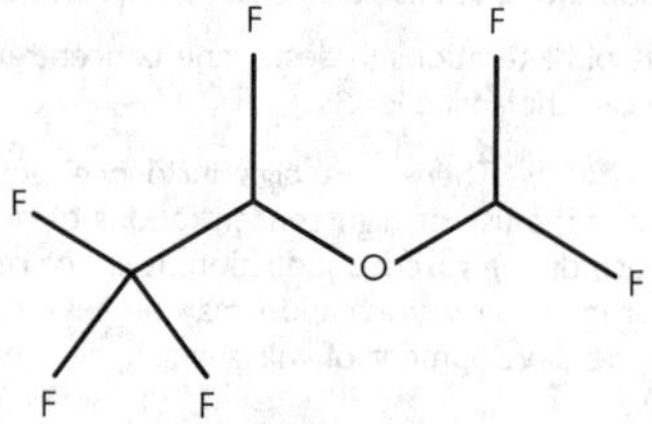

Fig. 1 Drug structure of desflurane.

Dexamethasone

Uses Dexamethasone is used:
1. as replacement therapy in congenital adrenocortical deficiency states and in the treatment of
2. allergic disorders
3. asthma
4. many autoimmune and rheumatologic disorders
5. eczema and contact sensitivity syndromes and
6. leukaemia and lymphoma chemotherapy regimes and
7. immunosuppression after organ transplantation
8. palliative treatment of tumours
9. prevention of post-operative and chemotherapy-induced nausea and vomiting
10. ophthalmic inflammatory diseases
11. acute exacerbations of inflammatory bowel disease
12. acute severe skin diseases
13. cerebral oedema
14. bacterial meningitis—prevents hearing loss
15. tests for Cushing's syndrome
16. hypercalcaemia of malignancy, sarcoidosis, and vitamin D toxicity
17. antenatal use in preterm labour
18. myasthenia gravis
19. autoimmune renal disease and
20. has been used for epidural injection.

Chemical A synthetic glucocorticosteroid.

Presentation As 0.5/2 mg tablets of dexamethasone, an oral solution and in vials as dexamethasone (sodium phosphate) 3.8 mg/mL, and as a variety of topical creams, some of which are fixed-dose combinations.

Main action Anti-inflammatory.

Mode of action Corticosteroids act by controlling the rate of protein synthesis; they react with cytoplasmic receptors to form a complex which directly influences the rate of RNA transcription. This directs the synthesis of lipocortins. Dexamethasone has approximately a seven-times higher anti-inflammatory potency than prednisolone and 30 times that of hydrocortisone. Adrenocorticoids act on the hypothalamic–pituitary–adrenal axis at specific receptors on the plasma membrane. In other tissues, the adrenocorticoids diffuse across cell membranes and form complexes with specific cytoplasmic receptors which enter the cell nucleus and stimulate protein synthesis. Adrenocorticoids have anti-allergic, antitoxic, antishock, antipyretic, and immunosuppressive properties.

Routes of administration/doses For oral administration, the initial dosage of dexamethasone varies from 0.75 to 9 mg daily, depending on the disease being treated.

Effects

CVS In the absence of corticosteroids, the capillary wall permeability increases; small blood vessels demonstrate an inadequate motor response, and the cardiac output decreases. Steroids have a positive effect on myocardial contractility and cause vasoconstriction by increasing the number of alpha-1 adrenoreceptors and beta-adrenoreceptors and stimulating their function. They prevent oedema formation.

CNS Corticosteroids increase the excitability of the CNS; the absence of glucocorticoids leads to apathy, depression, and irritability. In the CSF, they reduce the inflammatory response to anti-infective released bacterial endotoxins and cell wall components, including reduction of the release of cytokines (e.g. interleukin-1 (IL-1) beta, tumour necrosis factor (TNF)).

AS Dexamethasone increases the likelihood of peptic ulcer disease; it also decreases the gastrointestinal absorption of calcium.

GU The urinary excretion of calcium is increased by the drug, and it increases the glomerular filtration rate and stimulates tubular secretory activity. Dexamethasone has only minor mineralocorticoid activities and does not induce water and sodium retention.

Metabolic/other Dexamethasone exerts profound effects on carbohydrate, protein, and lipid metabolism. Glucocorticoids stimulate gluconeogenesis and inhibit the peripheral utilization of glucose; they cause a redistribution of body fat, enhance lipolysis, and also reduce the conversion of amino acids to protein, resulting in a negative nitrogen balance.

Dexamethasone is a potent anti-inflammatory agent, which inhibits all stages of the inflammatory process by inhibiting neutrophil and macrophage recruitment, blocking the effect of lymphokines, and inhibiting the formation of plasminogen activator. It decreases inflammation by stabilizing leucocyte lysosomal membranes, preventing the release of destructive acid hydrolases from leucocytes, or reducing leucocyte adhesion to the capillary endothelium. The drug antagonizes histamine activity and the release of kinin, and decreases immunoglobulin and complement concentrations and the passage of immune complexes through basement membranes. It depresses the reactivity of tissues to antigen–antibody interactions.

Corticosteroids stimulate erythroid cells of the bone marrow and increase neutrophil and red cell numbers, whilst causing eosinopenia and lymphocytopenia and reducing the activity of lymphoid tissue. It prolongs the survival time of erythrocytes and platelets.

Dexamethasone inhibits pituitary corticotropin (adrenocorticotrophin hormone, ACTH) release and decreases the output of endogenous corticosteroids.

It reduces fibroblast proliferation, collagen deposition, and subsequent scar tissue formation.

Short-course intramuscular therapy is used in selected women with preterm labour to hasten fetal maturation (e.g. lungs, cerebral blood vessels), including preterm premature rupture of membranes, pre-eclampsia, or third-trimester haemorrhage. It reduces the incidence and/or severity of neonatal respiratory distress syndrome (RDS), causing a reduction in the need for neonatal ventilatory support and surfactant therapy; these beneficial effects are additive with the surfactant. The combined effects on multiple organ maturation reduce neonatal mortality, with the beneficial effects extending over a wide range of gestational age (24–34 weeks).

Toxicity/side effects Consist of an acute withdrawal syndrome and a syndrome (Cushing's) produced by prolonged use of excessive quantities of the drug. Cushing's syndrome is characterized by growth arrest, a characteristic appearance consisting of central obesity, a moon face and buffalo hump, striae, acne, hirsutism, and skin and capillary fragility, together with the following metabolic derangements: altered glucose tolerance, fluid retention, a hypokalaemic alkalosis, and osteoporosis. A proximal myopathy, cataracts, and an increased susceptibility to peptic ulcer disease may also complicate the use of the drug. Neuropsychiatric symptoms, including psychosis, are well described.

Kinetics

Absorption After intravenous administration, dexamethasone sodium phosphate is rapidly hydrolysed to dexamethasone. After an intravenous dose of 20 mg dexamethasone, plasma levels peak within 5 minutes.

Distribution Dexamethasone is bound (up to 77%) by plasma proteins, mainly albumin. There is a high uptake of dexamethasone by the liver, kidney, and adrenal glands.

Metabolism Metabolism in the liver is slow, and excretion is mainly in the urine, largely as unconjugated steroids.

Excretion The plasma half-life is 3.5–4.5 hours, but, as the effects outlast the significant plasma concentrations of steroids, the plasma half-life is of little relevance, and the use of the biological half-life is more applicable. The biological half-life of dexamethasone is 36–54 hours; therefore, dexamethasone is especially suitable in conditions where continuous glucocorticoid action is desirable.

Special points It has been recommended that perioperative steroid cover be given:
1. to patients who have received high-dose steroid replacement therapy for 2 weeks in the preceding year prior to surgery
2. to patients undergoing pituitary or adrenal surgery.

Glucocorticoids antagonize the effects of anticholinesterase drugs.
  Injection of corticosteroids into the epidural space of the spine may result in rare, but serious, adverse events, including loss of vision, stroke, paralysis, and death.

Dexmedetomidine

Uses Dexmedetomidine is used as a sedative for post-surgical patients requiring mechanical ventilation.

Chemical An imidazole derivative.

Presentation As a clear, colourless isotonic solution containing 100 g/ml of dexmedetomidine base and 9 mg/ml of sodium chloride in water. The solution is preservative-free and contains no additives.

Main action Sedation, anxiolysis, and analgesia.

Mode of action Dexmedetomidine is a specific alpha-2 adrenoceptor agonist that acts via post-synaptic alpha-2 receptors primarily in the locus coeruleus to increase conductance through K^+ channels.

Routes of administration/dose The drug is administered by intravenous infusion, commencing at 1 mcg/kg over 10 minutes, then at 0.2–0.7 mcg/kg/hr. The duration of use should not exceed 24 hours. Dexmedetomidine has also been administered transdermally and intramuscularly.

Effects

CVS The drug causes a predictable decrease in the mean arterial pressure and heart rate.

RS Dexmedetomidine causes a slight increase in $PaCO_2$ and a decrease in minute ventilation, with minimal change in the respiratory rate—these effects are not clinically significant.

CNS The drug is sedative and anxiolytic—ventilated patients remain easily rousable and cooperative during treatment. Reversible memory impairment is an additional feature.

Metabolic/other Dexmedetomidine causes a decrease in plasma epinephrine and norepinephrine concentrations. It does not impair adrenal steroidogenesis when used in the short term.

Toxicity/side effects Hypotension, bradycardia, nausea, and a dry mouth are the most commonly reported side effects of the drug.

Kinetics

Distribution Dexmedetomidine is 94% protein-bound in the plasma; the V_D is 1.33 l/kg. The distribution half-life is 6 minutes.

Metabolism The drug undergoes extensive hepatic metabolism to methyl and glucuronide conjugates.

Excretion 95% of the metabolites are excreted in the urine. The elimination half-life is 2 hours, and the clearance is 39 l/hour.

Special points The drug shows a pharmacodynamic interaction with volatile agents and analgesic agents. The clearance is decreased in hepatic impairment, although renal impairment does not significantly alter its pharmacokinetics. Dexmedetomidine is currently licensed for use in the United States of America (USA), but not Europe.

Dextrans

Uses Dextrans are used:
1. for plasma volume replacement in haemorrhage, burns, or excessive fluid and electrolyte loss and
2. in the prophylaxis of post-operative thromboembolism.

Chemical Dextrans are polysaccharide derivatives of sucrose by the action of the bacterium *Leuconostoc mesenteroides*; the preparation is then further processed by hydrolysis and fractionation.

Presentation Dextrans are available as dextran 40 and dextran 70. Both agents are presented as clear, colourless solutions in either 5% glucose or 0.9% saline. Dextran 40 is a 10% solution containing molecules with an average molecular weight of 40 000; 90% of molecules have a molecular weight within the range of 10 000–75 000. Dextran 70 is a 6% solution containing molecules with an average molecular weight of 70 000; 90% of molecules have a molecular weight within the range of 20 000–115 000.

Main action Plasma volume expansion and an antithrombotic effect.

Mode of action Each gram of dextran in the circulation will retain approximately 20 ml of water by its osmotic effect; an infusion of 500 ml of dextran 40 will maximally increase the circulating plasma volume by approximately 1000 ml. An infusion of 500 ml of dextran 70 will increase the circulating plasma volume by approximately 750 ml. Molecules above the renal threshold for dextran elimination of 55 000 daltons are generally retained within the intravascular space, whereas those below 20 000 daltons have access to the interstitial space. Dextrans exert their antithrombotic action by reducing ADP-induced platelet aggregation and by decreasing the activating effect of thrombin on platelets. These agents also alter fibrinogen binding.

Routes of administration/doses The specific dose of an agent administered is dependent on the clinical indication, haemodynamic status of the patient, and particular agent being used. When used in the prophylaxis of post-operative thrombosis, the adult dose is 500 ml infused over 4–6 hours in the immediate post-operative period, repeated on the next day. For high-risk cases, this may be continued on alternate days for up to 2 weeks.

Effects

CVS The haemodynamic effects of dextrans are proportional to the prevailing circulating volume. The duration of action of these agents depends on the type of dextran used.

RS Dextran 70 appears to protect against the development of acute respiratory distress syndrome (ARDS) in patients with multiple trauma.

Metabolic/other Infusion of dextran reduces serum lipid levels and produces a reduction in the serum albumin concentrations.

Toxicity/side effects Severe hypersensitivity reactions occur in 1 in 3300—this is probably due to a cross-reaction with antibodies to a recent pneumococcal infection. Overtransfusion may lead to pulmonary oedema. Increased capillary oozing due to improved perfusion pressure and capillary flow may be noted perioperatively. Acute renal failure may complicate the use of dextran 40 when it is used in the management of profound hypovolaemia.

Kinetics Data are incomplete.

Distribution Chronic overdosage leads to the storage of dextrans in the liver. Dextrans are not significantly protein-bound.

Metabolism Occurs by the action of dextranases present in the lung, liver, kidney, and spleen to CO_2 and water.

Excretion Dextran 70 has a half-life of 23–25.5 hours, and dextran 40 has a half-life of 4–9 hours. Small molecules are excreted renally; the remainder are metabolized and excreted as CO_2 and water.

Special points Dextrans do not interfere with cross-matching if enzymatic methods are used (although older preparations did).

If a dextran of molecular weight of 1000 is administered prior to the administration of dextran 40/70, the incidence of anaphylaxis is reduced by 15- to 20-fold.

Diamorphine

Uses Diamorphine is used:
1. for premedication
2. as an analgesic in the management of moderate to severe pain
3. in the treatment of left ventricular failure
4. as an antitussive agent, and
5. to provide analgesia for palliative care.

Chemical A synthetic diacetylated morphine derivative.

Presentation As tablets containing 10 mg and as a lyophilized white powder in ampoules containing 5/10/30/100/500 mg of diamorphine hydrochloride for reconstitution with water. A number of non-proprietary elixirs and suppositories are also available.

Main action Analgesia, euphoria, and respiratory depression.

Mode of action Diamorphine is a pro-drug; it does not possess an unsubstituted phenolic hydroxyl group at the 3-position and acts via active derivatives (6-O-acetylmorphine and morphine) which are MOP receptor agonists. Opioids appear to exert their effects by increasing intracellular calcium concentration which, in turn, increases potassium conductance and hyperpolarization of excitable cell membranes. The decrease in membrane excitability that results may decrease both pre- and post-synaptic responses.

Routes of administration/doses The average adult dose by the intravenous or intramuscular route is 5–10 mg. The corresponding intrathecal or epidural dose is 2.5–5 mg. Due to its higher lipid solubility, the drug has a more rapid onset of action than morphine and has a duration of action of 90 minutes after intramuscular administration.

Effects

CVS Diamorphine has little effect on the CVS when used in normal doses. In high doses, it may cause bradycardia due to a combination of increased vagal activity and decreased sympathetic activity; hypotension resulting from a decrease in the systemic vascular resistance may occur.

RS The principal effect of the drug is respiratory depression in opioid-naive subjects, with a decreased ventilatory response to hypoxia and hypercapnia. Diamorphine also has a potent antitussive action. Bronchoconstriction may occur with the use of high doses of the drug.

CNS Diamorphine is 1.5–2 times as potent an analgesic agent as morphine. The drug tends to cause marked euphoria; there is a clinical impression that it causes less nausea and vomiting than morphine. Miosis is produced as a result of stimulation of the Edinger–Westphal nucleus. Seizures may occur with the use of high doses of the drug.

AS Diamorphine decreases gastrointestinal motility and gastric acid, biliary, and pancreatic secretions; it also increases the common bile duct pressure by causing spasm of the sphincter of Oddi. There is a clinical impression that the drug causes less constipation than does an equipotent dose of morphine.

GU The drug increases the tone of the ureters, bladder detrusor muscle, and sphincter, and may precipitate urinary retention.

Metabolic/other Mild diaphoresis and piloerection may occur with the use of diamorphine. Intrathecal diamorphine suppresses the metabolic response to surgery.

Toxicity/side effects Respiratory depression, nausea and vomiting, hallucinations, and dependence may complicate the use of diamorphine. Pruritus may occur after epidural or spinal administration of the drug.

Kinetics Data are incomplete due to the instability of the drug *in vivo* and difficulties in the assay methodology.

Absorption Diamorphine is extensively absorbed when administered orally; the bioavailability appears to be low due to an extensive first-pass metabolism.

Distribution The drug is 40% protein-bound in the plasma; the V_D is 350 l.

Metabolism Diamorphine undergoes rapid enzymatic hydrolysis in the plasma and in association with red blood cells, probably via pseudocholinesterase and at least three esterases located within red blood cells. The initial metabolic product is 6-O-acetylmorphine (which is the active form of the drug) which is, in turn, further metabolized to morphine, with subsequent glucuronidation.

Excretion 50–60% of an administered dose appears in the urine as a morphine derivative; 0.13% is excreted unchanged. The elimination half-life of diamorphine is 3 minutes. The clearance of the morphine component is 3.1 ml/min/kg.

Special points Late respiratory depression has not been reported following the use of epidural diamorphine. The actions of the drug are all reversed by naloxone.

Diamorphine is not removed by dialysis.

Diazepam

Uses Diazepam is used:
1. in the short-term treatment of anxiety
2. in the treatment of status epilepticus
3. for muscle spasm in tetanus and other spastic conditions
4. for alcohol withdrawal, and for
5. premedication and
6. sedation during endoscopy and procedures performed under local anaesthesia.

Chemical A benzodiazepine.

Presentation As tablets containing 2/5/10 mg, a syrup containing 0.4/1 mg/ml, as 10 mg suppositories, and as a solution for rectal administration containing 2/4 mg/ml of diazepam. The drug is also supplied as a clear, yellow solution and as a white oil-in-water emulsion for injection containing 5 mg/ml.

Main actions
1. Hypnosis
2. Sedation
3. Anxiolysis
4. Anterograde amnesia
5. Anticonvulsant, and
6. Muscular relaxation.

Mode of action Benzodiazepines are thought to act via specific benzodiazepine receptors found at synapses throughout the CNS, but concentrated especially in the cortex and midbrain. Benzodiazepine receptors are closely linked with GABA receptors and appear to facilitate the activity of the latter. Activated GABA receptors open chloride ion channels which then either hyperpolarize or short-circuit the synaptic membrane.

Diazepam has kappa-opioid agonist activity *in vitro*, which may explain the mechanism of benzodiazepine-induced spinal analgesia.

Routes of administration/doses The adult oral dose is 2–60 mg/day in divided doses; the initial intravenous dose is 10–20 mg, increasing according to clinical effect.

Effects

CVS A transient decrease in the blood pressure and a slight decrease in the cardiac output may occur, following the intravenous administration of diazepam. The coronary blood flow is increased, secondary to coronary arterial vasodilation; a decrease in myocardial oxygen consumption has also been reported.

RS Large doses cause respiratory depression; hypoxic drive is depressed to a greater degree than is hypercarbic drive.

CNS Diazepam is anxiolytic and decreases aggression, although paradoxical excitement may occur. Sedation, hypnosis, and anterograde amnesia occur after the administration of diazepam. The drug has anticonvulsant and analgesic properties, and depresses spinal reflexes.

Toxicity/side effects Depression of the CNS, including drowsiness, ataxia, and headache, may complicate the use of diazepam. Rashes, gastrointestinal upsets, and urinary retention have also been reported. Tolerance and dependence may occur with prolonged use of benzodiazepines; acute withdrawal of benzodiazepines in these circumstances may produce insomnia, anxiety, confusion, psychosis, and perceptual disturbances. Intravenous diazepam is highly irritant to veins; the oil-in-water preparation is less so.

Kinetics

Absorption Diazepam is rapidly absorbed after oral administration; the bioavailability is 86–100%. Absorption after intramuscular administration is slow and erratic.

Distribution The drug is 99% protein-bound in the plasma; the V_D is 0.8–1.4 l/kg.

Metabolism Diazepam is converted in the liver to active products; the major metabolite is desmethyldiazepam. Other metabolites are oxazepam (which is further metabolized by glucuronidation) and temazepam. These metabolites are active; desmethyldiazepam has a half-life of 100 hours.

Excretion The metabolites are excreted in the urine as oxidized and glucuronide derivatives; <1% is excreted unchanged. The clearance is 0.32–0.44 ml/min/kg (this is reduced by 42% by the concurrent administration of halothane), and the elimination half-life is 20–40 hours.

Special points Diazepam decreases the MAC of volatile agents and potentiates non-depolarizing muscle relaxants. Cimetidine decreases the clearance of co-administered diazepam and thereby increases the plasma levels of the latter. Diazepam is adsorbed onto plastic.

The drug is not removed by dialysis.

Diclofenac

Uses Diclofenac is used in the treatment of:
1. rheumatoid arthritis and osteoarthritis
2. musculoskeletal disorders
3. soft tissue injuries
4. ankylosing spondylitis
5. acute gout
6. renal and biliary colic
7. dysmenorrhoea
8. minor post-surgical pain and as an adjunct to systemic opioid therapy
9. as an antipyretic, and
10. to inhibit perioperative miosis and post-operative inflammation in cataract surgery.

Chemical A phenylacetic acid derivative.

Presentation As 25/50/100 mg tablets, 12.5/25/50/100 mg suppositories, and in ampoules containing either 25 mg/ml or 75 mg/2ml of diclofenac sodium for injection, depending on the nature of the preparation. An emulsified gel as diethylammonium and eye drops as a 0.1% solution of diclofenac sodium are also available. Modified-release/slow-release preparations are also available for oral administration, in addition to a dispersible formulation. Depending on the intravenous preparation, the following additives may be present: mannitol, sodium metabisulfite, benzyl alcohol, propylene glycol, sodium hydroxide, or hydroxypropylbetadex (a solubilizing agent).

Main actions Analgesic, anti-inflammatory, and antipyretic.

Mode of action Diclofenac is a non-specific inhibitor of COX (COX-2:COX-1 ratio = 1:1) which converts arachidonic acid to cyclic endoperoxidases, thus preventing the formation of prostaglandins, thromboxanes, and prostacylin. Prostaglandins are involved in the sensitization of peripheral pain receptors to noxious stimuli. The drug may also inhibit the lipo-oxygenase pathway by an action on hydroperoxy fatty acid peroxidase.

Route of administration/doses The adult oral dose is 75–150 mg/day in divided doses; the rectal dose is 100 mg, usually administered at night with further suppositories or tablets up to a maximum dose of 150 mg per 24 hours; it may also be given pre- or perioperatively. The intramuscular dose is 75 mg once or twice daily. The paediatric dose is 1 mg/kg three times a day. The intravenous dose is 25–75 mg, up to a maximum daily dose of 150 mg. Depending on the intravenous preparation, a bolus administration may or may not be recommended. Some preparations require dilution in 100–500 ml of 0.9% sodium chloride or 5% glucose solutions, with subsequent buffering with sodium bicarbonate solution.

Effects

AS Diclofenac causes less gastrointestinal damage than aspirin or indometacin. Dyspepsia, nausea, bleeding from gastric and duodenal vessels, mucosal ulceration, perforation, and diarrhoea are expected COX-1 effects. The drug may lead to disease exacerbation in patients with Crohn's disease or ulcerative colitis. Diclofenac may cause a rise in ALT in up to 15% of patients.

RS Bronchoconstriction and eosinophilia may occur in up to 20% of asthmatic patients.

GU The plasma renin activity and aldosterone concentrations are reduced by 60–70%.

Metabolic/other Diclofenac interferes with neutrophil function. The drug reversibly inhibits platelet aggregation but does not affect bleeding time, prothrombin time, plasma fibrinogen, or factors V and VII to XIII. Osteoblast activity is inhibited in animal studies and *in vitro*.

Toxicity/side effects Occur in 12%; complications are related to the duration of therapy, and risks increase markedly after >5 days of continuous therapy, especially in the elderly.

Disturbances of the gastrointestinal system and CNS occur occasionally.

Rashes and hepatic, renal, and haematological impairment have been reported.

As with other NSAIDs, prolonged use may lead to analgesic nephropathy, characterized by papillary necrosis and interstitial fibrosis. Acute renal failure may be precipitated when NSAIDs are administered to patients who have renal perfusion dependent on prostaglandin production (i.e. when there are high levels of circulating vasoconstrictors or hypovolaemia).

Intramuscular injection may be painful, and sterile abscesses have been reported.

The drug may inhibit uterine contraction.

Kinetics

Absorption The drug is well absorbed when administered by all routes. The oral bioavailability is 60%.

Distribution Diclofenac is 99.5% protein-bound in the plasma, predominantly to albumin. The V_D is 0.12–0.17 l/kg. The drug crosses the placenta in animal models. Diclofenac enters the synovial fluid and reaches maximum concentration 2–4 hours after peak plasma concentrations have been achieved. Drug levels within the synovial fluid may remain high for up to 12 hours, before being eliminated with a half-life of 3–6 hours.

Metabolism Diclofenac undergoes significant first-pass metabolism, principally in the liver by hydroxylation and methoxylation to phenolic metabolites, with subsequent conjugation to inactive glucuronide and sulfate metabolites. Two phenolic metabolites have biological activity, although much reduced, compared with the parent drug.

Excretion Approximately 65% of the dose is excreted in the urine and 35% in the bile. Less than 1% is excreted unchanged. The clearance is 263 ml/min, and the terminal elimination half-life in the plasma is 1–2 hours.

Special points Renal and hepatic impairment have little effect on the plasma concentration of diclofenac. The drug may increase plasma concentrations of co-administered digoxin and lithium by reducing renal clearance.

Diclofenac may increase the effect of co-administered oral anticoagulants, heparin, and sulfonylureas due to displacement from plasma proteins.

NSAIDs antagonize the antihypertensive effects of ACEIs via the inhibition of vasodilatory prostaglandin synthesis. The risk of renal impairment increases if NSAIDs and ACEIs are co-administered. NSAIDs inhibit the activity of diuretics.

Diclofenac should not be administered to aspirin-sensitive asthmatics.

In patients with severe renal impairment, the excipient hydroxypropylbetadex is subject to renal elimination and may accumulate if present in the intravenous preparation. The clinical relevance of this in man is unclear.

NSAIDs cause closure of the ductus arteriosus in the fetus.

Digoxin

Uses Digoxin is used in the treatment of:
1. atrial fibrillation and flutter
2. heart failure and may be of use
3. in the prevention of supraventricular dysrhythmias following thoracotomy.

Chemical A glycoside (sterol lactone and a sugar).

Presentation As 0.0625/0.125/0.25 mg tablets, an elixir containing 0.05 mg/ml, and as a clear, colourless solution for injection containing 0.25 mg/ml of digoxin.

Main action Positive inotropism and slowing of the ventricular response.

Mode of action Digoxin acts both directly and indirectly; its direct action is exerted by binding to, and inhibiting the action of, $Na^+K^+ATPase$ within the sarcolemma cell membrane. This produces an increase in the intracellular Na^+ concentration and a decrease in the intracellular K^+ concentration. The increase in the intracellular Na^+ concentration causes displacement of bound intracellular Ca^{2+}. This increased availability of Ca^{2+} results in a positive inotropic action. The decrease in the intracellular K^+ concentration leads to slowing of AV conduction and of the pacemaker cells. The drug also acts indirectly by modifying autonomic activity and increasing efferent vagal activity.

Routes of administration/doses The loading dose by both oral and parenteral routes is 10–20 micrograms/kg 6-hourly until the desired effect is achieved. Intravenous injection must be slow (at a rate not exceeding 0.025 mg/min)—the peak effects are observed 2 hours after intravenous administration. The maintenance dose is 10–20 micrograms/kg/day in divided doses; therapy should be adjusted according to response, guided (where appropriate) by measurement of serum levels of the drug. The therapeutic range is 1–2 micrograms/ml.

Effects

CVS The main action of digoxin is to increase the force of cardiac contraction; automaticity and contractility also increase. The heart rate is slowed due to a combination of improved haemodynamics, depression of sinus node discharge, slowing of AV nodal conduction, an increase in the AV nodal refractory period, and an indirect vagotonic effect. Rapid intravenous administration of digoxin may cause vasoconstriction, leading to hypertension and decreased coronary blood flow. The characteristic ECG changes produced by the drug include prolongation of the PR interval, ST-segment depression, T-wave flattening, and shortening of the QT interval.

GU Digoxin has a mild intrinsic diuretic effect.

Toxicity/side effects Side effects are common with digoxin, especially if the therapeutic range is exceeded. The gastrointestinal side effects include anorexia, nausea and vomiting, diarrhoea, and abdominal pain. The neurological side effects of the drug include headache, drowsiness, confusion, visual disturbances, muscular weakness, and coma. Digoxin may cause any form of dysrhythmia, especially junctional bradycardia, ventricular bigemini, and second- or third-degree heart block. Rashes and gynaecomastia occur uncommonly. Digoxin-specific antibody fragments are available for the treatment of digoxin toxicity.

Kinetics

Absorption Absorption from the gastrointestinal tract is highly variable, and the bioavailability by this route varies from 60% to 90%. Absorption after intramuscular injection is erratic.

Distribution Digoxin is 20–30% protein-bound in the plasma; the V_D is 5–11 l/kg. The concentrations achieved at steady state in cardiac tissue are 15–30 times that of plasma.

Metabolism Less than 10% of the dose undergoes hepatic metabolism via stepwise cleavage of the sugar moieties.

Excretion 50–70% of an administered dose of digoxin is excreted unchanged in the urine as a result of glomerular filtration and active tubular secretion. The clearance is dependent on renal function and may be calculated from the formula:

$$\text{Clearance} = (0.88 \times \text{creatinine clearance} + 0.33) \pm 52\%$$

The elimination half-life is 1.6 days. The dose interval should be increased in the presence of renal impairment.

Special points Patients receiving suxamethonium, pancuronium, or beta-adrenergic agonists concurrently with digoxin may exhibit an increased incidence of dysrhythmias.

The following states increase the likelihood of digoxin toxicity: hypokalaemia, hypernatraemia, hypercalcaemia, hypomagnesaemia, acid–base disturbances, hypoxaemia, and renal failure. Co-administered verapamil, nifedipine, amiodarone, and diazepam also increase plasma digoxin concentrations.

Digoxin is not removed by dialysis.

Diltiazem

Uses Diltiazem is recommended for use:
1. in the treatment of stable and variant angina and may be of use in the treatment of:
2. hypertension
3. supraventricular tachycardias
4. Raynaud's phenomenon
5. migraine, and
6. oesophageal motility disorders.

Chemical A benzothiapine.

Presentation As 60/90/120/180/240/300 mg tablets of diltiazem hydrochloride.

Main action Diltiazem increases myocardial oxygen supply and decreases myocardial oxygen demand by coronary artery dilation, possibly aided by direct and indirect haemodynamic alterations.

Mode of action Diltiazem acts via dose-dependent inhibition of the slow inward calcium current in normal cardiac tissue.

Routes of administration/doses The adult oral dose is 30–120 mg 6- to 8-hourly.

Effects

CVS Diltiazem is a potent peripheral and coronary arterial vasodilator, leading to a decrease in the systemic and pulmonary vascular resistances; the cardiac output increases due to a reduction in afterload. Little effect on the heart rate occurs in man; bradycardia tends to occur with chronic use. AV nodal conduction is decreased by the drug; diltiazem is thus of use in the treatment of supraventricular tachycardias.

RS The drug inhibits bronchoconstriction due to inhaled histamine in man.

AS A significant reduction in lower oesophageal pressure is produced in patients with achalasia, although no effect is seen in normal subjects.

GU Renal artery dilation, leading to an increased renal plasma flow and subsequent diuresis, occurs after the administration of diltiazem. Uterine activity is decreased *in vitro*.

Metabolic/other Platelet aggregation is decreased by diltiazem *in vitro*, although no significant effect on haemostasis can be demonstrated *in vivo*.

Toxicity/side effects Occur in 2–10% and include headaches, flushing, peripheral oedema, and bradycardia.

Kinetics

Absorption 90% of an oral dose is absorbed; the bioavailability by this route is 33–40% due to a significant first effect.

Distribution Diltiazem is 78–87% protein-bound in the plasma; the V_D is 5.3 l/kg.

Metabolism Occurs by deacetylation and demethylation in the liver, with subsequent conjugation to glucuronide and sulfates—the metabolites are active.

Excretion 1–4% is excreted unchanged in the urine. The clearance is 11.5–21.3 ml/kg/min, and the elimination half-life is 2–7 hours. Renal failure has no effect on the pharmacokinetics of diltiazem.

Special points Caution should be used if the drug is administered concurrently with a beta-adrenergic antagonist, as serious bradycardias may arise. All volatile agents in current use decrease Ca^{2+} release from the sarcoplasmic reticulum and decrease Ca^{2+} flux into cardiac cells; the negative inotropic effects of diltiazem are thus additive with those of the volatile agents. Experiments in animals have demonstrated an increased risk of sinus arrest if volatile agents and calcium antagonists are used concurrently. If withdrawn acutely (especially in the post-operative period) after chronic oral use, severe rebound hypertension may result. Calcium antagonists may also:
1. reduce the MAC of volatile agents by up to 20% and
2. increase the efficacy of NMB agents.

Diltiazem may increase the plasma concentration of co-administered digoxin by 20–60%. It also increases the toxicity of bupivacaine in animal models.

Dobutamine

Uses Dobutamine is used to provide inotropic support in patients with a low cardiac output, secondary to:
1. myocardial infarction
2. cardiac surgery
3. cardiomyopathy
4. positive end-expiratory pressure ventilation
5. in septic shock to increase oxygen transport to the tissues and
6. cardiac stress testing.

Chemical A synthetic isoprenaline derivative.

Presentation Dobutamine is presented in vials which hold a solution for injection containing 12.5/50 mg/ml of dobutamine hydrochloride, which needs to be diluted prior to infusion.

Main action Positive inotrope.

Mode of action Dobutamine acts directly on catecholamine receptors to activate adenylate cyclase, which catalyses the conversion of adenosine triphosphate (ATP) to cAMP. This results in increased cell membrane permeability to Ca^{2+} which are necessary for depolarization and completion of the contractile process.

Routes of administration/doses Dobutamine is infused intravenously, diluted in a suitable crystalloid to a volume of at least 50 ml. The dose range is 0.5–40 micrograms/kg/min, titrated against response; the drug acts within 1–2 minutes. Solutions should be used within 24 hours.

Effects

CVS The primary action of dobutamine is to increase cardiac contractility by a direct action on cardiac beta-1 adrenoceptors. Sinoatrial nodal automaticity is increased, leading to an increased heart rate; AV nodal conduction velocity is also increased by the drug. Dobutamine also has activity at alpha- and beta-2 adrenoceptors, and thus tends to have only moderate effect on the systemic vascular resistance. Myocardial perfusion may increase. The drug leads to a decrease in both the left ventricular end-diastolic pressure and systemic vascular resistance, and thus to an increase in the cardiac index in patients with severe congestive cardiac failure.

CNS Stimulation occurs at high dose ranges.

GU The urine output increases, secondary to an increase in the cardiac output; dobutamine is devoid of any specific renal vasodilatory effect.

Metabolic/other Dobutamine enhances natural killer cell activity. It decreases blood glucose and increases free fatty acid concentrations.

Toxicity/side effects Are uncommon at dose ranges below 10 micrograms/kg/min. Dysrhythmias, excessive tachycardia and hypertension, fatigue, nervousness, headache, and chest pain may occur. Allergic phenomena have been reported.

Kinetics

Distribution Due to a half-life of 2 minutes, steady-state concentrations occur within 8–10 minutes when the drug is given at a fixed rate. The V_D is 0.2 l/kg.

Metabolism The major route of metabolism is by methylation via catechol-O-methyl transferase to 3-O-methyldobutamine, with subsequent conjugation to glucuronide.

Excretion The (inactive) 3-O-methyl derivative is excreted in the urine, with 20% of the total dose appearing in the faeces. The clearance is 244 l/hour, and the elimination half-life is 2 minutes.

Special points Dobutamine should not be used in patients with cardiac outflow obstruction, e.g. cardiac tamponade or aortic stenosis. Tachyphylaxis may occur during prolonged infusion.

Domperidone

Uses Domperidone is used for the symptomatic treatment of nausea and vomiting from any cause.

Chemical A butyrophenone derivative.

Presentation As tablets containing 10 mg and a suspension containing 1 mg/ml of domperidone; 30 mg suppositories are also available.

Main action Increased gastrointestinal motility and tone, and a central antiemetic effect.

Mode of action The effects of domperidone on gastrointestinal mobility appear to be mediated by antagonism of peripheral dopaminergic (D2) receptors. Little else is known of the mechanism of action of the drug.

Routes of administration/doses The adult oral dose is 10–20 mg, and the rectal dose 60 mg 4- to 8-hourly.

Effects

CVS Domperidone has no significant effects on the cardiac output, heart rate, blood pressure, or conduction.

CNS The drug does not readily cross the blood–brain barrier and is thus essentially devoid of central effects.

AS The drug increases the lower oesophageal sphincter tone and the rate of gastric emptying. It has an antiemetic effect indistinguishable from that of metoclopramide in the prevention of post-operative vomiting but appears to be more effective in the treatment of established post-operative vomiting.

Metabolic/other The drug causes an increase in the serum prolactin concentration.

Toxicity/side effects Domperidone is generally very well tolerated; there are occasional reports of extrapyramidal reactions occurring with the use of the drug. Galactorrhoea and gynaecomastia have also been reported.

Kinetics

Absorption The bioavailability is 13–17% when administered orally due to first-pass metabolism in the gut wall and liver.

Distribution Domperidone is 92% protein-bound in the plasma; the V_D is 5.7 l/kg.

Metabolism 90% of the drug is metabolized by hydroxylation and oxidative N-dealkylation.

Excretion 30% appears in the urine, and 60% in the faeces; the elimination half-life is 7.5 hours. Accumulation appears not to occur in the presence of renal impairment.

Special points Cardiac arrest has been reported after the rapid intravenous administration of domperidone. This preparation is no longer available.

Dopamine

Uses Dopamine has been used in the management of:
1. low cardiac output states
2. septicaemic shock, and
3. impending renal failure to promote diuresis.

Chemical A naturally occurring catecholamine.

Presentation As a clear, colourless solution for injection containing 40/160 mg/ml of dopamine hydrochloride.

Main action Sympathomimetic and increased renal blood flow.

Mode of action In low doses (1–5 micrograms/kg/min), dopamine acts upon specific dopaminergic receptors, of which at least two types are recognized. D1 receptors are a form of adenylate cyclase; D2 receptors are not linked to adenylate cyclase and are involved in the central modulation of behaviour and movement. At higher dose ranges, the drug acts via direct and indirect stimulation of beta- and alpha-adrenergic receptors; at an infusion rate of 5–10 micrograms/kg/min, beta stimulation predominates, whereas, at infusion rates exceeding 15 micrograms/kg/min, alpha effects predominate.

Routes of administration/doses Dopamine is administered by intravenous infusion, diluted in glucose/saline or Hartmann's solution. A dedicated central vein is preferred for the administration of the drug. A dose of 1–20 micrograms/kg/min may be used, titrated according to response. The drug acts within 5 minutes and has a duration of action of 10 minutes.

Effects

CVS The cardiovascular effects of dopamine depend upon the rate of infusion. At low doses (5 micrograms/kg/min), beta-adrenergic effects predominate, leading to a positive inotropic effect, increased automaticity, and an increase in the cardiac output and coronary blood flow; the drug has little effect on the heart rate. Systolic and diastolic blood pressures may decrease slightly due to a decrease in the systemic vascular resistance (a beta-2 effect). With the use of high doses (15 micrograms/kg/min), peripheral vasoconstriction (an alpha-adrenergic effect) occurs, leading to an increased venous return and systolic blood pressure. Dopamine has variable effects on the PVR.

RS Dopamine activates the carotid bodies and may decrease the ventilatory response to hypoxia.

CNS Dopamine is a central neurotransmitter involved in the modulation of movement; exogenous dopamine does not cross the blood–brain barrier, except in its laevorotatory form. The drug causes marked nausea due to a direct action on the chemosensitive trigger zone (which lies outside the blood–brain barrier). Increased intraocular pressure occurs with dopamine administration in critically ill patients.

AS The drug causes vasodilation of the splanchnic circulation by an effect on dopaminergic receptors and decreases gastroduodenal motility in the critically ill.

GU In low doses (1–5 micrograms/kg/min), dopamine causes a marked decrease in the renal vascular resistance, with a corresponding increase in renal blood flow. Dopamine produces diuresis via the D1 receptors on the luminal and basal membranes of the proximal convoluted tubule. Natriuresis is produced by the inhibition of $Na^+K^+ATPase$. Creatinine clearance remains unaltered.

Metabolic/other Dopamine reduces the release of prolactin and aldosterone. The drug appears to induce or aggravate the sick euthyroid syndrome and partial hypopituitarism, and also depresses growth hormone secretion in the critically ill.

Toxicity/side effects Tachycardia, dysrhythmias, angina, hypertension, and nausea and vomiting may all follow the administration of the drug. Extravasation of dopamine may cause ischaemic tissue necrosis and skin sloughing. An increase in perioperative cardiac events may occur.

Kinetics

Absorption Dopamine is ineffective when administered orally.

Metabolism Exogenous dopamine is metabolized in the plasma, liver, and kidneys by monoamine oxidase and catechol-O-methyltransferase to homovanillic acid and 3,4-dihydroxyphenylacetic acid. Twenty-five percent of an administered dose is converted to noradrenaline within adrenergic nerve terminals.

Excretion Occurs principally in the urine as homovanillic acid and its sulfate and glucuronide derivatives; a small fraction is excreted unchanged. The clearance is 234–330 l/hour, and the elimination half-life is 2 minutes.

Special points As with all inotropes, correction of hypovolaemia should be ensured before use of the drug. A reduced dose should be used in patients who have recently received monoamine oxidase inhibitors (MAOIs). Halogenated volatile anaesthetic agents may increase the likelihood of dysrhythmias occurring during the concurrent use of dopamine. The dopaminergic stimulation is blocked by phenothiazines.

There is no evidence dopamine provides renal protection, and it may worsen renal ischaemia. It does not prevent the need for renal support nor does it delay the time for support.

The drug is inactivated by alkaline solutions (e.g. sodium bicarbonate).

Dopexamine

Uses Dopexamine is used in the treatment of:
1. low cardiac output states (including those complicating cardiac surgery)
2. acute heart failure
3. to increase splanchnic blood flow and
4. to prevent renal shutdown.

Chemical A synthetic dopamine analogue.

Presentation As a clear solution containing 10 mg/ml of dopexamine hydrochloride; the solution should be discarded if it becomes discoloured.

Main action Arterial vasodilatation, positive inotropism, and renal arterial vasodilatation.

Mode of action Dopexamine is an agonist at dopaminergic D1 and D2 receptors and thus leads to relaxation of vascular smooth muscle in the renal, mesenteric, cerebral, and coronary arterial beds (D1 effects) and stimulation of sympathetic pre-junctional receptors, thereby decreasing noradrenaline release (a D2 effect). The drug also inhibits uptake-1 of noradrenaline and has potent beta-2 adrenergic agonist activity.

Route of administration/doses Dopexamine should be diluted prior to administration in either glucose or saline and administered via a central vein using a controlled infusion device. The initial dose is 0.5 micrograms/kg/min which may be increased, as necessary, to a maximum dose of 6 micrograms/kg/min.

Effects

CVS Dopexamine has positive inotropic and chronotropic effects, and thus increases the cardiac output. The drug causes arteriolar vasodilation, leading to a mild decrease in the diastolic blood pressure with a slight increase in the systolic blood pressure; the left and right ventricular afterload, left ventricular end-diastolic pressure, and pulmonary artery pressure decrease following the administration of the drug. Dopexamine also causes a slight increase in the coronary artery blood flow, with no attendant alteration in myocardial oxygen extraction. The drug has a low propensity to cause dysrhythmias.

RS Dopexamine causes measurable bronchodilatation.

CNS The drug increases the cerebral blood flow, secondary to cerebral vasodilation. Nausea and vomiting may result from a weak D2 effect at the chemoreceptor trigger zone.

AS Splanchnic blood flow may increase due to mesenteric vasodilation.

GU Dopexamine reduces renal vascular resistance, leading to an increase in the renal plasma flow and an attendant diuresis and natriuresis.

Metabolic/other Beta-2 adrenergic stimulation may result in hypokalaemia and hyperglycaemia; the platelet count may also decrease due to temporary splenic sequestration of platelets.

Toxicity/side effects The use of the drug may be complicated by headache, flushing, tremor, angina, and dysrhythmias.

Kinetics Data are incomplete.

Distribution Dopexamine is 40% bound to red blood cells; the V_D is 317–446 ml/kg.

Metabolism The drug is rapidly cleared from blood by tissue uptake and is extensively metabolized by methylation and sulfate conjugation.

Excretion Dopexamine is excreted as metabolites in the urine and faeces; the clearance is 30–35 ml/min/kg, and the elimination half-life is 5–10 minutes.

Special points The use of dopexamine should be avoided in patients with uncorrected hypovolaemia, aortic stenosis, hypertrophic obstructive cardiomyopathy, or a phaeochromocytoma.

Dopexamine has an unexpected antioxidant effect.

Doxapram

Uses Doxapram is used:
1. as a respiratory stimulant for the treatment of post-operative respiratory depression and acute-on-chronic respiratory failure and has been used
2. in the treatment of laryngospasm
3. to facilitate blind nasal intubation and
4. in the treatment of post-operative shivering.

Chemical A monohydrated pyrrolidinone derivative.

Presentation As a clear, colourless solution containing 20 mg/ml and as a solution for infusion containing 2 mg/ml in 5% glucose of doxapram hydrochloride.

Main action Respiratory stimulation.

Mode of action Doxapram acts primarily by stimulating the peripheral chemoreceptors and secondarily by a direct action on the respiratory centre.

Routes of administration/doses The drug may be administered intravenously as a bolus of 1 mg/kg or as an infusion of 1.5–4 mg/min. Given intravenously, doxapram acts in 20–40 seconds; its peak effect is seen at 1–2 minutes, and the duration of action is 5–12 minutes, although pharmacological effects are detectable for 2 hours.

Effects

CVS Doxapram causes an increase in the cardiac output, primarily due to an increase in the stroke volume. A slight increase in the blood pressure and heart rate may be produced by the drug.

RS The minute volume is increased by doxapram due to an increase in the tidal volume; at higher doses, an increase in respiratory rate occurs. The CO_2 response curve is displaced to the left by the drug. The work of breathing is increased.

CNS The cerebral blood flow is increased, following the administration of doxapram; the drug has less convulsant activity than other analeptic agents.

AS In animals, salivation and gastrointestinal tone and motility are increased by the drug.

GU In animal models, doxapram increases both the urine output and motility within the genitourinary (GU) system.

Metabolic/other Catecholamine and steroid secretion are increased in animal models. The metabolic rate may increase by up to 30% and may lead to hypoxia due to increased oxygen consumption.

Toxicity/side effects Restlessness, dizziness, hallucinations, excessive sweating, and a sensation of perineal warmth have been described subsequent to the administration of doxapram.

Kinetics Data are incomplete.

Distribution The V_D is 1.5 l/kg.

Metabolism The metabolic pathway of doxapram in man is unknown.

Excretion 5% is excreted unchanged in the urine. The clearance is 370 ml/min, and the half-life is 2–4 hours.

Special points Doxapram has been shown:
1. to lead to a more rapid return to consciousness after inhalational anaesthesia
2. to reverse opioid-induced respiratory depression without reversing analgesia and
3. to prevent the necessity for mechanical ventilation in some patients.

The drug may possibly decrease the incidence of post-operative chest infections.

Oxygen must be given to patients receiving doxapram due to the increased metabolic rate and the increase in the work of breathing.

Droperidol

Uses Droperidol is used:
1. in premedication
2. in the technique of neuroleptanalgesia
3. in the treatment of nausea and vomiting occurring post-operatively or as a result of chemotherapy
4. in the treatment of psychosis and has been used
5. for the control of perioperative hiccuping.

Chemical A butyrophenone derivative.

Presentation As 10 mg tablets, a syrup containing 1 mg/ml, and as a clear solution for injection containing 5 mg/ml of droperidol.

Main action Antiemetic and neuroleptic.

Mode of action The antiemetic and neuroleptic effects of the drug appear to be mediated by:
1. central dopaminergic (D2) blockade, leading to an increased threshold for vomiting at the chemoreceptor trigger zone and
2. post-synaptic GABA antagonism.

Route of administration/doses The adult oral or intramuscular dose is 5–10 mg, and the intravenous dose when used as a neuroleptic agent is 5–15 mg, although the drug appears to be an effective antiemetic in doses as low as 0.5 mg. The onset of action after intravenous administration is 3–20 minutes, and the drug may act for up to 12 hours.

Effects

CVS Droperidol has minimal cardiovascular effects, but its antagonistic effects at alpha-adrenergic receptors may lead to hypotension in the presence of hypovolaemia.

RS The drug causes small decreases in the minute volume, functional residual capacity, and airways resistance.

CNS Droperidol induces neurolepsis, a state characterized by diminished motor activity, anxiolysis, and indifference to the external environment. The seizure threshold is raised by the drug.

AS The drug has a powerful antiemetic effect via a central effect at the chemosensitive trigger zone.

Metabolic/other Droperidol, in common with other dopamine antagonists, may cause hyperprolactinaemia. The drug reduces total body oxygen consumption.

Toxicity/side effects Extrapyramidal effects occur in 1%. Gastrointestinal disturbances, abnormalities of liver function tests, and allergic phenomena have been reported after the use of droperidol. Malignant neuroleptic syndrome may be precipitated by droperidol.

Kinetics

Absorption The drug is well absorbed after intramuscular administration. The pharmacokinetics of droperidol after oral administration has not been elucidated.

Distribution The drug is 85–90% protein-bound in the plasma; the V_D is 1.54–2.54 l/kg.

Metabolism Droperidol is extensively metabolized in the liver (the major metabolic pathway in animals being oxidative N-dealkylation); the only metabolite that has been identified in man is 2-benzimidazolinone.

Excretion 75% of the dose is excreted in the urine (1% unchanged), and 22% in the faeces. The clearance is 9.7–18.5 ml/min/kg, and the elimination half-life is 2–2.5 hours.

Special points Droperidol is pharmaceutically incompatible with thiopental and methohexital. The sedative effects of the drug are additive with those of other CNS depressants administered concurrently.

Edrophonium

Uses Edrophonium is used:
1. for the reversal of non-depolarizing neuromuscular blockade
2. in the diagnosis of suspected phase II block
3. in the diagnosis of myasthenia gravis (the 'Tensilon® test') and
4. in the differentiation of myasthenic and cholinergic crisis in myasthenic patients.

Chemical A synthetic quaternary ammonium compound.

Presentation As a clear, colourless solution for injection containing 10 mg/ml of edrophonium chloride.

Main action Cholinergic.

Mode of action Edrophonium is a synthetic reversible inhibitor of acetylcholinesterase; it competes with acetylcholine for the anionic site of the enzyme and reversibly binds to it. At least, part of the effect of the drug appears to be exerted pre-junctionally.

Route of administration/doses The drug is usually administered intravenously; it has a more rapid onset (its peak effect occurring at 0.8–2 minutes) and shorter duration of effect (10 minutes) than does neostigmine. The 'Tensilon® test' for the diagnosis of myasthenia gravis consists of the slow administration of 2 mg of edrophonium, followed by a further 8 mg if clinical deterioration does not occur. When used in the differentiation of a myasthenic and cholinergic crisis, a dose of 2 mg of edrophonium is used—weakness will increase if the crisis is cholinergic (and improve if myasthenic) in nature. An anticholinergic agent (e.g. atropine) must be immediately available when these tests are performed. The dose for reversal of competitive neuromuscular blockade is 0.5–0.7 mg/kg by slow intravenous injection, preceded by an appropriate dose of an anticholinergic agent to counter the peripheral muscarinic side effects of the drug.

Effects

CVS The drug may cause bradycardia, leading to a fall in the cardiac output; it decreases the effective refractory period of cardiac muscle and increases the conduction time.

RS Edrophonium increases bronchial secretion and may cause bronchoconstriction.

CNS Agitation and dreaming may occur; the drug has a predictable miotic effect. Weakness leading to fasciculation and paralysis may occur when edrophonium is administered to normal subjects.

AS The drug increases salivation, lower oesophageal and gastric tone, gastric acid output, and lower gastrointestinal tract motility. Nausea and vomiting may occur.

GU Edrophonium increases ureteric peristalsis and may lead to involuntary micturition.

Metabolic/other Sweating and lacrimation are increased by the drug.

Toxicity/side effects The side effects are manifestations of its pharmacological actions, as described above. Cardiac arrest has been reported after the use of edrophonium.

Kinetics Data are incomplete.

Distribution The V_D is 0.9–1.3 l/kg.

Metabolism The metabolic fate of edrophonium is uncertain; it is not hydrolysed by anticholinesterases.

Excretion Details of the excretory pathways of the drug are unknown. The clearance is 6.9–12.3 ml/min/kg, and the elimination half-life is 110 minutes.

Special points The potency of edrophonium is 12–16 times less than that of neostigmine; the muscarinic effects of the drug are correspondingly easier to counteract than those of neostigmine. Edrophonium is less predictable than neostigmine when used to reverse profound competitive neuromuscular blockade.

Enflurane

Uses Enflurane is used for the induction and maintenance of general anaesthesia.

Chemical A halogenated methylethyl ether which is a geometric isomer of isoflurane.

Presentation As a clear, colourless liquid (that should be protected from light) with a characteristic sweet smell. The commercial preparation contains no stabilizers or preservatives; it is non-flammable in normal anaesthetic concentrations. The molecular weight of enflurane is 184.5, the boiling point 56.5°C, and the saturated vapour pressure 23.3 kPa at 20°C. The MAC of enflurane is 1.68 (0.57 in 70% N_2O), the oil/water solubility coefficient 120, and the blood/gas solubility coefficient 1.91. The drug is readily soluble in rubber; it does not attack metals.

Main action General anaesthesia (reversible loss of both awareness and recall of noxious stimuli).

Mode of action The mechanism of general anaesthesia remains to be fully elucidated. General anaesthetics appear to disrupt synaptic transmission (especially in the area of the ventrobasal thalamus). This mechanism may include potentiation of the $GABA_A$ and glycine receptors and antagonism at NMDA receptors. Their mode of action at the molecular level appears to involve expansion of hydrophobic regions in the neuronal membrane, either within the lipid phase or within hydrophobic sites in cell membrane proteins.

Routes of administration/doses Enflurane is administered by inhalation, conventionally via a calibrated vaporizer. The concentration used for the inhalational induction of anaesthesia is 1–10% and for maintenance 0.6–3%.

Effects

CVS Enflurane is a negative inotrope; it also causes a decrease in the systemic vascular resistance, and these two effects produce a decrease in the mean arterial pressure. Unlike halothane, enflurane produces a slight reflex tachycardia. The drug decreases coronary vascular resistance; it also reduces the rate of phase IV depolarization, increases the threshold potential, and prolongs the effective refractory period. Enflurane is not markedly arrhythmogenic but does sensitize the myocardium to the effects of circulating catecholamines.

RS Enflurane is a powerful respiratory depressant, markedly decreasing the tidal volume, although the respiratory rate may increase during the administration of the drug. A slight increase in the $PaCO_2$ may result in spontaneously breathing subjects; the drug also decreases the ventilatory response to hypoxia and hypercapnia. Enflurane is non-irritant to the respiratory tract; it causes bronchodilatation and no increase in secretions. The drug inhibits pulmonary macrophage activity and mucociliary transport.

CNS The principal effect of enflurane is general anaesthesia; the drug has little analgesic effect. The drug increases the cerebral blood flow, leading to an increase in the intracranial pressure; it also decreases cerebral oxygen consumption. The drug may induce tonic/clonic muscle activity and may also produce epileptiform EEG traces, especially in the presence of hypocapnia. A marked decrease in skeletal muscle tone results from the use of enflurane, mediated by an effect on the post-junctional membrane.

AS Enflurane decreases the splanchnic blood flow as a result of the hypotension it produces.

GU Enflurane decreases the renal blood flow and glomerular filtration rate; a small volume of concentrated urine results. The drug reduces the tone of the pregnant uterus.

Metabolic/other Enflurane decreases plasma noradrenaline concentration and may increase blood sugar concentration. The drug causes a fall in the body temperature, predominantly by cutaneous vasodilation. Enflurane depresses white cell function for 24 hours post-operatively but has no effect on platelet function.

Toxicity/side effects Enflurane is a recognized trigger agent for the development of malignant hyperthermia. The drug may also cause the appearance of myocardial dysrhythmias, particularly in the presence of hypoxia, hypercapnia, or excessive catecholamine concentrations. Shivering ('the shakes') may occur post-operatively. There have been isolated reports of hepatotoxicity associated with the repeated use of enflurane; there is also the theoretical risk of fluoride ion toxicity occurring with the use of the drug, particularly in patients with renal failure.

Kinetics

Absorption The major factors affecting the uptake of volatile anaesthetic agents are solubility, cardiac output, and the concentration gradient between the alveoli and venous blood. Enflurane is less soluble in blood than is halothane; the alveolar concentration therefore reaches inspired concentration relatively rapidly, resulting in a rapid induction of anaesthesia. An increase in the cardiac output increases the rate of alveolar uptake and slows the induction of anaesthesia. The concentration gradient between alveoli and venous blood approaches zero at equilibrium; a large concentration gradient favours the onset of anaesthesia.

Distribution The drug is initially distributed to organs with a high blood flow (brain, heart, liver, and kidney) and later to less well-perfused organs (muscles, fat, and bone).

Metabolism 2.4% of an administered dose is slowly metabolized in the liver via cytochrome P450 2EI, principally by oxidation and dehalogenation; plasma fluoride ion concentrations may reach ten times those observed after the use of halothane or isoflurane.

Excretion More than 80% is exhaled unchanged; 2.4% of an administered dose is excreted in the urine as non-volatile fluorinated compounds. The remainder is excreted via the skin, sweat, and faeces.

Special points Enflurane markedly potentiates the action of co-administered non-depolarizing relaxants.

The dose of co-administered adrenaline should not exceed 10 ml of a 1:100 000 solution in a 10-minute period to guard against the development of ventricular dysrhythmias.

Enflurane is not recommended for use in epileptic patients.

Drug structure For the drug structure, please see Fig. 2.

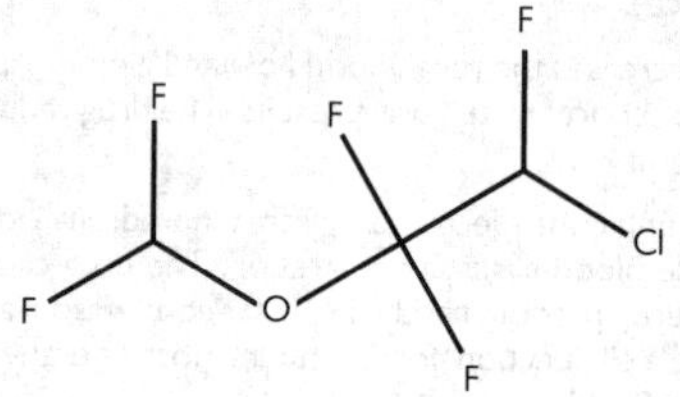

Fig. 2 Drug structure of enflurane.

Enoximone

Uses Enoximone is used:
1. in the treatment of acute-on-chronic heart failure
2. during and after the withdrawal of cardiopulmonary bypass, and
3. in the treatment of low-output states prior to cardiac transplantation.

Chemical An imidazolone derivative.

Presentation As a clear, yellow solution containing 5 mg/ml of enoximone.

Main action Positive inotropism and vasodilation.

Mode of action Enoximone acts by inhibiting type III phosphodiesterase, the enzyme responsible for the degradation of cAMP. The drug thus has a synergistic effect with those catecholamines, which directly activates adenylate cyclase and leads to an increase in the intracellular concentration of cAMP.

Route of administration/doses Enoximone is administered intravenously, diluted in a ratio of 1:1 with either water or saline, either by a slow bolus injection of 0.5–1 mg/kg to a maximum dose of 3 mg/kg every 3–6 hours or by infusion at the rate of 90 micrograms/kg/min over 10–30 minutes and thereafter at the rate of 5–20 micrograms/kg/min. The drug acts within 10–30 minutes after intravenous administration; the mean duration of effect is 4–6 hours.

Effects

CVS Enoximone has a positive inotropic action and leads to an increase in the cardiac output; the left ventricular stroke work index and cardiac index increase by 40–55% in patients with heart failure. Similarly, right atrial pressure, pulmonary capillary wedge pressure, PVR, and systemic vascular resistance all decrease by 30%. The drug has little effect on myocardial oxygen consumption; myocardial efficiency and coronary blood flow increase in animal models. Enoximone usually has little effect on the blood pressure or heart rate; dysrhythmias occur uncommonly.

Metabolic/other The drug has little effect on plasma renin activity or catecholamine concentrations. A decrease in the platelet count has been observed in a small percentage of patients receiving the drug.

Toxicity/side effects Dysrhythmias, hypotension, and CNS and gastrointestinal disturbances occur uncommonly with the use of enoximone.

Kinetics

Absorption Enoximone is readily absorbed but undergoes extensive first-pass metabolism to an active sulfoxide form.

Distribution The drug is 70% protein-bound in the plasma; the V_D is 2.1–8 l/kg.

Metabolism Enoximone is primarily metabolized in the liver to an active sulfoxide form.

Excretion The drug appears predominantly in the form of sulfoxide in the urine; trace amounts are excreted unchanged. The clearance is 3.7–13 ml/min/kg, and the elimination half-life is 6.2 hours. A decreased dose should be used in the presence of renal or hepatic impairment.

Enoximone appears to be partially removed by haemodialysis.

Ephedrine

Uses Ephedrine is used in the treatment of:
1. hypotension occurring in general, spinal, or epidural anaesthesia
2. nocturnal enuresis
3. narcolepsy
4. diabetic autonomic neuropathy
5. hiccups and
6. as a nasal decongestant.

Chemical A naturally occurring sympathomimetic amine.

Presentation As 15/30/60 mg tablets, an elixir containing 3 mg/ml, as 0.5/1% nasal drops, as a constituent of proprietary cold cures, and as a clear, colourless solution for injection containing 30 mg/ml of ephedrine hydrochloride. It has four isomers, with only the L-isomer being active.

Main action Sympathomimetic.

Mode of action Ephedrine acts both indirectly (by causing release of noradrenaline from sympathetic nerve terminals) and directly by stimulation of alpha- and beta-adrenoceptors.

Route of administration/doses The adult dose by the oral route is 30 mg 8-hourly; as a nasal decongestant, 1–2 drops may be administered every 4 hours. The parenteral preparation should be diluted before use in 0.9% sodium chloride. The recommended intravenous dose in adults is 3–7.5 mg (maximum 9 mg), administered slowly, repeated every 3–4 minutes to a maximum of 30 mg, titrated to response. When administered orally, the drug acts within 60 minutes and has a duration of action of 3–5 hours. When administered intravenously, the onset of the cardiovascular effects of the drug is rapid; the duration of action is up to 1 hour.

Effects

CVS The effects of ephedrine are similar to those of adrenaline but are more prolonged, as the drug is not metabolized by monoamine oxidase or catechol-O-methyl transferase. Ephedrine has positive inotropic and chronotropic actions, producing an increase in the cardiac output, myocardial work, and myocardial oxygen consumption. Myocardial irritability is increased by the drug. Ephedrine increases the coronary blood flow, systolic and diastolic blood pressures, and pulmonary artery pressure. An increase in the circulating volume may follow the use of the drug due to post-capillary vasoconstriction.

RS Ephedrine is a respiratory stimulant and causes marked bronchodilatation.

CNS Ephedrine has a stimulatory effect similar to amphetamine; the cerebral blood flow increases after the administration of the drug. Mydriasis occurs, but light reflexes remain unaffected. The drug has local anaesthetic properties.

AS The drug relaxes gastrointestinal smooth muscle and causes splanchnic vasoconstriction.

GU Ephedrine constricts renal blood vessels and may lead to a decrease in both renal blood flow and glomerular filtration rate. The drug contracts the bladder sphincter and relaxes the detrusor muscle which may precipitate acute retention of urine. Ephedrine decreases the uterine tone. The drug does not cause alpha-1-mediated vasoconstriction of uterine blood vessels.

Metabolic/other The drug increases the rate of hepatic glycogenolysis and may increase the basal metabolic rate. The drug has been shown to stimulate oxygen uptake and thermogenesis.

Toxicity/side effects Insomnia, anxiety, tremor, headache, dysrhythmias, nausea and vomiting, and chest pain may complicate the use of the drug. Ephedrine is irritant to mucous membranes. An acute hypertensive crisis may be precipitated when the drug is administered to patients receiving MAOIs, doxapram, beta-blockers, oxytocin, and ergot alkaloids.

Kinetics
Absorption Ephedrine is rapidly and completely absorbed when administered orally, intramuscularly, or subcutaneously.

Distribution Ephedrine is rapidly and extensively distributed throughout the body, with accumulation in the liver, lungs, kidneys, spleen, and brain. The V_D ranges from 122 to 320 l. Ephedrine crosses the placental barrier and is excreted into breast milk.

Metabolism The drug is resistant to metabolism by monoamine oxidase and catechol-O-methyl transferase. A small amount of drug is metabolized in the liver by N-demethylation to phenylpropanolamine (norephedrine), the major metabolite, which may produce central stimulant effects. The drug is also deaminated, yielding benzoic acid, hippuric acid, and 1-phenylpropane-1,2-diol.

Excretion 55–99% of an administered dose is excreted unchanged in the urine. The elimination half-life is 6.3 hours (the half-life of norephedrine is 1.5–4 hours). The clearance is 13.6–44.3 l/hour. Urinary excretion is pH-dependent; elimination is enhanced, and the half-life is accordingly shorter in acidic urine. Excretion is reduced to 20–35% in the presence of an alkaline urine. Renal disease is likely to impair the elimination of ephedrine.

Special points Tachyphylaxis occurs with prolonged use of the drug. Dysrhythmias occur with a greater frequency when ephedrine is used in the presence of halothane.

Clonidine premedication enhances the pressor effects of ephedrine.

Epoprostenol

Uses Epoprostenol is used:
1. as an anticoagulant during renal replacement therapy and cardiopulmonary bypass and may be of use in the treatment of
2. pre-eclampsia
3. Raynaud's disease
4. the haemolytic–uraemic syndrome, and
5. pulmonary hypertension.

Chemical A prostanoid (formerly called prostacyclin, PGI2).

Presentation As vials containing 500 micrograms of freeze-dried epoprostenol sodium, to be diluted before use in a mixture of sodium chloride and glycine.

Main action Inhibition of platelet aggregation and vasodilation.

Mode of action Epoprostenol stimulates adenylate cyclase, leading to an increase in the cAMP concentration within platelets; this, in turn, leads to inhibition of platelet phospholipase and COX, and ultimately of platelet aggregation.

Route of administration/doses The drug may be administered intravenously or into the extracorporeal circulation; an infusion of 5 ng/kg/min should be started 15–30 minutes before dialysis is commenced and continued throughout the procedure. The effects of epoprostenol may persist for 30 minutes after cessation of an infusion.

Effects

CVS The drug causes relaxation of vascular smooth muscle, leading to a decrease in the systemic vascular resistance, a slight tachycardia, and a decrease in the diastolic blood pressure.

RS Epoprostenol causes a decrease in the PVR and interferes with the mechanism of hypoxic pulmonary vasoconstriction.

CNS The drug produces cerebral vasodilation, leading to increased cerebral blood flow.

AS Epoprostenol inhibits gastric acid secretion.

Metabolic/other Epoprostenol is the most powerful inhibitor of platelet aggregation known; the bleeding time may double with high doses. It also appears to have a fibrinolytic effect and increases red cell deformability. The drug stimulates renin secretion and may cause an increase in blood sugar concentrations.

Toxicity/side effects Facial flushing and headache occur commonly after the administration of the drug. Gastrointestinal upsets and chest, abdominal, and jaw pain have also been reported.

Kinetics Data are incomplete.

Metabolism Epoprostenol is rapidly removed from the circulation by hydrolysis to 6-oxo-PGF1 alpha in the blood and by metabolism to a bicyclic 15-oxo derivative in the tissues.

Excretion The plasma half-life is 30 seconds to 3 minutes.

Special points Epoprostenol extends the life of filters during renal replacement therapy and decreases the incidence of bleeding in these critically ill patients, compared to heparin.

Eptacog alfa

Uses Eptacog alfa is used for the treatment of bleeding episodes and for the prevention of bleeding in the following patient groups undergoing surgery or an invasive procedure:
1. patients with congenital haemophilia with inhibitors to coagulation factors VIII or IX
2. patients with congenital haemophilia who may have an increased anamnestic response to factor VIII or IX administration
3. patients with acquired haemophilia
4. patients with congenital factor VII deficiency, and
5. patients with Glanzmann's thrombasthenia.

Chemical Activated coagulation factor VII produced using recombinant DNA technology from baby hamster kidney cells. The drug is a vitamin K-dependent glycoprotein consisting of 406 amino acid residues. It has a molecular weight of 50 000 daltons.

Presentation As a white, lyophilized powder together with a solvent for solution for injection. The solution formed has a pH of 6. Eptacog alfa (activated) is available in 1/2/5 mg vials equivalent to 50/100/250 kallikrein inhibitory units (KIU) (1 KIU equals to 1000 IU).

Main actions Activation of coagulation cascade, leading to thrombin production.

Mode of action Eptacog alfa (activated) binds to tissue factor, leading to activation of factors IX and X, resulting in the production of thrombin. In addition, the drug also causes the activation of factor X on the surface of platelets, independently of tissue factor.

Routes of administration/doses The drug is administered intravenously as a bolus at a variety of dosages, depending on the indication. Eptacog alfa (activated) should be given as early as possible after the start of a bleeding episode or immediately prior to an invasive procedure. In patients with haemophilia A or B who have inhibitors or acquired haemophilia, the dose is 90 micrograms/kg, repeated at 2–3 hours initially, with further dose intervals of increasing duration of 4/6/8 or 12 hours, depending on the duration of treatment that is required. In patients with factor VII deficiency, the recommended dose is 15–30 micrograms/kg.

Effects
Metabolic/other The main effect of the drug is its ability to increase the ability of the clotting cascade to produce thrombin.

Toxicity/side effects In conditions where tissue factor expression may be greater than considered normal, use of the drug may lead to the development of DIC or thrombotic events. Severe atherosclerotic disease, septicaemia, crush injury, or DIC may lead to increased tissue factor expression. Hypersensitivity reactions may occur in individuals who have antibodies that react with trace elements of mouse immunoglobulin G (IgG), bovine IgG, and trace culture proteins.

Kinetics Limited data are available on the pharmacokinetic properties of the drug. There appears to be a variation in values, depending on disease states.

Distribution The V_D is 130–165 ml/kg.

Metabolism The metabolism of the drug is unknown, although, in rat models, hepatic metabolism has been implicated.

Excretion The clearance is 33–37 ml/kg/hour. The terminal elimination half-life is in the range of 3.9–6 hours.

Special points The drug should not be used in conjunction with pro-thrombin complex concentrates due to the potential increased risk of thrombotic events.

Inhibitory antibody formation may occur in patients with factor VII deficiency. This may correlate with an *in vitro* inhibitory effect.

Erythropoietin

Uses Erythropoietin is used for the treatment of anaemia associated with:
1. chronic renal failure
2. cytotoxic chemotherapy
3. low birthweight prematurity and is also used
4. to increase the yield of autologous blood preoperatively.

Chemical A glycoprotein.

Presentation Two forms (alpha and beta) of the drug are available, which are clinically indistinguishable. Erythropoietin alpha is presented as a solution for injection containing 2000/4000/10 000 units/ml. Erythropoietin beta is presented as a solution for injection containing 500/1000/5000/10 000 units/ml and as a powder for reconstitution prior to injection.

Main action Enhancement of erythropoiesis.

Mode of action Erythropoietin specifically stimulates erythropoiesis by acting as a mitosis-stimulating factor and differentiation hormone.

Routes of administration/doses The drug is preferably administered subcutaneously initially as 50 units/kg three times a week; the dose is adjusted every 4 weeks in 25 units/kg increments. The maintenance dose is usually 25–100 units/kg three times weekly. The intravenous dose is usually 20–30% greater than the subcutaneous dose. For increasing the yield of autologous blood preoperatively, the usual dose is 600 units/kg once or twice weekly for 3 weeks, together with iron supplementation.

Effects

CVS The drug causes a dose-dependent increase in the blood pressure.

Metabolic/other The primary effect of erythropoietin is to enhance erythropoiesis. It causes a dose-dependent increase in the platelet count, but not thrombocytosis.

Toxicity/side effects Hypertension, influenza-like symptoms, and shunt thrombosis have been reported.

Kinetics Data are incomplete and available only for patients with renal impairment.

Absorption The bioavailability after subcutaneous administration is 23–42%.

Distribution The V_D is 5 l.

Excretion The elimination half-life is 8–15 hours.

Special points Erythropoietin is not removed by haemofiltration or haemodialysis.

Esmolol

Uses Esmolol is effective in the treatment of:
1. acute supraventricular dysrhythmias (atrial fibrillation or flutter)
2. perioperative hypertension, and
3. hypotensive anaesthesia.

Chemical An aryloxypropanolamine.

Presentation As a clear solution for injection containing 10 mg/ml as 10/250 ml of esmolol hydrochloride.

Main action Negative inotropism and chronotropism.

Mode of action Esmolol acts by competitive blockade of beta-adrenoceptors; the drug is relatively selective for beta-1 receptors and has little or no intrinsic sympathomimetic activity.

Routes of administration/doses The drug is administered by intra-venous infusion (preferably via a peripheral vein), diluted in any crystalloid, with the exception of sodium bicarbonate, at a rate of 50–150 micrograms/kg/min according to response. Esmolol has a major advantage over other currently available beta-adrenergic antagonists in that its peak effects are observed within 6–10 minutes of administration and are almost completely attenuated 20 minutes after cessation of the infusion. The advantages of this 'on–off' control are obvious.

Effects

CVS Esmolol causes a fall in the blood pressure and a dose-dependent fall in the heart rate; the cardiac output falls by about 20% (i.e. to a similar extent as with propranolol). It slows AV conduction at doses that have no effect on other haemodynamic or ECG variables. The drug will obtund the cardiovascular responses to intubation and sternotomy and protects against infarction in animal models of myocardial ischaemia.

RS Esmolol appears to have little effect on airways resistance.

Toxicity/side effects Hypotension, bradycardia, bronchospasm, nausea and vomiting, alteration of taste, and CNS disturbances may occur with use of the drug.

Kinetics

Distribution Esmolol is 56% protein-bound in the plasma; the V_D is 3.43 l/kg. Rapid, but limited, transplacental passage occurs in animal models.

Metabolism Occurs primarily by hydrolysis by esterases located in red cells to methanol and a (major) primary acid metabolite which has weak beta-adrenergic antagonist activity, but a long elimination half-life of 3.5 hours.

Excretion 70–80% appears in the urine as the major acid metabolite; 1% is excreted unchanged. The clearance is 285 ml/min/kg, and the elimination half-life is 9.2 minutes. The drug should be used with caution in patients with renal impairment; hepatic disease has no effect.

Special points The drug has no effect on the pharmacokinetics of co-administered morphine or digoxin; it has been shown to increase the recovery time from suxamethonium from 5.6 to 8.3 minutes.

Ether

Uses Ether is used for the induction and maintenance of general anaesthesia.

Chemical Diethyl ether.

Presentation As a clear, colourless liquid (that should be protected from light) with a characteristic sweet smell. Ether is flammable in air at concentrations of 1.83–48% and explosive in oxygen at concentrations of 2–82%. The molecular weight of ether is 74, the boiling point 35°C, and the saturated vapour pressure 56.7 kPa at 20°C. The MAC of ether is 1.92, the oil/water solubility coefficient 3.2, and the blood/gas solubility coefficient 12. Ether is relatively inert but decomposes on exposure to air, heat, and light to produce acetaldehyde and ether peroxide. Ether is no longer commercially available in the United Kingdom (UK).

Main action General anaesthesia (reversible loss of both awareness and recall of noxious stimuli) and analgesia.

Mode of action The mechanism of general anaesthesia remains to be fully elucidated. General anaesthetics appear to disrupt synaptic transmission (especially in the area of the ventrobasal thalamus). This mechanism may include potentiation of the $GABA_A$ and glycine receptors and antagonism at NMDA receptors. Their mode of action at the molecular level appears to involve the expansion of hydrophobic regions within the neuronal membrane, either within the lipid phase or within hydrophobic sites in cell membranes.

Routes of administration/doses Ether is administered by inhalation, conventionally via a calibrated vaporizer. The concentration used for the induction and maintenance of anaesthesia is 3–20%.

Effects

CVS Ether is a negative inotrope *in vitro*; *in vivo*, sympathetic stimulation and catecholamine release and a vagolytic effect tend to offset this effect. The cardiac output is increased by 20%; the heart rate and systemic vascular resistance also increase, and the blood pressure is well maintained as a result. The drug causes dilatation of coronary arteries. Dysrhythmias are rare, and the drug does not sensitize the myocardium to the effects of circulating catecholamines. Light ether anaesthesia produces peripheral vasoconstriction, whereas deeper anaesthesia results in vasodilation (due to an effect on the vasomotor centre), causing a decrease in both the cardiac output and blood pressure.

RS Ether is a respiratory stimulant; at light planes of anaesthesia the respiratory rate may exceed 30 breaths per minute; although the tidal volume decreases, the minute volume remains unaltered. The respiratory centre remains responsive to CO_2 at light planes, and the $PaCO_2$ remains constant. At deeper planes of anaesthesia, respiratory depression occurs, and intubation becomes possible without the aid of muscle relaxants. Ether vapour is irritant and may cause breath-holding and coughing if the inspired concentration is increased too rapidly. The drug causes bronchodilatation with no increase in bronchial secretions.

CNS The principal effect of ether is general anaesthesia; the drug also has an analgesic effect. The drug causes cerebral vasodilation, leading to an increased cerebral blood flow and intracranial pressure. Ether decreases the intraocular pressure and causes progressive pupillary dilatation. Clonus may occur at light planes due to increased stretch receptor reflexes. Skeletal muscle tone decreases as anaesthesia deepens, as a result of both depression of spinal reflexes and a direct action on the neuromuscular junction. Depression of the medulla is a late event, occurring at very deep planes of anaesthesia.

AS The drug increases both salivation and lacrimation. Ether decreases gastrointestinal motility; hepatic function and biliary secretion are also transiently decreased. Splenic contraction may also occur, resulting in an elevated haematocrit and white cell count.

GU Ether causes renal arterial vasoconstriction and therefore decreases renal blood flow and the glomerular filtration rate; a small volume of concentrated urine results; albuminuria may also occur. The drug reduces the tone of the pregnant uterus.

Metabolic/other Ether stimulates gluconeogenesis and may cause an increase in the blood sugar concentration. The drug occasionally causes metabolic acidosis in young children and patients unable to tolerate an increased lactate load.

Toxicity/side effects The predominant disadvantages of ether are its inflammability and the high incidence of PONV (which occurs in 50% of patients who receive the agent). The dramatic increase in salivation produced by the drug necessitates the use of antisialogogue premedication. Convulsions and post-operative shivering may complicate the use of ether.

Kinetics

Absorption The major factors affecting the uptake of volatile anaesthetic agents are solubility, cardiac output and the concentration gradient between the alveoli and venous blood. Ether is relatively soluble in blood; the alveolar concentration therefore reaches the inspired concentration relatively slowly, resulting in a slow induction of, and recovery from, anaesthesia. The irritant properties of the drug compound the slow induction. An increase in the cardiac output increases the rate of alveolar uptake and slows the induction of anaesthesia. The concentration gradient between alveoli and venous blood approaches zero at equilibrium; a large concentration gradient favours the onset of anaesthesia.

Distribution The drug is initially distributed to organs with a high blood flow (brain, heart, liver, and kidney) and later to less well-perfused organs (muscles and fat).

Metabolism 2–3% of an administered dose is metabolized in the liver, to yield acetaldehyde, alcohol, acetic acid, and CO_2.

Excretion 85–90% is exhaled unchanged; the metabolites are excreted in the urine.

Special points Ether potentiates the action of co-administered non-depolarizing relaxants. Diathermy should be used with extreme caution (if at all) in the presence of ether. Ether is cheap and has a wide safety margin; it therefore retains a useful role for anaesthesia in difficult circumstances.

Etomidate

Uses Etomidate is used:
1. for the intravenous induction of general anaesthesia
2. in treatment prior to surgery for Cushing's syndrome.

Chemical A carboxylated imidazole derivative.

Presentation As a clear, colourless solution for injection containing 2 mg/ml of etomidate in an aqueous vehicle of 35% propylene glycol and water. Etomidate is a weak base with a pKa of 4.2. The pH of the aqueous solution is 8.1.

Main action Hypnotic.

Mode of action Etomidate appears to act upon GABA type A receptors to modulate fast inhibitory synaptic transmission within the CNS. In animal models, the beta-3 subunit of the $GABA_A$ receptor appears to have a role in etomidate-induced anaesthesia. It has a chiral centre resulting in enantiomers. The R(+) isomer of etomidate is ten times more potent than its S(−) isomer at potentiating $GABA_A$ receptor activity.

Routes of administration/dose Etomidate is administered intravenously in a dose of 0.3 mg/kg; the drug acts in 10–65 seconds, with a duration of action of 6–10 minutes. In elderly patients, the dose should be reduced to 0.15–0.2 mg/kg. Etomidate is non-cumulative with repeated administration.

Effects

CVS Etomidate is notable for its relative cardiovascular stability. Recommended doses of the drug may produce a slight decrease in the cardiac output and systemic vascular resistance, resulting in a mild degree of hypotension; tachycardia is produced only by high doses of the drug. Etomidate has little effect on myocardial or cerebral oxygen delivery and consumption. It does not alter sympathetic or baroreceptor reflexes, and therefore the haemodynamic responses may not be obtunded, unless concomitant administration of an opioid is given.

RS The drug causes a dose-related decrease in the respiratory rate and tidal volume; transient apnoea, coughing, and hiccuping may occur. There are case reports of laryngospasm occurring, following the administration of etomidate.

CNS Induction of anaesthesia with etomidate may be accompanied by the development of involuntary muscle movements (up to 50%), tremor, and hypertonus. The drug decreases the intracranial and intraocular pressures, the cerebral blood flow (by 20–30%), and the cerebral metabolic rate. Twenty percent of patients demonstrate generalized epileptiform EEG activity, following the administration of etomidate.

AS 2–15% of patients who have received the drug experience nausea and vomiting post-operatively; this is increased to 40% if an opiate is used.

Metabolic/other Etomidate is a potent inhibitor of steroidogenesis. The drug inhibits adrenal 11-beta-hydroxylase and 17-alpha-hydroxylase, resulting in depression of cortisol and aldosterone synthesis for 24–48 hours. This effect is seen after single doses and infusions. Etomidate has significant antiplatelet activities. Prolongation of the bleeding time may occur, together with inhibition of ADP- and collagen-induced platelet aggregation.

Toxicity/side effects 25–50% of patients who receive etomidate experience pain on injection; the incidence of this is decreased by the addition of lignocaine, the use of larger veins, or an intravenous dose of fentanyl 1–2 minutes prior to the administration of the drug. Venous thrombosis and thrombophlebitis may occur. Myoclonus may occur in unpremedicated patients. Skeletal muscle movements appear to be commoner in patients who experience pain on injection. Most movements are bilateral. Histamine release and allergic phenomena are rare with the use of etomidate. *In vitro* studies have shown the drug to be an inhibitor of microsomal enzymes. Limited *in vivo* studies have demonstrated only minimal inhibition of hepatic metabolism.

The use of etomidate infusions for the sedation of critically ill patients is associated with an increased mortality and is contraindicated. There is no conclusive evidence that anaesthetic doses of etomidate have any effect on morbidity or mortality. However, recent data have questioned the safety of using etomidate for single-bolus administration in patients at risk of adrenal insufficiency. The results of a double-blind randomized controlled trial comparing etomidate with midazolam for intubation of patients with sepsis is awaited.

Kinetics

Distribution Etomidate is 76.5% protein-bound in the plasma; the V_D is approximately 4.5 l/kg. The relatively brief duration of action of a bolus of the drug is due to the rapid redistribution to muscle and later to fat.

Metabolism Occurs rapidly by plasma and hepatic esterases to yield inactive carboxylic metabolites.

Excretion Between 75% and 87% of an administered dose is excreted in the urine (80% of which comprise the chief metabolite R-(+)-1-(1-phenyethyl)-1H-imidazole-5-carboxylic acid). Two to 3% is excreted unchanged in the urine. The remainder is excreted in the bile. The clearance is 870–1700 ml/min (this is reduced by 31% in the presence of 67% N_2O); the elimination half-life is 1–4.7 hours, reflecting the slow distribution of etomidate from the deep peripheral compartment. Data suggest that, in patients with cirrhosis and oesophageal varices, etomidate has a V_D and elimination half-life approximately twice those of healthy subjects.

Special points Etomidate is porphyrinogenic in animal models and *in vitro*. The drug may cross the placenta during obstetric anaesthesia. The drug should not be mixed with pancuronium.

Etomidate has been formulated as a lipid emulsion which appears to be less irritant on injection. The lipid formulation has also been shown to have a faster onset of action, compared with the standard preparation.

Fentanyl

Uses Fentanyl is used:
1. to provide the analgesic component in general anaesthesia
2. in combination with a major tranquillizer to produce neuroleptanalgesia
3. to provide analgesia during labour when regional anaesthesia is not in use
4. as an agent used for patient-controlled analgesia
5. in premedication and
6. for palliative care.

Chemical A tertiary amine which is a synthetic phenylpiperidine derivative.

Presentation As a clear, colourless solution for injection containing 50 micrograms/ml fentanyl citrate; as transdermal patches which deliver 12/25/50/75/100 micrograms/hour over a 72-hour period; as sublingual tablets containing 100/200/400/600/800 micrograms; as lozenges containing 200/400/600/800/1200/1600 micrograms; and as fentanyl hydrochloride in an iontophoretic transdermal system. The pKa of fentanyl is 8.4, is 9% unionized at a pH of 7.4, has a molecular weight of 286, and is highly lipid-soluble, having an octanol:water partition coefficient of 717.

Main actions Analgesia and respiratory depression.

Mode of action Fentanyl is a highly selective mu-agonist (or MOP agonist); the MOP receptor appears to be specifically involved in the mediation of analgesia. Opioids appear to exert their effects by interacting with presynaptic Gi-protein receptors, leading to hyperpolarization of the cell membrane by increasing K^+ conductance. Inhibition of adenylate cyclase, leading to reduced production of cAMP, and closure of voltage-sensitive calcium channels also occur. The decrease in membrane excitability that results may decrease both pre- and post-synaptic responses.

Routes of administration/doses The adult dose for premedication by the intramuscular route is 50–100 micrograms. For the induction or supplementation of general anaesthesia, an intravenous dose of 1–100 micrograms/kg may be used. The drug may be administered by intravenous infusion. Fentanyl may also be administered via the epidural route—a dose of 50–100 micrograms is usually employed—or via the spinal route at doses of 5–25 micrograms. The drug acts rapidly in 2–5 minutes due to its high lipid solubility when administered intravenously; a small dose has a duration of action of 30–60 minutes, whereas high (>50 micrograms/kg) doses may be effective for 4–6 hours. Following application of a transdermal patch, serum fentanyl concentrations only increase gradually, with equilibrium occurring at between 12 and 24 hours. Transdermal fentanyl patches should be replaced every 72 hours, whilst iontophoretic transdermal system devices should be replaced or stopped after 24 hours. Administration of fentanyl reduces the amount of hypnotic/volatile agent required to maintain anaesthesia.

Effects

CVS The most significant cardiovascular effect of fentanyl is bradycardia of vagal origin; cardiac output, mean arterial pressure, pulmonary and systemic vascular resistance, and pulmonary capillary wedge pressure are unaffected by the administration of the drug. Fentanyl obtunds the cardiovascular responses to laryngoscopy and intubation.

RS Fentanyl is a potent respiratory depressant, causing a decrease in both the respiratory rate and tidal volume; it also diminishes the ventilatory response to hypoxia and hypercarbia. The drug is a potent antitussive agent. Chest wall rigidity (the 'wooden chest' phenomenon) may occur after the administration of fentanyl—this may be an effect of the drug on mu-receptors located on GABA-ergic interneurones. Fentanyl causes minimal histamine release; bronchospasm is thus rarely produced by the drug.

CNS Fentanyl is 50–80 times more potent an analgesic than morphine and has little hypnotic or sedative activity. Miosis is produced as a result of stimulation of the Edinger–Westphal nucleus. There have been several reports of seizure-like motor activity occurring in patients receiving fentanyl; however, no epileptic spike-wave patterns are demonstrable on the EEG (although beta activity is initially decreased, and alpha activity is increased; subsequently alpha activity disappears, and delta activity predominates).

AS The drug decreases gastrointestinal motility and decreases gastric acid secretion; it also doubles the common bile duct pressure by causing spasm of the sphincter of Oddi.

GU Fentanyl increases the tone of the ureters, bladder detrusor muscle, and vesicular sphincter.

Metabolic/other High doses of fentanyl will obtund the metabolic 'stress response' to surgery, although the drug has no effect on white cell function. Unlike morphine, fentanyl does not increase the activity of ADH.

Toxicity/side effects Respiratory depression may occur postoperatively, possibly related to the appearance of a secondary peak in the plasma fentanyl concentration due to elution from muscle. Nausea, vomiting, and dependence may also complicate the use of the drug.

Kinetics There is large inter-individual variability in pharmacokinetics.

Absorption Fentanyl is absorbed orally and has a bioavailability of 33%. Orally administered fentanyl may become highly ionized in the stomach (99.9%), leading to slow absorption in the alkaline small bowel and subsequent first-pass metabolism. Transdermal delivery produces 47% absorption at 24 hours, 88% at 48 hours, and 94% by 72 hours. Drug delivery continues after patch removal.

Distribution Fentanyl is 81–94% bound to plasma proteins; the V_D is 0.88–4.41 l/kg. The short duration of action of a single dose of the drug is due to redistribution (cf. thiopental), whereas continuous administration leads to saturation of tissues and a significantly prolonged duration of action. Fentanyl is more lipid-soluble than morphine and thus crosses the blood–brain barrier more easily; it thus has a more rapid onset of action than morphine. Additionally, intrathecal fentanyl does not cause delayed respiratory depression, unlike morphine, as, due to its high lipid solubility, it is rapidly absorbed into the spinal cord.

Metabolism Fentanyl appears to be metabolized primarily by N-dealkylation to norfentanyl, with subsequent hydroxylation of this and the parent compound to hydroxypropionyl derivatives. The drug may also undergo hydroxylation and amide hydrolysis. Cytochrome P450 3A4 plays the predominant role in fentanyl metabolism. As well as the liver, this is also found in the human intestine. Some enterosystemic cycling of the drug may occur as does first-pass metabolism (see above). The metabolites are not pharmacologically active.

Excretion 10% of an administered dose is excreted in the urine. The clearance of fentanyl is 13 ml/kg/min, and the elimination half-life range is 141–853 minutes. Halothane decreases the clearance of fentanyl by 48%; a similar effect occurs with enflurane. The clearance of fentanyl is decreased in surgical patients with renal impairment and in patients with hepatic impairment. Oral ritonavir (a potent CYP3A4 inhibitor) prolongs the clearance of intravenously administered fentanyl by two-thirds.

Special points Fentanyl decreases the apparent MAC of co-administered volatile agents and increases the effect of non-depolarizing muscle relaxants to a similar extent as does halothane. The drug is pharmacologically incompatible with thiopental or methohexital.

It is unknown whether fentanyl is removed by haemodialysis.

The physical and chemical properties of fentanyl make it a suitable agent for transdermal administration. The fentanyl iontophoretic transdermal system works by generating a low-intensity electrical current (activated by the patient) which causes positively charged fentanyl molecules held within a positively charged hydrogel reservoir to be repelled and delivered transdermally into the systemic circulation.

Flecainide

Uses Flecainide is an antiarrhythmic agent used:
1. for the suppression of irritable foci, e.g. ventricular tachycardia and ventricular ectopics
2. in the treatment of re-entry dysrhythmias, e.g. the Wolff–Parkinson–White syndrome and
3. in the treatment of symptomatic paroxysmal atrial fibrillation intolerant of other medication.

Chemical An amide type local anaesthetic.

Presentation As 50/100 mg tablets and as a 10 mg/ml solution of flecainide acetate for intravenous administration.

Main action A class Ic antiarrhythmic.

Mode of action Flecainide reduces the maximum rate of depolarization in heart muscle and thereby slows conduction, particularly in the His–Purkinje system. It has a profound effect on conduction in accessory pathways, especially on retrograde conduction, and markedly suppresses ventricular ectopic foci. It is a local anaesthetic agent which depresses membrane responsiveness and conduction velocity, with no effect on the duration of the action potential.

Routes of administration/doses The adult oral dose is 100–200 mg 12-hourly. Intravenously, flecainide may be administered as a bolus dose of 2 mg/kg over 10 minutes, followed by an infusion of 1.5 mg/kg/hour for 1 hour, reducing to 0.25 mg/kg/hour.

Effects

CVS Flecainide is generally well tolerated; the blood pressure and heart rate usually remain unchanged. The drug has negative inotropic potential.

CNS Visual disturbances may occur and are probably a central effect of the drug.

Toxicity/side effects Reversible liver damage, dizziness, paraesthesiae, headaches, and nausea may complicate the use of the drug.

Kinetics

Absorption Flecainide is rapidly and completely absorbed after oral administration; the bioavailability is 85–90%.

Distribution Flecainide is 37–58% protein-bound in the plasma; the V_D is 5.8–10 l/kg.

Metabolism Occurs in the liver to two major metabolites—meta-O-dealkylated flecainide and its lactam.

Excretion 10–50% of the dose is excreted unchanged in the urine. The clearance is 10 ml/min/kg, and the elimination half-life is 7–15 hours after intravenous administration and 12–27 hours after oral administration.

Special points Flecainide increases plasma digoxin levels by 15% when the two drugs are administered concurrently. Hypokalaemia reduces the effectiveness of the drug; a reduced dose should be used in renal or hepatic failure.

Flecainide is not removed by haemodialysis.

Flucloxacillin

Uses Flucloxacillin is used in the treatment of:
1. respiratory tract infections as an adjunct
2. skin and soft tissue infections
3. osteomyelitis
4. staphylococcal endocarditis and for
5. prophylaxis during surgery.

Chemical A semi-synthetic isoxazolyl penicillin.

Presentation As 250/500 mg capsules, in vials containing 250/500/1000 mg of flucloxacillin sodium, and as a syrup containing 25/50 mg/ml of flucloxacillin magnesium.

Main action Flucloxacillin is an acid-stable, penicillinase-resistant, narrow-spectrum bactericidal antibiotic active against *Staphylococcus aureus*, group A beta-haemolytic streptococci, and pneumococci.

Mode of action Flucloxacillin acts in a manner typical of penicillins, by binding to a cell wall PBP, and thereby interfering with the activity of the enzymes which are involved in the cross-linking of bacterial cell wall peptidoglycans.

Routes of administration/doses The adult oral and intramuscular dose is 250–500 mg 6-hourly; the corresponding intravenous dose is 250 mg to 2 g 6-hourly.

Toxicity/side effects Gastrointestinal and CNS disturbances, rashes, sore throat, and glossitis may complicate the use of the drug. Flucloxacillin may cause both pseudomembranous colitis and jaundice in the critically ill.

Kinetics
Absorption Flucloxacillin is 50–70% absorbed when administered orally.

Distribution The drug is 95% protein-bound in the plasma; the V_D is 6.8–9.4 l.

Metabolism 8–13% is metabolized to an active form 5-hydroxymethyl-flucloxacillin, and 4% is hydrolysed in the liver to penicilloic acid which is inactive.

Excretion Excretion of the drug occurs by glomerular filtration and tubular secretion, 35–75% of the dose appearing in the urine, according to the dose and route of administration. The clearance is 3 ml/min/kg, and the elimination half-life is 46 minutes.

Special points Reduction of the dose of flucloxacillin should be considered if the creatinine clearance is 10 ml/min; the drug is not significantly removed by haemodialysis.

Precipitation occurs if flucloxacillin is co-administered with an aminoglycoside.

Flucloxacillin is not active against MRSA.

Flumazenil

Uses Flumazenil is used:
1. as an aid to weaning and neurological assessment of ventilated patients who have received benzodiazepine sedation during intensive care
2. as part of the 'wake-up' test during scoliosis surgery
3. to reverse oversedation after endoscopy and
4. for diagnosis of, and assessment after, benzodiazepine overdose.

Chemical An imidazobenzodiazepine.

Presentation As a clear, colourless solution containing 100 micrograms/ml of flumazenil.

Main action Reversal of the actions of benzodiazepines.

Mode of action Flumazenil is a competitive antagonist at central benzodiazepine receptors.

Routes of administration/doses Flumazenil is administered intravenously, titrated in 100 micrograms increments to a total maximum adult dose of 1 mg. It acts in 30–60 seconds and lasts 15–140 minutes. It may also be infused intravenously at 100–400 micrograms/hour.

Toxicity/side effects Hypertension, dysrhythmias, dizziness, nausea and vomiting, facial flushing, anxiety, and headache have been described. Resedation after prior administration of a benzodiazepine and convulsions in epileptics have also been reported.

Kinetics

Absorption Flumazenil is well absorbed when administered orally but undergoes significant first-pass hepatic metabolism.

Distribution The drug is 50% protein-bound in the plasma; the V_D is 0.9 l/kg.

Metabolism Flumazenil is extensively metabolized in the liver to a carboxylic acid and glucuronide, both of which are inert.

Excretion 95% is excreted in the urine, 0.1% unchanged. The clearance is 700–1100 ml/min, and the elimination half-life is 53 minutes.

Special points Flumazenil improves the quality of emergence from anaesthesia and reduces post-operative shivering.

Fluoroquinolones

Uses Fluoroquinolones are used in the treatment of infections of:
1. the respiratory tract
2. skin, soft tissue, bone, and joints
3. ocular, ear, nose, and oral infections
4. gastrointestinal infections
5. GU infections
6. pelvic and intra-abdominal infections
7. gonorrhoea
8. septicaemia and
9. in the prophylaxis/treatment of organisms with the potential for use in bioterrorism.

Chemical Fluorinated quinolones derived from nalidixic acid.

Presentation Fluoroquinolones in clinical use include ciprofloxacin, levofloxacin, moxifloxacin, norfloxacin, and ofloxacin, and all are available for intravenous administration aside from norfloxacin. Ciprofloxacin is available as eye drops and as an eye ointment, as a powder for oral suspension, and in tablet formulations. Ofloxacin is available in an eye drop preparation.

Main action Fluoroquinolones are bactericidal antibiotics that are active against:
1. Gram-positive bacteria
2. Gram-negative bacteria
3. Gram-positive and negative anaerobes.

There is emerging resistance to fluoroquinolones from a number of species, including *Escherichia coli*, *Shigella*, *Neisseria gonorrhoeae*, *Acinetobacter*, and *Pseudomonas* spp.

Mode of action Fluoroquinolones act by inhibiting bacterial DNA gyrase, topoisomerase IV, and type II topoisomerases, thereby inhibiting bacterial DNA replication.

Routes of administration/doses Fluoroquinolones may be administered topically as ointments, orally, or intravenously. The specific dose, route, and frequency of an agent administered are dependent on the clinical indication, age of the patient, and particular agent being used.

Toxicity/side effects Common side effects include abdominal pain, nausea, and vomiting. Neuropsychiatric disturbances have been reported, including anxiety, insomnia, seizures, and hallucinations. Fluoroquinolone use is associated with Achilles tendon rupture, particularly when co-administered with corticosteroids. Allergic reactions, photosensitivity, and transient elevations of liver enzymes have all been reported. The use of these antibiotics is associated with an increased risk of *Clostridium difficile* and MRSA infection.

Kinetics

Absorption Fluoroquinolones are generally well absorbed, depending on the specific agent: ciprofloxacin (70–80%), levofloxacin (100%), moxifloxacin (91%). Norfloxacin has a lower bioavailability of 30–40%. Ciprofloxacin undergoes first-pass metabolism. Co-administration of sucralfate or calcium/magnesium/iron salts reduces the amount of drug absorbed.

Distribution Protein binding of 30–40% is typical of this group of drugs. Norfloxacin has lower protein binding of <15%. The V_D for ciprofloxacin is 2–3 l/kg. Fluoroquinolones demonstrate high CSF and tissue penetration.

Metabolism Fluoroquinolones undergo little hepatic metabolism in man.

Excretion The majority of fluoroquinolones undergo renal excretion. Ciprofloxacin undergoes active tubular secretion, as demonstrated by a higher clearance rate of 416–650 ml/min, compared to other fluoroquinolones: moxifloxacin (179–246 ml/min) and norfloxacin (275 ml/min). The half-life for these drugs are as follows: ciprofloxacin (3–6.9 hours), levofloxacin (6–8 hours), moxifloxacin (12 hours), norfloxacin (3–4 hours).

Special points Dose reduction is required in severe renal impairment. 25–30% of an administered dose of ciprofloxacin is removed during haemodialysis.

Ciprofloxacin significantly increases the half-life of co-administered theophylline, necessitating monitoring of plasma concentrations of the latter.

Ciprofloxacin is used in combination therapy in the treatment of *Bacillus anthracus* infection and as a single agent against *Yersinia pestis*. The drug is also used for post-exposure prophylaxis to the following potential bioterrorism organisms: *Bacillus anthracus* (anthrax), *Yersinia pestis* (plague), and *Francisella tularensis* (tularaemia).

Antimicrobial agents should always be administered, following consideration of local pharmacy and microbiological policies.

Fondaparinux

Uses Fondaparinux is used in the treatment of:
1. acute pulmonary embolism
2. acute DVT, and
3. in the prophylaxis of DVT.

Chemical Synthetic and specific inhibitor of activated factor X (Xa)

Presentation Fondaparinux sodium solution is provided in a single-dose, sterile, preservative-free prefilled syringes with an automatic needle protection system, containing 2.5/5/7.5/10 mg. The packaging (needle guard) contains latex.

Main action Prevention of thrombus formation.

Mode of action The antithrombotic activity of fondaparinux is the result of antithrombin III (ATIII)-mediated selective inhibition of factor Xa. By selectively binding to ATIII, fondaparinux potentiates (about 300 times) the innate neutralization of factor Xa by ATIII. Neutralization of factor Xa interrupts the blood coagulation cascade and so inhibits thrombin formation and thrombus development. Fondaparinux does not inactivate thrombin (activated factor II), has no effect on platelet function, and does not affect fibrinolytic activity or bleeding time.

Routes of administration/dose 2.5/5/7.5/10 mg dose. It is administered by subcutaneous injection, according to the patient's weight and desired treatment.

Effects
Metabolic/other May be excreted in breast milk.

Toxicity/side effects Fondaparinux should be used with extreme caution in conditions with an increased risk of haemorrhage—rates of 1–2% of bleeding if the risk is low, and thrombocytopenia (moderate 3% and severe 1%) are reported. Local irritation (injection site bleeding, rash, and pruritus) may occur, following subcutaneous injection. Asymptomatic increases in AST and ALT have been described.

Kinetics
Absorption Fondaparinux administered by subcutaneous injection is rapidly and completely absorbed; bioavailability is 100%, with a maximum plasma concentration at 2 hours.

Distribution It distributes mainly in blood and, only to a minor extent, in extravascular fluid; hence, the V_D is 7–11 l. Fondaparinux is >94% protein-bound to ATIII.

Metabolism This has not been investigated, as it is excreted unchanged in the urine.

Excretion In healthy individuals up to 75 years of age, up to 77% of a single fondaparinux dose is eliminated in the urine as unchanged drug in 72 hours. The elimination half-life is 17–21 hours.

Special points Routine coagulation tests, such as prothrombin time and activated partial thromboplastin time (APTT), are relatively insensitive measures of the activity of fondaparinux. Fondaparinux increases the risk of bleeding in patients with impaired renal function due to reduced clearance and should not be used with a creatinine clearance of <30 ml/min.

Epidural or spinal haematomas may occur in patients who are anticoagulated with LMWHs, heparinoids, or fondaparinux. These haematomas may result in long-term or permanent paralysis. Factors that can increase the risk of developing epidural or spinal haematomas include:

1. use of indwelling epidural catheters
2. concomitant use of other drugs that affect haemostasis such as NSAIDs, platelet inhibitors, or other anticoagulants
3. history of traumatic or repeated epidural or spinal puncture
4. history of spinal deformity or spinal surgery
5. the optimal timing between the administration of fondaparinux and neuraxial procedures is not known.

Patients need to be monitored frequently for signs and symptoms of neurologic impairment, and, if discovered, urgent treatment is necessary.

Furosemide

Uses Furosemide is used in the treatment of:
1. oedema of cardiac, renal, or hepatic origin
2. chronic renal insufficiency
3. hypertension
4. raised intracranial pressure
5. symptomatic hypercalcaemia, and
6. conversion of oliguric to polyuric renal failure.

Chemical An anthranilic acid (sulfonamide) derivative.

Presentation As a clear solution (which must be protected from light) for injection containing 10 mg/ml and as 20/40/500 mg tablets of furosemide. A syrup containing 20/40/50 mg in 5 ml is available. A number of fixed-dose combinations with amiloride, triamterene, spironolactone, and potassium chloride are also available.

Main action Diuresis.

Mode of action Furosemide acts by inhibition of active chloride ion reabsorption in the proximal tubule and ascending limb of the loop of Henle—by reducing the tonicity of the renal medulla, a hypotonic or isotonic urine is produced. The mechanism of action at a cellular level may be exerted via inhibition of $Na^+K^+ATPase$ or by inhibition of glycolysis.

Routes of administration/doses The adult oral dose is 20–2000 mg daily; the intramuscular dose is 20–50 mg. Intravenous administration is titrated according to response—a range of 10–1000 mg is recommended. The infusion rate should not exceed 4 mg/min, as ototoxicity may result.

Effects

CVS/RS Pulmonary and systemic vasodilation occur, leading to symptomatic relief of breathlessness prior to diuresis.

GU A diuresis occurs within a few minutes and lasts 2 hours when furosemide is administered intravenously; correspondingly, diuresis starts 1 hour after oral administration and lasts 4–6 hours. Free water clearance is increased by the drug. The renal blood flow is increased and redistributed in favour of inner corticomedullary flow. Oxygen consumption in the loop of Henle is reduced to basal levels and may protect the kidney from ischaemia.

Metabolic/other The drug causes a metabolic alkalosis and may be diabetogenic; the serum urate concentrations are increased.

Toxicity/side effects Hypokalaemia, hypocalcaemia, hypomagnesaemia, and metabolic alkalosis may occur after the administration of furosemide. Transient auditory nerve damage, pancreatitis, skin rashes, and bone marrow depression have been reported. Furosemide causes interstitial nephritis in high doses; this is a common cause of acute renal failure when co-administered with an aminoglycoside—the two drugs are synergistic in this respect. Deafness is also more likely to result when furosemide and an aminoglycoside are co-administered.

Kinetics

Absorption Furosemide is 60–70% absorbed after oral administration; the bioavailability by this route is 43–71%.

Distribution The drug is 96% protein-bound in the plasma, almost exclusively to albumin. The V_D is 0.11–0.13 l/kg.

Metabolism Furosemide appears to be metabolized primarily in the kidney to a glucuronide.

Excretion 80% is excreted in the urine as unchanged and glucuronidated furosemide; the rest appears in the faeces. The clearance is 2.2 ml/min/kg, and the elimination half-life is 45–92 minutes.

Special points The effects of non-depolarizing muscle relaxants may be enhanced by furosemide, probably due to hypokalaemia. The response to concurrently administered vasopressors may be diminished and that to vasodilators enhanced, both phenomena being manifestations of a contracted circulating blood volume.

The drug is not removed by haemodialysis.

Gabapentin

Uses Gabapentin is used in the treatment of:
1. post-herpetic neuralgia
2. painful diabetic neuropathy
3. partial seizures with or without secondary generalization, and
4. neuropathic pain.

Chemical An acetic acid derivative which is a structural analogue of GABA.

Presentation As 600/800 mg tablets and 100/300/400 mg capsules.

Main actions Anticonvulsant and analgesic.

Mode of action Gabapentin is structurally related to GABA but does not interact with GABA receptors. The binding site for the drug is the alpha-2-delta subunit of voltage-gated calcium channels. Gabapentin does not interact with sodium channels *in vitro* (cf. phenytoin, carbamazepine). It may also:
1. partially reduce the response to the glutamate agonist NMDA
2. reduce the release of monoamine neurotransmitters *in vitro*
3. stimulate glutamate decarboxylase (the enzyme which converts glutamate to GABA), and
4. increase the synaptic release of GABA.

Routes of administration/doses The drug is administered orally and for all indications; a titration scheme can be employed during the initiation of therapy. Alternatively, an initially dose of 300 mg three times daily may be used. Dosage required for long-term epilepsy treatment is determined on an individual basis, although clinical trial data demonstrate the effective dosing range of between 900 and 3600 mg/day. Typically, dosage for treatment of neuropathic pain is up to 1800 mg/day, although a maximum dose of 3600 mg/day can be used. If discontinuation of gabapentin therapy is to be undertaken, this should be performed gradually over a minimum of 1 week, regardless of the indication. The total daily dose of the drug should be reduced in patients with renal impairment.

Effects

CNS Gabapentin has analgesic and anticonvulsant properties and improves sleep in patients with neuropathic pain.

Toxicity/side effects Dizziness, ataxia, nystagmus, somnolence, tremor, diplopia, nausea, and vomiting occur with a frequency >5%. Leucopenia, erectile dysfunction, and weight gain have all been reported, following use of the drug.

Kinetics

Absorption Gabapentin is well absorbed orally and has a bioavailability of 60%. Peak plasma levels of the drug occur within 2–3 hours of administration.

Distribution The drug is not bound to plasma proteins; the V_D is 0.85 l/kg. In patients with epilepsy, gabapentin concentrations in the CSF are approximately 20% of the corresponding steady-state trough plasma concentrations. The drug is present in the breast milk of breastfeeding women.

Metabolism Gabapentin is not metabolized in man and does not induce hepatic mixed function oxidase enzymes.

Excretion The drug is excreted unchanged by renal excretion. The elimination half-life is 5–7 hours. The clearance is directly proportional to creatinine clearance.

Special points Gabapentin enhances the analgesic effect of co-administered morphine. It is removed by haemodialysis. The bioavailability of the drug decreases with increasing dose which may minimize toxicity resulting from overdose. Co-administration of gabapentin with antacids containing aluminium and magnesium may reduce bioavailability of the drug by up to 24%.

Gelatins

Uses Gelatins are used as plasma volume substitutes to expand and maintain circulating blood volume.

Chemical Animal collagen derivatives. Two types of gelatin are available: succinylated gelatins (molecular weight: 30 000 daltons) and urea-linked gelatins (molecular weight: 35 000 daltons). They are produced by the thermal degradation of bovine gelatin.

Presentation A number of agents are available in the UK for intravenous administration. Examples of commercially available products include:

• Gelofusine® 4%, a succinylated gelatin
• Volplex® 4%, a succinylated gelatin
• Haemaccel® 3.5%, a urea-linked gelatin.

The above agents are presented in 0.9% sodium chloride for intravenous administration. Haemaccel® also contains the following electrolytes: K^+ 5.1 mmol/l, Ca^{2+} 6.25 mmol/l.

Main action Intravascular volume expansion.

Mode of action Temporary increase in plasma oncotic pressure.

Routes of administration/doses The specific dose of an agent administered is dependent on the clinical indication, the haemodynamic status of the patient, and the particular agent being used.

Effects

CVS The haemodynamic effects of gelatins are proportional to the prevailing circulating volume. The duration of action of these agents depends on the specific agent in use.

Toxicity/side effects The most important side effect is that of overtransfusion, leading to pulmonary oedema. Administration of gelatins dissolved in saline containing solvents may lead to a hypernatraemic, hyperchloraemic metabolic acidosis. Hyperkalaemia and hypercalcaemia may complicate the use of agents containing solvents that include the electrolytes potassium and calcium. Allergic reactions have been reported, following the use of these agents.

Kinetics Data are incomplete.

Distribution Gelatin-containing solutions are initially distributed into the plasma but later equilibrate with the extracellular fluid compartment, following excretion of the gelatin component.

Metabolism In vitro studies suggest that gelatins are degraded by proteolytic enzymes into smaller peptides and amino acids.

Excretion Approximately 75% is excreted via the urine. Gelatins have a half-life of approximately 4 hours.

Special points Following renal excretion, gelatins have an osmotic diuretic effect within the renal tubules. Agents containing calcium should not be administered immediately following a blood transfusion through the same intravenous line, without the giving-set being flushed with saline. The ionic calcium component may enhance digoxin toxicity if administered concurrently.

Glucagon

Uses Glucagon is recommended for use:
1. in the treatment of hypoglycaemia and
2. to facilitate radiological investigation of the gastrointestinal tract and has been used in the management of
3. cardiogenic shock
4. renal colic
5. acute diverticulitis, and
6. propranolol overdose.

Chemical A polypeptide hormone extracted from the alpha cells of the pancreatic islets of Langerhans.

Presentation As vials containing 1/10 mg of lyophilized glucagon hydrochloride with lactose—this is reconstituted in glycerol and water prior to use and in prefilled syringes containing 1 mg glucagon.

Main action Elevation of blood sugar concentration, positive inotropism and chronotropism, and relaxation of smooth muscle.

Mode of action Glucagon acts via cell membrane receptors which stimulate adenylate cyclase activity, leading to an increase in the intracellular concentrations of cAMP. The final effects of the hormone are mediated via a cascade of protein kinases.

Routes of administration/doses Glucagon may be administered intravenously, intramuscularly, or subcutaneously in a dose of 1–5 mg for an adult. The drug may also be infused intravenously (diluted in 5% glucose) at a rate of 1–20 mg/hour. Glucagon acts within 1 minute when administered intravenously and in 8–10 minutes when administered intramuscularly or subcutaneously—the ensuing increase in the blood sugar concentration lasts 10–30 minutes.

Effects

CVS Glucagon has marked positive inotropic and somewhat less marked positive chronotropic effects, and acts synergistically with beta-adrenergic agonist drugs in this respect. The drug does not increase myocardial irritability.

AS The drug reduces tone throughout the entire gastrointestinal tract, including the common bile duct; gastric and pancreatic secretions are simultaneously inhibited.

GU Glucagon decreases the ureteric tone and has a small effect in improving the renal blood flow and urine output.

Metabolic/other Glucagon increases gluconeogenesis, glycogenolysis, lipolysis, proteolysis, and ketogenesis, leading to an increase in the blood sugar concentration. It also stimulates the release of endogenous catecholamines and may cause hypokalaemia secondary to an increase in the rate of insulin secretion.

Toxicity/side effects The drug is usually well tolerated; nausea and vomiting, hypo- or hyperglycaemia, diarrhoea, and allergic phenomena may complicate the use of glucagon.

Kinetics

Absorption Glucagon is inactive when administered orally. The bioavailability appears to be similar when administered intramuscularly or subcutaneously.

Metabolism The drug is degraded by proteolysis in approximately equal quantities by splanchnic, hepatic, and renal routes. The precise metabolic pathways are unknown.

Excretion The clearance is 8–12 ml/min/kg, and the elimination half-life is 3–6 minutes.

Special points The clearance of glucagon is halved in patients with renal failure; the drug is not removed by haemodialysis.

Glucagon potentiates the anticoagulant effect of warfarin, but not that of heparin.

Glucose

Uses Glucose solutions are used:
1. to provide a source of water (5% solutions) and
2. calories (10/20/50% solutions) and
3. in the treatment of hypoglycaemia.

Chemical Glucose is D-glucopyranose D-glucose monohydrate, a monosaccharide obtained by the hydrolysis of cornstarch.

Presentation As a clear, colourless sterile solution containing 5/10/20/50% glucose in water in ampoules or bags containing 500/1000 ml. The preparations are sterile and contain no buffers or bacteriostatic agents. The pH varies from 3.5 to 6.5, according to concentration. The 5% solution contains 170 kcal/l and has an osmolarity of 250 mOsm/l; the 10/20/50% solutions are appropriate multiples of these figures.

Main action An increase in the blood sugar concentration and glycogen deposition; ketosis and nitrogen loss are decreased.

Routes of administration/doses Glucose solutions are administered intravenously; the 20% and 50% solutions should preferably be administered via a central vein. The dose depends upon the state of hydration, nutritional requirements, and blood sugar concentration of the individual patient.

Effects

CVS The haemodynamic effects of glucose solutions are proportional to the prevailing volaemic status; infusion of the crystalloid will temporarily restore cardiovascular parameters towards normal.

GU Renal perfusion is temporarily restored towards normal in hypovolaemic subjects transfused with the crystalloid.

Toxicity/side effects Overhydration leading to water intoxication, hyponatraemia, mental confusion, and fits may occur with injudicious use of isotonic solutions (5%). This may produce central pontine myelinolysis. Hyperglycaemia and venous thrombosis may occur with the 10/20/50% solutions.

Kinetics Data are incomplete.

Absorption Glucose is rapidly and completely absorbed when administered orally.

Distribution Glucose solutions are initially distributed within the intravascular compartment and rapidly equilibrate within the intra- and extravascular space.

Metabolism Glucose is completely metabolized to CO_2 and water.

Excretion The metabolic products are excreted via the lungs and kidneys.

Special points Use of excessive quantities of glucose solutions (especially in premenopausal women and prepubertal children) may result in cerebral oedema and respiratory arrest, a condition associated with poor neurological outcome.

Glyceryl trinitrate

Uses Glyceryl trinitrate is used in the treatment of:
1. stable, unstable, and variant angina
2. left ventricular failure secondary to myocardial infarction and
3. in the perioperative control of blood pressure and
4. for the prophylaxis of phlebitis associated with venous cannulation and may be of use in
5. decreasing infarct size in patients with acute myocardial infarction and used
6. to promote venodilation when administering peripheral total parenteral nutrition (TPN).

Chemical An organic nitrate which is an ester of nitric acid.

Presentation As 300/500/600 micrograms tablets for sublingual administration, 1/2/3/5 mg tablets for buccal administration, an oral spray delivering 400 micrograms per metered dose, a slow-release transdermal patch delivering 5/10 mg per 24 hours, and as a clear solution for injection (which must be protected from light) containing 0.5/1/5 mg/ml of glyceryl trinitrate.

Main action Vasodilation of both arteries and veins.

Mode of action Glyceryl trinitrate is metabolized to nitric oxide (NO) which then stimulates guanylate cyclase in the vascular smooth muscle cells, resulting in the relaxation of smooth muscles.

Routes of administration/doses The adult dose is 0.3 mg by the sublingual route, 0.4–0.8 mg when delivered by buccal spray, 1–5 mg when delivered by the buccal route in tablet form, 5–10 mg/24 hours when administered transdermally, and (diluted in glucose or saline) at the rate of 10–400 micrograms/min when administered intravenously. The maximum effect occurs in 15–30 minutes when administered buccally or sublingually, and 90–120 seconds after intravenous administration.

Effects

CVS At low dose ranges, glyceryl trinitrate causes venodilation and, at higher concentrations, venous and arterial vasodilation. The systolic blood pressure decreases more than does the diastolic blood pressure; the central venous pressure, pulmonary artery pressure, left ventricular end-diastolic pressure, and myocardial oxygen consumption all decrease with the use of glyceryl trinitrate. The cardiac output is usually unaltered or decreased slightly by administration of the drug; it may increase in patients with heart failure who have a high systemic vascular resistance. The coronary blood flow may decrease or remain unchanged. A reflex tachycardia occurs in normal subjects; no effect is observed on the heart rate in patients with heart failure. Glyceryl trinitrate reduces venous return (preload) and facilitates subendocardial blood flow with redistribution into ischaemic areas. It relieves coronary vasospasm and dilates arterioles, reducing afterload, and is thought to relieve angina primarily by reducing myocardial oxygen demand (secondarily to a fall in left ventricular end-diastolic pressure and myocardial wall tension); myocardial oxygen supply is simultaneously increased by redistribution of the coronary blood flow to the subendocardium.

RS The drug causes bronchodilatation; intrapulmonary shunting may increase, but the mechanism of hypoxic pulmonary vasoconstriction appears to be unaffected in man.

CNS The intracranial pressure may increase due to cerebral vasodilation.

AS Glyceryl trinitrate relaxes the smooth muscle of the gastrointestinal and biliary tracts.

GU The renal blood flow may decrease in patients with congestive cardiac failure, secondary to a fall in blood pressure, with no accompanying change in renal vascular resistance.

Toxicity/side effects Hypotension, sinus tachycardia, and occasionally bradycardia, nausea, and vomiting may result from administration of the drug. Headaches occur more commonly with oral or sublingual than with intravenous administration.

Kinetics The data vary widely.

Absorption Absorption is rapid and efficient after sublingual administration, but slow after oral or transdermal administration; the bioavailability is 3% after oral administration due to a significant first-pass effect.

Distribution Glyceryl trinitrate is 60% protein-bound in the plasma in animal models; the V_D is 0.04–2.9 l/kg.

Metabolism The drug is rapidly metabolized in the liver and red blood cells by reduction to dinitrates, mononitrates, and nitrites, all of which are less active than the parent compound.

Excretion 80% is excreted in the urine; trace amounts are exhaled as CO_2. The clearance after intravenous administration is 0.3–1 l/min/kg, and the elimination half-life is 1–3 minutes.

Special points 40–80% of the dose of intravenous glyceryl trinitrate is adsorbed onto plastic giving-sets. The drug has been shown to increase the duration of pancuronium-induced neuromuscular blockade and may also slow the catabolism of opioids. Clinically important tolerance does not occur with continued intravenous administration of the drug.

The drug is not removed by dialysis.

Excess cardiovascular mortality has been noticed with the use of nitrates and sildenafil.

Glycopyrronium bromide

Uses Glycopyrronium bromide is used:
1. in premedication where an antisialogogue action is desired
2. to protect against the peripheral muscarinic effects of anticholinesterases
3. for the treatment of bradycardias in anaesthetized patients
4. for the treatment of hyperhydrosis (via topical administration) and
5. for symptom control in palliative care.

Chemical A quaternary ammonium compound.

Presentation As a clear solution for injection containing 0.2 mg/ml of glycopyrronium bromide and as a powder for topical application. It is also supplied in a fixed-dose combination containing 0.5 mg of glycopyrronium bromide and 2.5 mg of neostigmine per ml.

Main action Anticholinergic; glycopyrronium bromide has a particularly profound anti-secretory action.

Mode of action Glycopyrronium bromide acts by competitive antagonism of acetylcholine at peripheral muscarinic receptors.

Routes of administration/doses The adult intravenous and intramuscular dose is 0.2–0.4 mg; the paediatric dose is 4–10 micrograms/kg. The peak effect occurs 3 minutes after intravenous injection.

Effects

CVS Glycopyrronium bromide has little effect on the blood pressure when used in normal doses and causes less dysrhythmias than atropine. Tachycardia occurs when the drug is administered intravenously in doses >0.2 mg to anaesthetized patients. Glycopyrronium bromide is protective against bradycardias due to the oculocardiac reflex or suxamethonium when administered intravenously. The vagolytic effects of the drug last approximately 2–3 hours.

RS The drug has a significant and long-lasting bronchodilator effect and causes an increase in the physiological dead space.

CNS Glycopyrronium bromide is unable to cross the blood–brain barrier and is theoretically devoid of any central effects; however, headache and drowsiness are well-recognized sequelae of the drug. Post-anaesthetic recovery appears to be significantly more rapid with glycopyrronium bromide than with atropine. Glycopyrronium bromide has no effect on pupil size or accommodation.

AS The drug has a powerful antisialogogue effect that lasts approximately 8 hours after intravenous or intramuscular injection—the drug is five times as potent as atropine in this respect. Glycopyrronium bromide reduces gastric volume by 90% for 4 hours after administration and reduces antral motility. The drug reduces lower oesophageal sphincter tone.

Metabolic/other The drug inhibits sweat gland activity, but little effect is produced on body temperature. Glycopyrronium bromide has a weak local anaesthetic action.

Toxicity/side effects Typical anticholinergic side effects are produced by the drug: dry mouth, difficulty in micturition, and inhibition of sweating.

Kinetics

Absorption Oral absorption is poor and erratic; bioavailability by this route is 5%. The drug seems to be absorbed in comparable amounts when administered by either the intramuscular or intravenous route.

Distribution Redistribution of the drug occurs rapidly—90% disappears from the plasma in 5 minutes. The drug crosses the placenta and may cause fetal tachycardia. The V_D is 0.2–0.64 l/kg.

Metabolism In animals, glycopyrronium bromide occurs by hydroxylation and oxidation in the liver; very little biotransformation of the drug occurs in man.

Excretion Excretion occurs in the urine (85%) and bile (15%), and 80% unchanged. The clearance of glycopyrronium bromide is 0.89 l/min, and the elimination half-life is 0.6–1.1 hours.

Special points When used in combination with neostigmine to reverse non-depolarizing neuromuscular blockade, glycopyrronium bromide causes less initial tachycardia and less anticholinesterase-induced late bradycardia than atropine (and control of secretions is superior) due to the fact that the time courses of action of neostigmine and glycopyrronium bromide are better matched.

The drug is physically incompatible with thiopental, methohexital, and diazepam.

Haloperidol

Uses Haloperidol is used in the treatment of:
1. schizophrenia and related psychoses
2. nausea and vomiting
3. motor tics and hiccuping
4. acute confusional states and delirium in critical care and
5. for premedication and
6. palliative care.

Chemical A butyrophenone derivative.

Presentation As 0.5/1.5/5/10/20 mg tablets, 0.5 mg capsules, a syrup containing 2/10 mg/ml, and as a clear solution for injection containing 5 mg/ml of haloperidol. A depot preparation containing 50/100 mg/ml of haloperidol decanoate is also available.

Main action Antiemetic and neuroleptic.

Mode of action The antiemetic and neuroleptic effects of the drug appear to be mediated by:
1. central dopaminergic (D2) blockade, leading to an increased threshold for vomiting at the chemoreceptor trigger zone, and
2. post-synaptic GABA antagonism.

Routes of administration/doses The adult oral dose is 1–15 mg daily in divided doses. The initial intramuscular dose is 2–30 mg, with additional doses of 5 mg until the symptoms are controlled. The intravenous dose is 1–5 mg. The drug has a longer duration of action than droperidol.

Effects

CVS Haloperidol has minimal cardiovascular effects, but its antagonistic effects at alpha-adrenergic receptors may lead to hypotension in the presence of hypovolaemia.

RS The drug has minimal effect on respiration.

CNS Haloperidol induces neurolepsis, a state characterized by diminished motor activity, anxiolysis, and indifference to the external environment. The seizure threshold is raised by the drug.

AS The drug has a powerful antiemetic effect via a central effect at the chemosensitive trigger zone.

Metabolic/other Haloperidol, in common with other dopamine antagonists, may cause hyperprolactinaemia.

Toxicity/side effects Extrapyramidal effects occur relatively commonly during the use of haloperidol; these include the neuroleptic malignant syndrome (a complex of symptoms that include catatonia, cardiovascular lability, hyperthermia, and myoglobinaemia) which has a mortality in excess of 10%. Gastrointestinal and haemopoietic disturbances, abnormalities of liver function tests, and allergic phenomena have been reported after the use of the drug.

Kinetics

Absorption The drug is well absorbed after oral administration; the bioavailability by this route is 50–88%.

Distribution The drug is 92% protein-bound in the plasma; the V_D is 18–30 l/kg.

Metabolism Haloperidol is extensively metabolized in the liver; a reduced metabolite may be active.

Excretion The clearance is 11.3 ml/min/kg, and the elimination half-life is 10–38 hours, dependent upon the route of administration.

Special points Haloperidol is the preferred agent for the treatment of delirium in the critically ill adult. The sedative effects of the drug are additive with those of other CNS depressants administered concurrently. Hypotension resulting from the administration of the drug should not be treated using adrenaline, as a further decrease in the blood pressure may result.

Haloperidol is not removed by dialysis.

Halothane

Uses Halothane is used for the induction and maintenance of general anaesthesia.

Chemical A halogenated hydrocarbon containing bromine, chlorine, and fluorine.

Presentation As a clear, colourless liquid (that should be protected from light) with a characteristic sweet smell. The commercial preparation contains 0.01% thymol which prevents decomposition on exposure to light; it is non-flammable at normal anaesthetic concentrations. The molecular weight of halothane is 197.4, the boiling point 50.2°C, and the saturated vapour pressure 32 kPa at 20°C. The MAC of halothane is 0.75 (0.29 in the presence of 70% N_2O), the oil/water solubility coefficient 220, and the blood/gas solubility coefficient 2.5. The drug is readily soluble in rubber; it does not attack metals in the absence of water vapour but will attack brass, aluminium, and lead in the presence of water vapour.

Main actions General anaesthesia (reversible loss of both awareness and recall of noxious stimuli).

Mode of action The mechanism of general anaesthesia remains to be fully elucidated. General anaesthetics appear to disrupt synaptic transmission (especially in the area of the ventrobasal thalamus). This mechanism may include potentiation of the $GABA_A$ and glycine receptors and antagonism at NMDA receptors. Their mode of action at the molecular level appears to involve the expansion of hydrophobic regions in the neuronal membrane, either within the lipid phase or within hydrophobic sites in cell membranes.

Routes of administration/doses Halothane is administered by inhalation, conventionally via a calibrated vaporizer. The concentration used for the inhalational induction of anaesthesia is 2–4% and for maintenance 0.5–2%.

Effects

CVS Halothane causes a dose-related decrease in myocardial contractility and cardiac output, with an attendant decrease in cardiac work and myocardial oxygen consumption, possibly by inhibition of Ca^{2+} flux within myocardial cells and of the interaction between Ca^{2+} and the contractile proteins. The heart rate decreases as a result of vagal stimulation; the systemic vascular resistance is decreased by 15–18%, leading to a decrease in systolic and diastolic blood pressures; halothane also obtunds the baroreceptor reflexes. The drug has little effect on coronary vascular resistance. The threshold potential and refractory period of myocardial cells are increased; the drug also decreases the rate of phase IV repolarization. Halothane causes marked sensitization of the myocardium to catecholamines, although it does not itself increase the concentration of circulating catecholamines.

RS Halothane is a respiratory depressant, markedly decreasing the tidal volume, although the respiratory rate may increase. A slight increase in $PaCO_2$ may result in spontaneously breathing subjects; the drug also decreases the ventilatory response to hypoxia and hypercapnia, and inhibits the mechanism of hypoxic pulmonary vasoconstriction. Halothane is non-irritant to the respiratory tract; it causes bronchodilatation by a direct effect on the bronchial smooth muscle and also inhibits histamine-induced bronchoconstriction. Bronchial secretions are reduced by the drug.

CNS The principal effect of halothane is general anaesthesia; the drug has little, if any, analgesic effect. The drug causes cerebral vasodilation, leading to an increase in both the cerebral blood flow and intracranial pressure; it also decreases cerebral oxygen consumption. A centrally mediated decrease in the skeletal muscle tone results from the use of halothane.

AS The drug decreases salivation and gastric motility; splanchnic blood flow decreases as a result of the hypotension the drug produces.

GU Halothane decreases renal blood flow by 40% and the glomerular filtration rate by 50%; a small volume of concentrated urine results. The drug reduces the tone of the pregnant uterus.

Metabolic/other Halothane decrease plasma noradrenaline concentration, whilst increasing the concentrations of thyroxine and growth hormone. It also inhibits leucocyte phagocytosis. The drug causes a fall in the body temperature, predominantly by cutaneous vasodilation. Halothane causes a significant decrease in NO synthase activity.

Toxicity/side effects Halothane is a potent trigger agent for the development of malignant hyperthermia. The drug may also cause the appearance of myocardial dysrhythmias, particularly in the presence of hypoxia, hypercapnia, or excessive catecholamine concentrations. Shivering ('halothane shakes') may occur post-operatively. The most serious side effect halothane hepatitis occurs (rarely) after repeated use of the drug in the same individual. Halothane hepatitis is thought to be the result of an immune reaction to a metabolite formed by a reductive metabolic pathway. The risk of this complication is increased by obesity, perioperative hypoxaemia, and a short interval between consecutive exposures. It has been recommended that a period of at least 6 months should elapse prior to repeated administration of the drug to any individual.

Kinetics
Absorption The major factors affecting the uptake of volatile anaesthetic agents are solubility, cardiac output, and the concentration gradient between the alveoli and venous blood. Halothane is relatively insoluble in blood; the alveolar concentration therefore reaches inspired concentration relatively rapidly, resulting in a rapid induction of anaesthesia. An increase in the cardiac output increases the rate of alveolar uptake and slows the induction of anaesthesia. The concentration gradient between alveoli and venous blood approaches zero at equilibrium; a large concentration gradient favours the onset of anaesthesia.

Distribution The drug is initially distributed to organs with a high blood flow (brain, heart, liver, and kidney) and later to less well-perfused organs (muscles, fat, and bone).

Metabolism 20% of an administered dose is metabolized in the liver via cytochrome P450 2EI, principally by oxidation and dehalogenation, to yield trifluoroacetic acid, trifluoroacetyl ethanolamide, chloro bromo difluoroethylene, and chloride and bromide radiscals.

Excretion 60–80% is exhaled unchanged; the metabolites are excreted in the urine. Excretion of metabolites may continue for up to 3 weeks after the administration of halothane.

Special points Halothane potentiates the action of co-administered non-depolarizing relaxants. The dose of co-administered adrenaline should not exceed 10 ml of a 1:100 000 solution in a 10-minute period, to guard against the development of ventricular dysrhythmias.

Drug structure For the drug structure, please see Fig. 3.

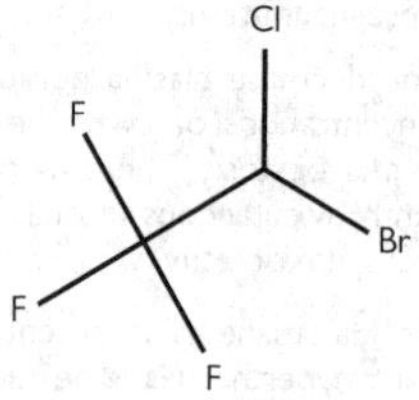

Fig. 3 Drug structure of halothane.

Hartmann's solution

Uses Hartmann's solution is used:
1. in the treatment of dehydration
2. for the acute expansion of intravascular volume and
3. to provide maintenance fluid and electrolyte requirements in the perioperative period.

Chemical Compound sodium lactate.

Presentation As a clear, colourless sterile solution in 500/1000 ml bags containing 131 mmol of Na^+, 111 mmol of chloride ions, 2 mmol of Ca^{2+}, 5 mmol of K^+, and 29 mmol of lactate ions (which are converted to bicarbonate ions in the liver) per litre. The pH of the solution is 6–7.3.

Main action Intravascular volume expansion.

Routes of administration/doses Hartmann's solution is administered intravenously at a rate titrated against the patient's clinical status.

Effects

CVS The haemodynamic effects of Hartmann's solution are proportional to the prevailing circulating volume and are short-lived.

GU Renal perfusion is temporarily restored towards normal in hypovolaemic patients transfused with the crystalloid.

Metabolic/other 1 l of one-sixth molar sodium lactate is potentially equivalent to 290 ml of 5% sodium bicarbonate in its acid-neutralizing effect and to 600 ml of 5% glucose in its antiketogenic effect.

Toxicity/side effects The predominant hazard is that of overtransfusion, leading to hypernatraemia, pulmonary oedema, and metabolic alkalosis.

Kinetics Data are incomplete.

Distribution Hartmann's solution is initially distributed into the plasma but later equilibrates with the extracellular fluid.

Metabolism The lactate component is oxidized in the liver to bicarbonate and glycogen over a period of about 2 hours. This is dependent on cellular oxidative activity, and the mechanism may be depressed by hypoxia and liver dysfunction.

Excretion Via the urine.

Heparins

Uses Heparin is used for:
1. the prevention of venous thromboembolic disease
2. the priming of haemodialysis and cardiopulmonary bypass machines and for maintaining the patency of indwelling lines and the treatment of
3. DIC
4. fat embolism, and
5. in the treatment of acute coronary syndromes.

Chemical Commercial heparin is a mixture of acid mucopolysaccharides (molecular weight 3000–60 000 daltons) extracted from bovine lung or porcine intestinal mucosa.

Presentation LMWHs are also available. These agents consist of short polysaccharide chains, which have an average molecular weight of <8000 daltons.

Main action Anticoagulant.

Mode of action The drug acts by binding reversibly to ATIII and enhancing its ability to inhibit certain proteases in the coagulation cascade (XIII, XII, XI, X, IX, plasmin, and thrombin). It also binds directly to several coagulation proteases and thereby facilitates their reaction with ATIII. LMWH acts via ATIII to inhibit factor Xa.

Routes of administration/dose The intravenous dose of heparin is titrated (at approximately 1000 IU/hour) to maintain APTT at 1.5–2 times the control value. The subcutaneous dose is 5000 IU 8- to 12-hourly. One IU of heparin will prevent 1 ml of citrated sheep plasma from clotting for 1 hour after the addition of 0.2 ml of 1:100 calcium chloride solution. Heparin sodium contains at least 120 IU/mg. LMWHs are available for subcutaneous and intravenous use. The dose and route of LMWH administration is dependent on the clinical indication and specific agent being used.

Effects

Metabolic/other In addition to its anticoagulant effects, heparin inhibits platelet aggregation by fibrin. Heparin increases hepatic triglyceride and other lipase activities in plasma, leading to an increase in plasma free fatty acid concentration.

Toxicity/side effects Excessive bleeding is the most commonly reported side effect; osteoporosis and aldosterone suppression have also been reported. Thrombocytopenia occurs in approximately 5% of patients who receive the drug and occurs more commonly when bovine heparin is used. Heparin-induced thrombocytopenia (HIT) predisposes to thrombosis, and, when thrombosis is identified, the condition is called heparin-induced thrombocytopenia and thrombosis (HITT). This may be asymptomatic or be associated with life-threatening arterial and venous thromboses, a condition which carries a mortality of 30%. HIT is caused by the formation of abnormal antibodies that activate platelets. HIT can be confirmed with specific blood tests. The treatment of HIT requires both protection from thrombosis and the choice of an agent that will not reduce the platelet count further.

Kinetics

Absorption There are no data concerning oral administration. The bio-availability appears to be the same for intravenous or subcutaneous administration.

Distribution One-third is bound in the plasma to ATIII, and the rest to albumin, fibrinogen, and proteases. The V_D is 40–100 ml/kg.

Metabolism Heparin appears to be desulfated and depolymerized (by heparinases) in the liver, kidneys, and reticulo-endothelial system.

Excretion Small amounts are excreted unchanged in the urine; renal impairment has little effect on the pharmacokinetics of heparin. The clearance is 0.5–2 ml/kg/min, and the elimination half-life is 0.5–2.5 hours. Heparin elimination is markedly decreased during hypothermia, e.g. during cardiopulmonary bypass.

Special points During heparin therapy, the thrombin time, whole blood clotting time, and APTT (kaolin cephalin time) are all prolonged. The bleeding time is unaffected by heparin, and the drug has no fibrinolytic activity. Specific antagonism of the effects of heparin may be achieved by the use of protamine (cf. protamine).

Neuroaxial anaesthesia and heparin therapy require careful consideration. Data suggest that at least 4 hours should elapse from the discontinuation of an unfractionated heparin infusion to the initiation of neuroaxial anaesthesia. If a patient has received LMWH for thromboembolism prophylaxis, then at least 12 hours should elapse prior to spinal/epidural insertion. If a treatment dose has been administered, then neuroaxial anaesthesia should be delayed by 24 hours.

LMWHs may be partially reversed using protamine (maximum effect <60%). Limited data suggest that, in the first 8 hours following administration of LMWH, 1 mg of protamine 'reverses' 1 mg of LMWH, up to the maximum dose of protamine that can be safely given. The effect of LMWH decreases over time, with a 50% reduction in effect by approximately 8 hours, and <33% effect after 12 hours.

LMWH has the apparent advantages of once-daily administration, safety during pregnancy, and causing thrombocytopenia less frequently.

Heparin is not removed by haemodialysis.

Human albumin solution

Uses Human albumin solution (HAS) is used:
1. for plasma volume replacement in haemorrhage, burns, or excessive fluid and electrolyte loss
2. for the priming of extracorporeal circuits
3. in the treatment of hypoalbuminaemic states and
4. as a replacement fluid during therapeutic plasma exchange.

Chemical A protein solution.

Presentation As a clear, straw-coloured fluid for infusion containing 4.5/5/20/25% of protein (of which 96% is albumin); the solutions contain sodium carbonate, sodium bicarbonate, and/or acetic acid to adjust the pH to 6.4–7.4 and stabilizers, but no preservatives. The solutions are prepared from pooled venous plasma from healthy subjects who are hepatitis B surface antigen (HepBsAg)- and human immunodeficiency virus (HIV)-negative; the solutions are pasteurized at 60°C for 10 hours. The sodium content of HAS is 130–160 mmol/l.

Main actions Plasma volume expansion and reversal of hypoalbuminaemia.

Mode of action Albumin is intimately involved in the regulation of plasma volume due to its colloid oncotic pressure; 5% HAS is iso-oncotic, but 20/25% HAS will draw 3/3.5 times the administered volume into the circulation from the tissues within 15 minutes.

Routes of administration/doses HAS is administered by intravenous infusion, according to clinical requirements; the haematocrit should be monitored and maintained above 25%—circulatory overload must be avoided.

Effects

CVS The haemodynamic effects of HAS are proportional to the prevailing volaemic status; in the face of hypovolaemia, HAS infusion restores cardiovascular parameters towards normal. Myocardial depression has been reported with HAS. Although it contains no clotting factors, HAS does not interfere with the mechanism of blood clotting.

GU Renal perfusion is restored towards normal in hypovolaemic subjects transfused with the colloid.

Toxicity/side effects The major concern with the use of HAS is circulatory overload. Allergic reactions and aluminium toxicity occur infrequently.

Kinetics Data are incomplete.

Metabolism Exogenous albumin enters the amino acid pool and undergoes biotransformation within the liver.

Excretion The elimination half-life is 16–18 days.

Special points HAS does not inhibit endothelial activation in sepsis. There is little evidence to support the use of albumin to improve outcome in the critically ill. Its effects on plasma volume are not predictable, especially in pathological states associated with leaky capillary membranes.

Hydralazine

Uses Hydralazine is used in the treatment of:
1. chronic moderate to severe hypertension
2. acute, severe hypertension
3. pre-eclampsia and
4. congestive heart failure.

Chemical A phthalazine derivative.

Presentation As 25/50 mg tablets of hydralazine hydrochloride, in ampoules containing 20 mg of hydralazine hydrochloride, as a white lyophilized powder which is reconstituted prior to use in water.

Main action Peripheral vasodilation.

Mode of action Hydralazine appears to act directly on vascular smooth muscle by interfering either with calcium entry into the cell or the release of calcium from intracellular stores; this leads to electromechanical decoupling and inhibition of contraction.

Routes of administration/doses The adult oral dose is 50–200 mg/day in divided doses; the intravenous dose is 20–40 mg administered slowly. The drug takes 15–20 minutes to act when administered intravenously and has a duration of action of 2–6 hours.

Effects

CVS Hydralazine causes predominantly arteriolar vasodilation, leading to a decrease in the systemic vascular resistance; a compensatory tachycardia develops, and the cardiac output increases.

CNS Cerebral blood flow increases after the administration of hydralazine.

GU The renal blood flow increases, secondary to the increased cardiac output; however, hydralazine usually produces sodium retention and a decrease in urine volume.

Metabolic/other Plasma renin activity is increased by the drug.

Toxicity/side effects Minor side effects, such as headache, flushing, sweating, nausea, and vomiting, are common. The drug may precipitate angina in patients with myocardial ischaemia. A lupus-like syndrome may occur when high doses are used. Peripheral neuropathies and blood dyscrasias occur rarely with the use of hydralazine.

Kinetics

Absorption The bioavailability of oral hydralazine is dependent on the acetylator status and thus the extent of first-pass metabolism; average values are 16–35%.

Distribution Hydralazine is 87% protein-bound in the plasma; the V_D is 4.2 l/kg.

Metabolism The drug is primarily metabolized by acetylation and oxidation, with subsequent conjugation. Phenotypically determined populations of fast and slow acetylators exist.

Excretion 50–90% is excreted in the urine, 1–2% unchanged. Up to 10% may appear in the faeces. The clearance is 1.4 l/kg/hour, and the elimination half-life is 0.67–3.6 hours.

Special points The drug is commonly used in combination with a beta-adrenergic antagonist to obtund the compensatory tachycardia and increased plasma renin activity caused by hydralazine.

The hypotensive effects of volatile agents and hydralazine are additive. A dose of 0.4 mg/kg has been recommended 10 minutes prior to induction in order to obtund the pressor response to intubation.

The drug crosses the placenta and may produce fetal tachycardia when used in pregnancy or labour.

The addition of hydralazine to glucose solutions is not recommended.

Hydralazine is not removed by haemodialysis.

Hydrocortisone

Uses Hydrocortisone is used:
1. as replacement therapy in adrenocortical deficiency states and in the treatment of
2. allergy and anaphylaxis
3. asthma
4. panoply of autoimmune disorders
5. eczema and contact sensitivity syndromes and
6. in leukaemia chemotherapy regimes and
7. for immunosuppression after organ transplantation.

Chemical A glucocorticosteroid.

Presentation As 10/20 mg tablets of hydrocortisone, in vials containing a white lyophilized powder which is diluted in water to yield a solution containing 100 mg of hydrocortisone sodium succinate, and as a variety of topical creams and retention enemas, some of which are fixed-dose combinations.

Main action Anti-inflammatory.

Mode of action Corticosteroids act by controlling the rate of protein synthesis; they react with cytoplasmic receptors to form a complex which directly influences the rate of RNA transcription. This directs the synthesis of lipocortins.

Routes of administration/doses The adult dose by the intravenous route is 100–500 mg 6- to 8-hourly; the drug acts within 2–4 hours and has a duration of action of 8 hours when administered intravenously. The corresponding oral dose is 10–20 mg/day, using the lowest dose that is effective and on alternate days, if possible, to limit the development of side effects. The intra-articular dose is 5–50 mg daily.

Effects

CVS In the absence of corticosteroids, vascular permeability increases; small blood vessels demonstrate an inadequate motor response, and cardiac output decreases. Steroids have a positive effect on myocardial contractility and cause vasoconstriction by increasing the number of alpha-1 adrenoreceptors and beta-adrenoreceptors and stimulating their function.

CNS Corticosteroids increase the excitability of the CNS; the absence of glucocorticoids leads to apathy, depression, and irritability.
AS Hydrocortisone increases the likelihood of peptic ulcer disease; it also decreases the gastrointestinal absorption of calcium.

GU Hydrocortisone has weak mineralocorticoid effects and produces sodium retention and increased potassium excretion; the urinary excretion of calcium is also increased by the drug. The drug increases the glomerular filtration rate and stimulates tubular secretory activity.

Metabolic/other Hydrocortisone exerts profound effects on carbohydrate, protein, and lipid metabolism. Glucocorticoids stimulate gluconeogenesis and inhibit the peripheral utilization of glucose; they cause a redistribution of body fat, enhance lipolysis, and also reduce the conversion of amino acids to protein. Hydrocortisone is a potent anti-inflammatory agent which inhibits all stages of the inflammatory process by inhibiting neutrophil and macrophage recruitment, blocking the effect of lymphokines, and inhibiting the formation of plasminogen activator. Corticosteroids increase red blood cell, neutrophil, and haemoglobin concentrations, whilst depressing other white cell lines and the activity of lymphoid tissue.

Toxicity/side effects Consist of an acute withdrawal syndrome and a syndrome (Cushing's) produced by prolonged use of excessive quantities of the drug. Cushing's syndrome is characterized by growth arrest, a characteristic appearance consisting of central obesity, a moon face and buffalo hump, striae, acne, hirsutism, and skin and capillary fragility, together with the following metabolic derangements: altered glucose tolerance, fluid retention, a hypokalaemic alkalosis, and osteoporosis. A proximal myopathy, cataracts, and an increased susceptibility to peptic ulcer disease may also complicate the use of the drug.

Kinetics

Absorption Hydrocortisone is well absorbed when administered orally or rectally; the oral bioavailability is 54%, and the rectal bioavailability is 30–90%.

Distribution The drug is reversibly bound in the plasma to albumin (20%) and a specific corticosteroid-binding globulin (70%); the drug is 90% protein-bound at low concentrations, but only 60–70% protein-bound at higher concentrations. The V_D is 0.3–0.5 l/kg, according to the dose.

Metabolism Occurs in the liver to tetrahydrocortisone.

Excretion The clearance of hydrocortisone is dose-dependent and ranges from 167 to 283 ml/min; the elimination half-life is 1.2–1.8 hours.

Special points Cortisone and hydrocortisone (cortisol) are metabolically interconvertible; only the latter is active. The conversion of cortisone to hydrocortisone is rapid and extensive, and occurs as a first-pass effect in the liver. Hydrocortisone is one-quarter as potent as an anti-inflammatory agent as prednisolone. It has been recommended that perioperative steroid cover be given:
1. to patients who have received high-dose steroid replacement therapy for 2 weeks in the preceding year prior to surgery
2. to patients undergoing pituitary or adrenal surgery. Glucocorticoids antagonize the effects of anticholinesterase drugs.

Relative adrenal insufficiency is reported in the critically ill, and low-dose hydrocortisone and mineralocorticoid replacement have been shown to decrease the time to 'shock' reversal and may decrease mortality.

Hyoscine

Uses Hyoscine is used:
1. in premedication
2. in the prophylaxis of motion sickness
3. as an antispasmodic and
4. in palliative care.

Chemical Hyoscine is an alkaloid derived from *Scopolia carniolica* and is an ester of tropic acid and scopine. Scopolamine is l-hyoscine.

Presentation Hyoscine hydrobromide is presented as a clear solution for injection containing 0.4 mg/ml and as a fixed-dose combination with papaveretum. Hyoscine butylbromide is presented as a clear solution containing 20 mg/ml and in 10 mg tablet form. A transdermal preparation delivering 1 mg/72 hours of hyoscine is also available.

Main actions Anticholinergic with marked sedative effects.

Mode of action The drug acts by competitive antagonism of acetylcholine at muscarinic receptors (hyoscine has little effect at nicotinic receptors).

Routes of administration/doses Hyoscine may be administered intramuscularly, intravenously, subcutaneously, transdermally, or orally. The intramuscular dose for premedication is 8–15 micrograms/kg. The adult oral dose is 20 mg 6-hourly.

Effects

CVS Hyoscine has less effect than atropine on cardiovascular parameters. When administered intravenously, an initial tachycardia may be followed by a bradycardia.

RS The drug causes a marked decrease in bronchial secretions, mild bronchodilatation, and mild stimulation of respiration.

CNS Hyoscine is a CNS depressant, causing 'twilight sleep' and amnesia. It has antanalgesic, antiemetic, and anti-parkinsonian properties. Hyoscine may also cause the central anticholinergic syndrome.

AS A marked antisialogogue, hyoscine is also antispasmodic throughout the gut and biliary tree.

GU The tone of the bladder and ureters is reduced, following administration of the drug.

Metabolic/other Hyoscine has a more marked effect on the eye and sweat gland activity than atropine.

Toxicity/side effects The central anticholinergic syndrome is the main side effect and may be prolonged, especially in the elderly; peripheral anticholinergic side effects may also occur, following the use of hyoscine.

Kinetics

Absorption Hyoscine is poorly absorbed after oral administration; the bio-availability is 10% by this route. The drug is well absorbed, following subcutaneous or intramuscular administration.

Distribution Hyoscine is 11% protein-bound in the plasma; the V_D is 2.0 l/kg.

Metabolism The drug is extensively metabolized in liver and tissues to scopine and scopic acid.

Excretion 2% of an oral dose is excreted unchanged in the urine, and 5% in the bile. The clearance is 45 l/hour, and the elimination half-life is 2.5 hours.

Special points The drug may induce acute clinical and biochemical manifestations in patients with porphyria.

Ibuprofen

Uses Ibuprofen is used in the treatment of:
1. rheumatoid arthritis and osteoarthritis
2. musculoskeletal disorders
3. soft tissue injuries
4. ankylosing spondylitis
5. acute gout
6. renal and biliary colic
7. dysmenorrhoea
8. migraine
9. post-surgical pain as an adjunct to other analgesic agents, including opioids, and
10. as an antipyretic.

Chemical A phenylpropanoic acid derivative.

Presentation Ibuprofen is available in multiple forms, including capsules, tablets, suspensions, suppositories, and topical gels. It may be presented as a sole agent or in combination with other drugs. The drug is often a component in proprietary cold cures. It has a pKa of 4.91.

Main actions Analgesic, anti-inflammatory, and antipyretic.

Mode of action Ibuprofen is a non-specific inhibitor of COX which converts arachidonic acid to cyclic endoperoxidases, thus preventing the formation of prostaglandins, thromboxanes, and prostacyclin. Prostaglandins are involved in the sensitization of peripheral pain receptors to noxious stimuli.

Routes of administration/doses The adult oral dose is 1200–1800 mg daily in divided doses. In severe conditions, the daily dose may be increased to 2400 mg. The paediatric oral dose is 20 mg/kg in divided doses. The drug may be administered orally, rectally, or topically.

Effects

RS Bronchoconstriction may occur in 20% of asthmatic patients.

AS Dyspepsia, nausea, bleeding from gastric and duodenal vessels, mucosal ulceration, perforation, and diarrhoea are expected COX-1 effects. The drug may lead to disease exacerbation in patients with Crohn's disease or ulcerative colitis.

Metabolic/other Ibuprofen reduces platelet aggregation.

Toxicity/side effects Disturbances of the gastrointestinal system occur commonly. Rashes, and hepatic, renal, and haematological impairment have been reported. As with other NSAIDs, prolonged use may lead to analgesic nephropathy, characterized by papillary necrosis and interstitial fibrosis. Acute renal failure may be precipitated when NSAIDs are administered to patients who have the renal perfusion dependent on prostaglandin production (i.e. when there are high levels of circulating vasoconstrictors or hypovolaemia).

Kinetics

Absorption The bioavailability of the drug is 80%.

Distribution Ibuprofen is 90–99% protein-bound in the plasma to albumin. The V_D is 0.14 l/kg. The drug crosses the placenta.

Metabolism Ibuprofen undergoes hepatic metabolism via oxidation to two inactive metabolites.

Excretion The drug is excreted in the urine. The half-life of ibuprofen is 2 hours.

Special points NSAIDs antagonize the antihypertensive effects of ACEIs via the inhibition of vasodilatory prostaglandin synthesis. The risk of renal impairment increases if NSAIDs and ACEIs are co-administered. NSAIDs inhibit the activity of diuretics. Ibuprofen may cause premature closure of the ductus arteriosus in the fetus when administered during the third trimester of pregnancy.

Imipramine

Uses Imipramine is used for the treatment of:
1. depression and
2. nocturnal enuresis.

Chemical A dibenzazepine derivative.

Presentation As 10/25 mg tablets and a syrup containing 5 mg/ml of imipramine hydrochloride.

Main action Antidepressant.

Mode of action Tricyclic antidepressants may potentiate the action of biogenic amines within the CNS by preventing their reuptake at nerve terminals. They also antagonize muscarinic cholinergic, alpha-1 adrenergic, and H1 and H2 histaminergic receptors.

Routes of administration/doses The adult oral dose is 25–50 mg 6- to 8-hourly.

Effects

CVS Imipramine causes postural hypotension as a result of peripheral alpha-adrenergic blockade; a compensatory tachycardia may develop. The tricyclic antidepressants are also negatively inotropic; they also have characteristic effects on ECG morphology, including T-wave flattening and inversion.

RS Imipramine has little effect on respiratory function when normal doses are used.

CNS The predominant effect of the drug is an antidepressant action which may take several weeks to develop; sedation, weakness, and fatigue are also commonly produced.

AS High doses of imipramine increase the gastric emptying time.

Metabolic/other The drug may produce excessive sweating by an unknown mechanism.

Toxicity/side effects Occur in 5% and include palpitations, dysrhythmias, tremor, confusion, mania, and hepatic dysfunction. Anticholinergic side effects (blurred vision, dryness of the mouth, constipation, and urinary retention) may also occur. Overdose of the drug may result in fits, coma, and fatal dysrhythmias.

Kinetics

Absorption The drug is well absorbed when administered orally; the bioavailability is 19–35%.

Distribution Imipramine is 95% protein-bound in the plasma; the V_D is 15–31 l/kg.

Metabolism/other The drug is demethylated to an active form desimipramine; this is inactivated by hydroxylation, with subsequent conjugation to glucuronide.

Excretion The glucuronide conjugates are excreted in the urine. The clearance is 11–19 ml/min/kg, and the elimination half-life is 11–25 hours.

Special points Hyoscine and the phenothiazines displace tricyclic antidepressants from their binding sites on plasma proteins and thus increase the activity of the latter; barbiturates increase the rate of hepatic metabolism of tricyclic antidepressants and decrease their activity.

Imipramine accentuates the cardiovascular effects of adrenaline; care should be exercised when local anaesthetic agents containing adrenaline are used in patients receiving the drug. Imipramine also increases the likelihood of dysrhythmias occurring during general anaesthesia.

Imipramine is not removed by haemodialysis.

Insulin

Uses Insulin is used in the management of:
1. type I diabetes mellitus
2. diabetic emergencies
3. the perioperative control of blood sugar concentration
4. hyperkalaemia and
5. to improve glucose utilization during TPN and
6. in provocation tests for growth hormone.

Chemical A polypeptide hormone. Human insulin is produced commercially by recombinant DNA techniques; bovine insulin differs by three, and porcine insulin by one, amino acid from human insulin.

Presentation A wide variety of insulin preparations are available; the standard preparations contain 100 units/ml. The source may be human recombinant, bovine, or porcine, and each may be modified by the addition of zinc or protamine to retard absorption.

Main actions Stimulation of carbohydrate metabolism, protein synthesis, and lipogenesis.

Mode of action Insulin binds to and activates a specific membrane-bound receptor; the effects of this may be mediated by alterations in the intracellular concentrations of cyclic nucleotides. Insulin exerts a direct effect on lipoprotein lipase, increases the rate of transcriptional and translational events during protein synthesis, and controls membrane polarization and ion transport by activating $Na^+K^+ATPase$.

Routes of administration/doses Insulin may be administered intravenously, intramuscularly, and subcutaneously in a dose titrated according to the blood sugar estimations. It may be diluted for intravenous infusion in saline/glucose. The apparent dose requirement is increased by 20% when bovine or porcine insulin is used in place of human insulin.

Rapidly acting insulins act within 1 hour and have a duration of action of 5–7 hours; slow-acting preparations act within 4 hours and have a duration of action of 18–36 hours.

Continuous insulin infusion devices are also available for patients.

Effects

Metabolic/other Insulin has profound effects upon carbohydrate, fat, and protein metabolism. The drug increases the rate of diffusion of glucose into all cells and specifically into hepatocytes by enhancing the activity of glucokinase (which causes the initial phosphorylation of glucose, thereby 'trapping' glucose intracellularly). The drug increases the rate of glycogen synthesis by enhancing the activity of phosphofructokinase (which is involved in glucose phosphorylation) and glycogen synthetase (which polymerizes monosaccharides to form glycogen). Insulin simultaneously inhibits glycogenolysis by an action on phosphorylase and inhibits gluconeogenesis. It also facilitates diffusion of glucose into muscle cells.

Insulin causes fat deposition in adipose tissue by increasing the hepatic synthesis of fatty acids; these are utilized within the liver to form triglycerides which are released into the bloodstream; insulin simultaneously activates lipoprotein lipase in adipose tissue which splits triglycerides into fatty acids, enabling them to be absorbed into adipose tissue where they are stored. The drug also inhibits a hormone-sensitive lipase, thereby preventing hydrolysis of triglycerides, and facilitates glucose transport into fat cells, leading to an increased supply of glycerol which is used in the manufacture of storage triglycerides.

Insulin causes active transport of amino acids into cells and increases mRNA translation and DNA transcription; in addition, it inhibits the catabolism of proteins.

The drug also causes an increase in the rate of potassium and magnesium transport into cells.

Toxicity/side effects The commonest acute side effect of insulin is hypoglycaemia. Chronic use may be complicated by localized allergic reactions, lipodystrophy, and insulin resistance due to antibody formation.

Kinetics

Absorption Insulin is inactive when administered orally, since it is destroyed by gastrointestinal proteases.

Distribution The drug exhibits little protein binding; the V_D is 0.075 l/kg (0.146 l/kg in the diabetic subject).

Metabolism Insulin is rapidly metabolized in the liver, muscle, and kidney by glutathione insulin transhydrogenase.

Excretion The metabolites appear in the urine. The clearance is 33.3 ml/min/kg (18.5 ml/min/kg in the diabetic subject), and the elimination half-life is 1.6–3.4 minutes (5.3–7.8 minutes in the diabetic subject).

Special points The co-administration of steroids, levothyroxine, thiazide diuretics, and sympathomimetic agents tends to counteract the effects of insulin on carbohydrate metabolism. Many regimes of insulin administration have been described for the perioperative management of diabetic patients.

Insulin is not removed by dialysis.

Tight blood sugar control in critical illness has been shown to decrease mortality, especially in surgical patients.

Intralipid® 20%

Uses Intralipid® 20% is used:
1. in the preparation of TPN mixtures
2. in the treatment of local anaesthetic toxicity with or without circulatory arrest and
3. in the prevention of essential fatty acid deficiency syndrome.

Chemical A fat emulsion.

Presentation As a white, oil–water emulsion containing 20% soybean oil, 1.2% egg yolk phospholipids, 2.25% glycerin, sodium hydroxide, and water. It has a pH of approximately 8 and contains emulsified fat particles of 0.5 micrometres in size. Soybean oil consists of long-chain unsaturated fatty acids in the following proportions: linoleic (44–62%), oleic (19–30%), palmitic (7–14%), linolenic (4–11%), stearic (1.4–5.5%). Intralipid® 20% has an osmolality of approximately 350 mOsm/kg water equivalent to 260 mOsm/l of emulsion.

Main action As an energy substrate. Intralipid® 20% appears to reverse local anaesthetic cardiotoxicity.

Mode of action The mechanism of action remains to be fully elucidated but may involve the establishment of a concentration gradient away from the primary site of action of the local anaesthetic.

Routes of administration/doses Intralipid® 20% is administered by intravenous infusion when given as part of TPN therapy. The various doses with regard to this indication are beyond the scope of this book. For the treatment of local anaesthetic toxicity with or without circulatory arrest, together with advanced life support measures as indicated, an initial intravenous bolus dose of 1.5 ml/kg should be administered over 1 minute, together with the commencement of an intravenous infusion at 15 ml/kg/hour. If cardiovascular stability has not been achieved or circulation deteriorates further, two subsequent bolus doses may be given 5 minutes apart. The continuous infusion rate should be doubled to 30 ml/kg/hour at any point after 5 minutes if identical criteria are met. The maximum cumulative dose is 12 ml/kg.

Effects

Metabolic/other The principal effect of the drug is to act as an energy substrate, 2 kcal/ml, resulting in an increase in heat production and oxygen consumption.

Toxicity/side effects Pancreatitis may occur, secondary to hyperlipidaemia, following administration of the drug. Hepatic dysfunction has been described after prolonged use.

Kinetics Data are incomplete. The emulsified fat particles are cleared from the bloodstream by a mechanism thought to be similar to the removal of chylomicrons.

Special points Following the administration of Intralipid® 20% (or another intravenous lipid emulsion) in the management of suspected local anaesthetic toxicity, serum amylase or lipase should be monitored for 2 days to assist in excluding the development of pancreatitis. Cases should be reported to the appropriate national regulatory organization governing patient safety (in the UK, this is the National Patient Safety Agency), and the use of lipid reported to the international registry at http://www.lipidrescue.org.

Ipratropium

Uses Ipratropium is used in the treatment of asthma and chronic obstructive airways disease.

Chemical A synthetic quaternary ammonium compound which is a derivative of atropine.

Presentation As an isotonic solution of ipratropium bromide containing 0.25 mg/ml for nebulization or as a metered-dose aerosol delivering 200 micrograms/dose (18 micrograms of which is available to the patient).

Main action Bronchodilatation.

Mode of action Ipratropium acts by competitive inhibition of cholinergic receptors on bronchial smooth muscle, thereby blocking the bronchoconstrictor action of vagal efferent impulses. It may also inhibit acetylcholine enhancement of mediator release by blocking cholinergic receptors on the surface of mast cells.

Routes of administration/doses The drug is administered by inhalation of a nebulized solution or aerosol in an adult dose of 100–500 micrograms 6-hourly or 1–2 puffs 6-hourly, respectively. The maximum effect is achieved in 1.5–2 hours and lasts 4–6 hours.

Effects

CVS No effect on cardiovascular function is observed after administration by inhalation. When administered intravenously, tachycardia with an increase in blood pressure and cardiac output and a fall in central venous pressure may result.

RS Bronchodilatation is the principal effect of the drug. No effect is seen on the viscosity or volume of secretions or the effectiveness of mucociliary clearance. The oxygen saturation remains unaltered, following the administration of ipratropium.

CNS The drug has no effect, since ipratropium is unable to cross the blood–brain barrier.

AS When given orally in large doses, gastric secretion and salivation are decreased by the drug.

Toxicity/side effects None of the typical anticholinergic side effects are observed if ipratropium is administered by inhalation. Twenty to 30% of patients receiving the drug experience transient local effects: dryness or unpleasant taste in the mouth. Local deposition of the nebulized drug on the eye may cause mydriasis and difficulty with accommodation.

Kinetics

Absorption The bioavailability of the drug when administered orally is 3–30%, and 5% by the inhaled route.

Distribution The V_D is 0.4 l/kg.

Metabolism Ipratropium is metabolized to eight inactive metabolites.

Excretion Occurs in approximately equal proportions in the urine and faeces. The clearance is 11.8 l/hour, and the elimination half-life is 3.2–3.8 hours.

Special points Ipratropium is less effective than beta-adrenergic agonists in the treatment of asthma, although its effectiveness in the treatment of bronchitis appears to be equal to that of the beta-adrenergic agonists. An additive effect with the latter drugs is difficult to prove.

Isoflurane

Uses Isoflurane is used:
1. for the induction and maintenance of general anaesthesia and has been used
2. for sedation during intensive care.

Chemical A halogenated methyl ether which is a structural isomer of enflurane.

Presentation As a clear, colourless liquid with a pungent smell, which is non-flammable; the commercial preparation contains no additives or stabilizers and is supplied in amber-coloured bottles. The molecular weight of isoflurane is 184.5, the boiling point 48.5°C, and the saturated vapour pressure 32 kPa at 20°C. The MAC of isoflurane is 1.15 (0.50 in 70% N_2O), although it is age-dependent and ranges from 1.05 in elderly patients to 1.6 in neonates; the blood:gas partition coefficient is 1.4, and the fat:blood partition coefficient is 50. The oil:gas partition coefficient is 97.

Main action General anaesthesia (reversible loss of both awareness and recall of noxious stimuli).

Mode of action The mechanism of general anaesthesia remains to be fully elucidated. General anaesthetics appear to disrupt synaptic transmission (especially in the area of the ventrobasal thalamus). This mechanism may include potentiation of the $GABA_A$ and glycine receptors and antagonism at NMDA receptors. Their mode of action at the molecular level appears to involve the expansion of hydrophobic regions in the neuronal membrane, either within the lipid phase or within hydrophobic sites in cell membranes.

Routes of administration/dose Isoflurane is administered by inhalation; the agent has a pleasant, non-irritant odour. The concentration used for induction of anaesthesia is quoted as 5–8%. Maintenance of anaesthesia is usually achieved using between 0.5 and 3%.

Effects

CVS Isoflurane causes a dose-related decrease in myocardial contractility and mean arterial pressure; the systolic pressure decreases to a greater degree than the diastolic pressure. The drug does not affect the heart rate, and myocardial sensitization to catecholamines does not occur. The drug does not appear to cause the 'coronary steal' phenomenon in man.

RS Isoflurane is a respiratory depressant, causing dose-dependent decreases in the tidal volume and an increase in the respiratory rate. The drug depresses the ventilatory response to CO_2 and inhibits hypoxic pulmonary vasoconstriction. Isoflurane appears to relax bronchial smooth muscle constricted by histamine or acetylcholine.

CNS The principal effect of isoflurane is general anaesthesia. The drug causes cerebral vasodilation, leading to an increase in cerebral blood flow; the cerebral metabolic rate is decreased. As with other volatile anaesthetic agents, isoflurane may increase the intracranial pressure in a dose-related manner. Isoflurane use is not associated with epileptiform activity.

GU Isoflurane reduces renal blood flow and leads to an increase in fluoride ion concentrations (12 micromoles/l to 90 micromoles/l in anaesthesia lasting 1 to 6 hours, respectively). There is no evidence that isoflurane causes gross changes in human renal function. The drug causes uterine relaxation.

Metabolic/other In animal models, the drug decreases liver synthesis of fibrinogen, transferrin, and albumin.

Toxicity/side effects Isoflurane may cause PONV. Isoflurane is a trigger agent for the development of malignant hyperthermia. There are no reports of renal toxicity occurring in patients who have received the drug.

Kinetics

Absorption The major factors affecting the uptake of volatile anaesthetic agents are solubility, cardiac output, and the concentration gradient between the alveoli and venous blood. Due to the low blood:gas partition coefficient of isoflurane, it is exceptionally insoluble in blood; the alveolar concentration therefore reaches inspired concentration very rapidly (fast wash-in rate), resulting in a rapid induction of (and emergence from) anaesthesia. An increase in the cardiac output increases the rate of alveolar uptake and slows the induction of anaesthesia. The concentration gradient between the alveoli and venous blood approaches zero at equilibrium; a large concentration gradient favours the onset of anaesthesia.

Distribution The drug is initially distributed to organs with a high blood flow (brain, heart, liver, kidney) and later to less well-perfused organs (muscle, fat, bone).

Metabolism 0.2% of an administered dose undergoes hepatic metabolism, principally by oxidation and dehalogenation.

Excretion Isoflurane is principally exhaled unchanged; 0.2% of an administered dose is excreted in the urine as non-volatile fluorinated compounds.

Special points Isoflurane potentiates the action of co-administered depolarizing and non-depolarizing muscle relaxants to a greater extent than either halothane or enflurane.

As with other volatile anaesthetic agents, the co-administration of N_2O, benzodiazepines, or opioids lowers the MAC of isoflurane.

Drug structure For the drug structure, please see Fig. 4.

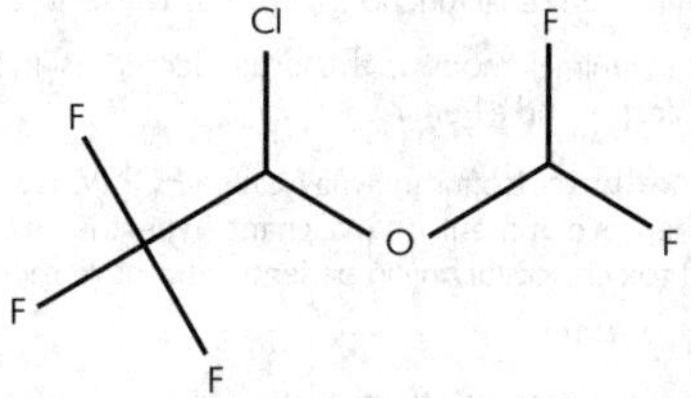

Fig. 4 Drug structure of isoflurane.

Isoprenaline

Uses Isoprenaline is used in the treatment of:
1. complete heart block (whilst awaiting transvenous pacing)
2. asthma
3. torsades de pointes and is used to provide
4. inotropic support.

Chemical A synthetic catecholamine.

Presentation As a clear solution for injection containing 0.02/1 mg/ml of isoprenaline hydrochloride. An aerosol delivering 80/400 micrograms of isoprenaline sulfate per metered dose is also available.

Main actions Positive inotropism, positive chronotropism, and bronchodilatation.

Mode of action Isoprenaline is a beta-adrenergic agonist; its actions are mediated by membrane-bound adenylate cyclase and the subsequent formation of cAMP.

Routes of administration/doses Isoprenaline may also be administered as an infusion, diluted in water or 5% glucose, at the rate of 0.5–8 micrograms/min, according to response. The positive chronotropic effect becomes apparent after 20 minutes.

Effects

CVS Isoprenaline is a powerful positive inotrope and chronotrope, and thus causes an increase in the cardiac output and systolic blood pressure. The drug causes a decrease in the peripheral vascular resistance (a beta-2 effect); as a result, the diastolic blood pressure tends to decrease. The drug increases automaticity and enhances AV nodal conduction; it also increases the coronary blood flow which tends to offset the increase in myocardial oxygen consumption that it produces.

RS The drug is a potent bronchodilator, and increases anatomical dead space and ventilation/perfusion mismatching which may lead to hypoxia.

CNS Isoprenaline is a CNS stimulant.

AS Isoprenaline decreases gastrointestinal tone and motility; the mesenteric blood supply is increased by the drug.

GU The administration of isoprenaline reduces the renal blood flow in normotensive subjects but may increase renal perfusion in shock states. The drug also reduces the uterine tone.

Metabolic/other In common with adrenaline, isoprenaline increases the plasma concentration of free fatty acids and may cause hyperglycaemia. Isoprenaline inhibits antigen-induced histamine release and the formation of slow-releasing substance of anaphylaxis.

Toxicity/side effects The use of isoprenaline may be complicated by excessive tachycardia, palpitations, angina, dysrhythmias, hypotension, and sweating. The use of isoprenaline inhalers by asthmatic patients has been associated with an excess mortality.

Kinetics Quantitative data are lacking.

Absorption The drug is well absorbed when administered orally but is subject to an extensive first-pass metabolism in the intestinal mucosa and liver.

Distribution Isoprenaline is 65% protein-bound in the plasma.

Metabolism Isoprenaline is a relatively poor substrate for the action of monoamine oxidase; the drug is predominantly metabolized by catechol-O-methyl transferase in the liver to sulfated conjugates.

Excretion 15–75% of an administered dose of isoprenaline is excreted unchanged in the urine, the remainder as sulfated conjugates. The plasma half-life is 1–7 minutes.

Special points Hypoxia, hypercapnia, and the co-administration of halothane, trilene, or cyclopropane increase the likelihood of the development of dysrhythmias during the use of isoprenaline. Tachyphylaxis may occur with prolonged use.

Ketamine

Uses Ketamine is used:
1. for the induction of anaesthesia, especially in poor-risk patients with hypotension or asthma
2. as a sole agent for short procedures such as change of burns dressings
3. for pre-hospital care and mass casualties
4. for analgesia both post-operatively and in patients receiving intensive care
5. for pain relief in patients with chronic pain, and
6. for the reversal of severe unresponsive asthma.

Chemical A phencyclidine derivative

Presentation Ketamine has a molecular weight of 238 and is presented as a colourless solution containing 10/50/100 mg/ml of racemic ketamine hydrochloride. It has a pH of between 3.5 and 5.5, with a pKa of 7.5. The racemic mixture contains in equal proportions two enantiomers due to its chiral centre of the cyclo-hexanone ring ([S-(+)-ketamine] and [R-(−)-ketamine]). All preparations now contain 0.1 mg/ml of benzethonium chloride as a preservative. S-(+)-ketamine is available in 5 and 25 mg/ml concentrations.

Main actions Dissociative anaesthesia (a combination of profound analgesia with superficial sleep).

Mode of action Ketamine is a non-competitive antagonist of the NMDA receptor Ca^{2+} channel pore and also inhibits NMDA receptor activity by interaction with the phencyclidine binding site. Inhibition of glutamate-gated NMDA receptors by ketamine provides a mechanism of a predominant analgesic profile. It reduces the pre-synaptic release of glutamate, in addition to complex interactions with opioid receptors. There is some evidence suggesting that ketamine acts as an antagonist at monoaminergic, muscarinic, and nicotinic receptors. Ketamine has local anaesthetic activity at high doses which may be the result of sodium channel inhibition.

S-(+)-ketamine has four times greater affinity for the NMDA receptor than R-(−)-ketamine. It is twice as potent as the racemic mixture and three times as potent as the R(−) form.

Routes of administration/doses The intramuscular dose for induction of anaesthesia is 4–10 mg/kg; the onset of action is 2–8 minutes, and the duration of action is 10–20 minutes. The corresponding intravenous dose is 0.5–2 mg/kg, administered over a period of 60 seconds; the onset of action occurs within 30 seconds, and the duration of action is 5–10 minutes. Ketamine may be used for the maintenance of anaesthesia, using an intravenous infusion at a rate of between 10 and 50 micrograms/kg/min. For sedation and analgesia, an intramuscular dose of 2–4 mg/kg or an intravenous dose of 0.2–0.75 mg/kg may be used, followed by an infusion of 5–20 micrograms/kg/min. Ketamine may also be administered orally, rectally, nasally, intrathecally, or extradurally. When used neuroaxially, the preservative-free solution must be used (not currently produced in the UK). Tolerance develops with repeated drug exposure.

Effects

CVS Ketamine causes tachycardia, and an increase in the blood pressure, central venous pressure, and cardiac output, secondary to an increase in the sympathetic tone. These effects mask the mild direct myocardial depressant effect ketamine exerts (reduced effect with S-(+)-ketamine). Baroreceptor function is well maintained, and dysrhythmias are uncommon.

RS Ketamine causes mild stimulation of respiration, with relative preservation of airway reflexes. It acts as a bronchial smooth muscle relaxant and improves pulmonary compliance. The R-(−) isomer has greater activity against acetylcholine bronchial smooth muscle contraction, compared with the S-(+) form. Therefore, the racemic mixture may be a more suitable choice in patients with bronchospasm.

CNS The dissociative state may be produced by separation functionally and electrophysiologically of the thalamo-neocortical and limbic systems. The eyes remain open; pupillary dilatation, nystagmus, and hypertonus occur. Cerebral blood flow, cerebral metabolic rate, and intracranial and intraocular pressures are all increased. Visceral pain is poorly obtunded by ketamine. The EEG demonstrates dominant theta activity with loss of the alpha rhythm. S-(+) ketamine has a faster recovery time.

AS Salivary secretions are increased. Gastric motility is unaffected.

GU Ketamine increases the uterine tone.

Metabolic/other Circulating levels of adrenaline and noradrenaline are increased. Ketamine significantly reduces leucocyte activation during sepsis or hypoxaemia, and *in vitro* tests suggest it suppresses pro-inflammatory cytokine production.

Toxicity/side effects PONV is common. Transient rashes occur in 15% of patients. Emergence delirium, unpleasant dreams, and hallucinations are common but may be alleviated by the use of a benzodiazepine premedication. Pain on injection (especially intramuscularly) can be reduced by combination with lidocaine. Bladder dysfunction is reported in chronic abusers.

Kinetics

Absorption The bioavailability of ketamine is: 20–25% (oral), 25–50% (nasal), and 93% (intramuscular).

Distribution Ketamine is 20–50% protein-bound in the plasma; the V_D is 3 l/kg. The distribution half-life is 11 minutes. Recovery occurs due to redistribution across lipid membranes.

Metabolism Ketamine is metabolized in the liver by N-demethylation and hydroxylation via the cytochrome P450 enzyme system of the cyclohexylamine ring. Norketamine, a metabolite, which is 30% as potent as ketamine, is metabolized to an inactive glucuronide.

Excretion The conjugated metabolites are excreted in the urine. The plasma clearance is 17 ml/kg/min, and the elimination half-life is 2.5 hours.

Special points Antisialogogue premedication is recommended prior to the use of ketamine. Emergence phenomena are less frequent in the young and elderly. Premedication can reduce the incidence of these reactions, as does leaving the patient in an undisturbed state during the recovery phase. Low-dose ketamine reduces tourniquet hypertension under general anaesthesia. Ketamine reduces inotropic requirements in septic patients. In animal models of endotoxic shock, ketamine reduces pulmonary drainage by enhancing haemodynamic stability and reducing pulmonary hypertension and extravasation. Ketamine may be harmful in patients with limited right ventricular reserve and increased PVR. Ketamine and thiopental are incompatible. Ketamine is a drug of misuse and is a Class C drug in the UK.

Drug structure For the drug structure, please see Fig. 5.

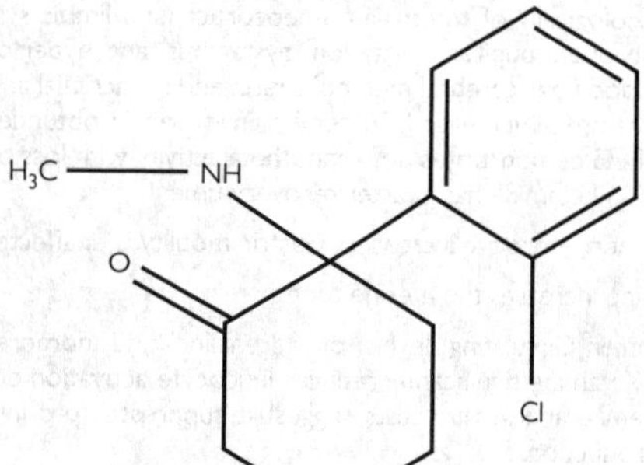

Fig. 5 Drug structure of ketamine.

Ketorolac

Uses Ketorolac is used for the management of moderate to severe post-operative pain.

Chemical Ketorolac trometamol is a dihydropyrrolizine carboxylic acid derivative. It is structurally related to indometacin.

Presentation As topical eye drops in a concentration of 5 mg/ml, and as a clear or pale yellow solution for injection in a concentration of 30 mg/ml.

Main actions Analgesia.

Mode of action Ketorolac is a non-specific inhibitor of COX which converts arachidonic acid to cyclic endoperoxidases, thus preventing the formation of prostaglandins, thromboxanes, and prostacyclin.

Routes of administration/doses Ketorolac may be administered by intramuscular injection or by intravenous bolus administration at an initial dose of 10 mg. Subsequent doses of 10–30 mg may be administered every 4–6 hours for up to 2 days.

The topical ophthalmic dose is one drop to the affected eye three times a day.

Effects

RS Bronchospasm may occur in up to 20% of asthmatic patients.

AS Dyspepsia, nausea, bleeding from gastric and duodenal vessels, mucosal ulceration, perforation, and diarrhoea are expected COX-1 effects. Ketorolac may exacerbate gastrointestinal symptoms in patients with ulcerative colitis and Crohn's disease.

GU Fluid retention may occur in some patients due to salt and water retention, and hence weight gain.

Metabolic/other Ketorolac inhibits platelet aggregation, decreases thromboxane concentrations, and prolongs the bleeding time.

Toxicity/side effects Gastrointestinal side effects are most commonly reported by patients. As with all NSAIDs, ketorolac use may lead to impaired renal function (especially in those patients who are dependent on renal prostaglandin production to maintain renal perfusion), and prolonged use may result in analgesic nephropathy.

All NSAIDs should be used with caution in patients with a history of, or risk factors for, cardiovascular disease, as there is an association between prolonged use of these drugs and arterial thrombotic events.

Kinetics

Absorption Following an intramuscular injection of ketorolac, the drug is rapidly absorbed. A mean peak plasma concentration of 2.2 micrograms/ml occurs 50 minutes after a 30 mg intramuscular injection. Intravenous administration of 30 mg of the drug results in a mean peak plasma concentration of 2.4 micrograms/ml 5.4 minutes after dosing.

Distribution Ketorolac is 99% protein-bound to albumin. The V_D is 13 l.

Metabolism The drug undergoes hepatic metabolism via hydroxylation and conjugation.

Excretion 91.4% of an administered dose is excreted renally; 6.1% of the dose is found in faeces. The total clearance of ketorolac in patients with normal renal function is 0.023 l/hour/kg, with a total half-life of 5.3 hours. In patients with impaired renal function, the half-life is prolonged to 10.3 hours.

Labetalol

Uses Labetalol is used in the treatment of:
1. all grades of hypertension
2. hypertensive emergencies and has been used
3. to produce controlled hypotension during anaesthesia
4. for the control of the reflex cardiovascular responses to intubation and
5. in the management of acute myocardial infarction.

Chemical A synthetic salicylamide derivative.

Presentation As a clear solution for injection containing 5 mg/ml and as 50/100/200/400 mg tablets of labetalol hydrochloride.

Main action Antihypertensive.

Mode of action Labetalol acts by selective antagonism of alpha-1, beta-1, and beta-2 adrenoceptors (the ratio of alpha:beta effects is 1:3 when administered orally, and 1:7 when administered intravenously). The drug has some intrinsic sympathomimetic activity at beta-2 adrenoceptors and may cause some vasodilation directly by stimulation of beta-2 receptors in vascular smooth muscle.

Routes of administration/doses The adult oral dose is 100–800 mg 12-hourly. The drug may also be administered intravenously as a 5–20 mg bolus injected over 2 minutes, with subsequent increments to a maximum adult dose of 200 mg, or by infusion (diluted in glucose or glucose saline) at the rate of 20–160 mg/hour. When administered intravenously, labetalol acts in 5–30 minutes and has a mean duration of action of 50 minutes.

Patients should remain supine, whilst receiving the drug via the intravenous route, and subsequently assume the upright position cautiously, as profound postural hypotension may occur.

Effects

CVS Intravenous labetalol causes a 20% (greater in hypertensive patients) decrease in the systolic and diastolic blood pressure; the heart rate and cardiac output may decrease by 10%. The drug reduces the systemic vascular resistance by 14%; limb blood flow increases, and coronary vascular resistance may decrease. Labetalol inhibits platelet aggregation *in vitro*.

RS With single doses, the drug has no effect on forced expiratory volume in 1 second (FEV$_1$), forced vital capacity (FVC), or specific airways resistance in patients with obstructive airways disease. Chronic use of the drug has no clinically significant effect on respiratory function.

CNS Labetalol has no effect on cerebral blood flow; autoregulation is well maintained.

GU Labetalol decreases renal vascular resistance by 20%, leading to an increase in the renal blood flow. The glomerular filtration rate, however, remains unchanged.

Metabolic/other The concentrations of adrenaline, noradrenaline, and prolactin increase acutely in hypertensive patients given labetalol intravenously. The drug may also decrease plasma renin activity and the concentration of angiotensin II. The erythrocyte sedimentation rate (ESR) and serum transaminase concentration may increase, following the administration of the drug; labetalol has no effect on plasma lipid concentration.

Toxicity/side effects The side effects of beta-blockade (asthma, Raynaud's phenomenon, heart failure, cramps, nightmares, etc.) occur less frequently during the use of labetalol than do the side effects of alpha-blockade (dizziness, formication, nasal congestion, etc.). Gastrointestinal disturbances may also complicate the use of labetalol.

Kinetics

Absorption Labetalol is rapidly absorbed when administered orally, but, due to a significant first-pass metabolism, the bioavailability shows an 8-fold variation (11–86%).

Distribution The drug is 50% protein-bound in the plasma; the V_D is 2.5–15.7 l/kg.

Metabolism Labetalol is extensively metabolized in the liver (and possibly in the gut wall) to several inactive conjugates.

Excretion Occurs predominantly as inactive conjugates in the urine (5% is excreted unchanged), with some appearing in the faeces. The clearance is 13–31 ml/min/kg, and the elimination half-life is 3–8 hours. Renal impairment has no effect on the kinetics of labetalol; the dose should be reduced in the presence of hepatic impairment.

Special points In the presence of concentrations of halothane 3%, labetalol causes a significant decrease in cardiac output, stroke volume, mean arterial pressure, and central venous pressure.

Haemodialysis will remove 1% of a dose of labetalol.

Levetiracetam

Uses Levetiracetam is used:
1. as a single agent for partial seizures
2. as an adjuvant therapy in the treatment of myoclonic epilepsy and generalized epilepsy.

Chemical A pyrrolidone derivative.

Presentation Levetiracetam is available as tablets containing 250, 500, 750, or 1000 mg. The drug is also available as an oral solution containing 100 mg/ml. An intravenous concentrate is available at a concentration of 100 mg/ml presented in a glass vial. The latter must be further diluted into 100 ml of compatible fluid prior to administration.

Main actions Antiepileptic.

Mode of action Levetiracetam acts in a different way to other antiepileptic medications. The mode of action remains to be fully elucidated, but the drug appears to reduce intracellular calcium release. In a rodent model, the drug binds to synaptic vesicle protein 2A, which is involved in excitatory neurotransmitter release. The interaction of levetiracetam and this protein may also contribute to its antiepileptic properties.

Routes of administration/doses Levetiracetam may be administered orally or by intravenous infusion. The recommended adult dose is 500 mg twice daily. The maximum dose is 1500 mg twice daily.

Effects

CNS Somnolence and headache occur in 10% of patients.

AS Levetiracetam causes nasopharyngitis in up to 10% of patients.

Toxicity/side effects Tremors, dizziness, and cutaneous rashes have been reported.

Kinetics

Absorption Very high bioavailability approaching 100%.

Distribution Data incomplete. Very little of the drug is protein-bound.

Metabolism 24% of an administered does undergoes hepatic hydrolysis of the acetamide group to an inactive metabolite.

Excretion 95% of an administered dose is excreted in the urine. The half-life of levetiracetam is 7 hours.

Special points A dose reduction is recommended for patients with moderate to severe renal failure. Levetiracetam does not interact with the cytochrome P450 enzyme system.

Levosimendan

Uses Levosimendan is used in the treatment of acute heart failure syndromes resulting from a variety of aetiologies.

Chemical A propanedinitrile derivative.

Presentation As a clear, yellow, or orange solution for injection containing 2.5 mg/ml of levosimendan in 5 and 10 ml ampoules which needs to be diluted prior to administration.

Main action Positive inotrope and vasodilatation.

Mode of action Levosimendan increases calcium sensitivity by binding to myocardial troponin C, leading to stabilization and increased duration of calcium binding. This results in increased myocardial contractility, without impairment of myocardial relaxation or increased oxygen demand. The drug also stimulates ATP-sensitive K^+ channels, leading to vasodilatation, in addition to myocardial anti-stunning/ischaemic effects.

Routes of administration/doses Levosimendan is administered by intravenous infusion either by peripheral or central routes. An initial loading dose of 6–12 micrograms/kg should be administered over a 10-minute period, followed by an intravenous infusion at a rate of 0.1–0.2 micrograms/kg/min.

Effects

CVS The primary action of levosimendan is to increase myocardial contractility via increased calcium sensitivity, without a corresponding increase in myocardial oxygen demand. The drug also causes coronary and peripheral vasodilatation. This may lead to anti-stunning and anti-ischaemia myocardial effects.

GU The urine output and glomerular filtration rate increase, secondary to the increase in cardiac output.

Metabolic/other Human data have demonstrated a reduction in lactate concentrations, following administration of the drug in patients with septic shock.

Toxicity/side effects Hypotension, headache, nausea, and vomiting are the commonest side effects reported, secondary to the vasodilatory effects of the drug. Hypokalaemia and arrhythmias have also been reported in small numbers of patients.

Kinetics

Distribution Levosimendan is 97–98% bound to albumin; the V_D at steady state is 0.2 l/kg.

Metabolism 95% of an administered dose undergoes hepatic conjugation to cyclic or N-acetylated cysteinylglycine and cysteine conjugates. Five percent of administered levosimendan undergoes intestinal reduction to aminophenylpyridazinone (OR-1855), followed by reabsorption into the plasma where further metabolism occurs by N-acetyltransferase to the active metabolite OR-1896. The rate of metabolism of the drug is genetically determined, although there is no evidence that any clinically significant therapeutic effect occurs between individuals who are rapid or slow acetylators. Levosimendan does not induce or inhibit the cytochrome P450 isoenzyme system.

Excretion 54% of an administered dose is renally excreted, and 44% is found in the faeces. The elimination half-life is approximately 3 hours, and the clearance is 3 ml/kg/hour. Less than 0.05% of levosimendan is excreted unchanged in the urine. The circulating metabolites (OR-1855 and OR-1896) are formed and excreted in a delayed pharmacokinetic profile, reaching a peak plasma concentration approximately 2 days after termination of an infusion of the drug. The metabolites of levosimendan have a half-life of 75–80 hours and are excreted predominantly in the urine.

Special points The drug is not removed by haemodialysis.

Levosimendan may produce a clinical improvement which continues beyond the termination of the treatment period.

There are human data to suggest that administration of the drug may lead to reduced levels of circulating pro-inflammatory cytokines (interleukin-6, IL-6) and soluble apoptosis mediators, in addition to lower concentrations of B-type natriuretic peptide.

Levothyroxine

Uses Thyroid hormones are used in the treatment of:
1. hypothyroidism
2. myxoedema coma, and
3. goitre.

Chemical Both hormones are iodine-containing amino acid derivatives of thyronine.

Presentation Levothyroxine is presented as tablets containing 25/50/100 micrograms of levothyroxine sodium. Triiodothyronine is presented as 20 micrograms tablets and a white lyophilized powder for reconstitution in water containing 20 micrograms of triiodothyronine.

Main action Modulation of growth and metabolism.

Mode of action The thyroid hormones, probably predominantly triiodothyronine, combine with a 'receptor protein' within the cell nucleus and thereby activate the DNA transcription process, leading to an increase in the rate of RNA synthesis and a generalized increase in protein synthesis.

Routes of administration/doses The adult oral dose of levothyroxine is 25–300 micrograms daily in divided doses, titrated according to the clinical response and results of thyroid function tests. The corresponding dose of triiodothyronine is 10–60 micrograms daily; the dose by the intravenous route is 5–20 micrograms 4- to 12-hourly; close monitoring is essential during intravenous administration. There is a 24-hour latency period, before the effects of levothyroxine are manifested; the peak effect occurs in 6–7 days. Triiodothyronine acts in 6 hours, and the peak effect is observed within 24 hours.

Effects

CVS The thyroid hormones are positively inotropic and chronotropic; these effects may be mediated by an increase in the number of myocardial beta-adrenergic receptors. The systolic blood pressure is increased by 10–20 mmHg; the diastolic blood pressure decreases, and the mean arterial pressure remains unchanged. Vasodilation results from the increase in peripheral oxygen consumption; the circulating blood volume also increases slightly.

RS The thyroid hormones increase the rate and depth of respiration, secondary to the increase in the basal metabolic rate.

CNS The hormones have a stimulatory effect on CNS function; tremor and hyperreflexia may result. Their physiological function also includes mediation of negative feedback on the release of thyroid-stimulating hormone from the pituitary.

AS Appetite is increased, following the administration of levothyroxine or triiodothyronine; the secretory activity and motility of the gastrointestinal tract are also increased.

GU The thyroid hormones are involved in the control of sexual function and menstruation.

Metabolic/other Thyroid hormones promote gluconeogenesis and increase the mobilization of glycogen stores. Lipolysis is stimulated, leading to an increase in the concentration of free fatty acids; hypercholesterolaemia may result from increased cholesterol turnover. The rate of protein synthesis is enhanced.

Toxicity/side effects Excessive administration of the thyroid hormones results in the clinical state of thyrotoxicosis.

Kinetics

Absorption Both levothyroxine and triiodothyronine are completely absorbed when administered orally.

Distribution Both hormones are bound to thyroid-binding globulin and thyroid-binding pre-albumin in the plasma; levothyroxine is 99.97% bound, and triiodothyronine is 99.5% bound. The V_D of levothyroxine is 0.2 l/kg, and that of triiodothyronine is 0.5 l/kg.

Metabolism 35% of levothyroxine is converted to triiodothyronine in the periphery (predominantly in the liver and kidney), and some to inactive reverse T3. Both levothyroxine and triiodothyronine undergo conjugation to glucuronide and sulfate, and are excreted in the bile; some enterohepatic circulation occurs.

Excretion 20–40% of an administered dose is excreted in the faeces unchanged. The clearance of levothyroxine is 1.7 ml/min, and the elimination half-life is 6–7 days; the clearance of triiodothyronine is 17 ml/min, and the elimination half-life is 2 days.

Special points The thyroid hormones increase the anticoagulant activity of co-administered warfarin. Beta-adrenergic antagonists interfere with the conversion of levothyroxine to triiodothyronine and lead to a relative increase in the inactive reverse T3 fraction.

Lidocaine

Uses Lidocaine is used:
1. as a local anaesthetic and
2. in the treatment of ventricular tachydysrhythmias, acting as a class Ib antiarrhythmic.

Chemical A tertiary amine which is an amide derivative of diethylaminacetic acid.

Presentation As a clear, colourless solution in concentrations of 0.5/1/1.5/2% solution of lidocaine hydrochloride (with or without 1:200 000 adrenaline); a gel containing of 21.4 mg/ml of lidocaine hydrochloride (with or without chlorhexidine gluconate); a 5% ointment, a 10% spray, and a 4% aqueous solution for topical application; and as a cream/suppositories (in combination with hydrocortisone) for rectal administration. The 1% and 2% preparations are available with or without the preservatives methylhydroxybenzoate (1.7 mg/ml) and propylhydroxybenzoate (0.3 mg/ml). Hydrochloric acid and sodium hydroxide are also present in some formulations (the latter to a maximum of 1%). The pKa of lidocaine is 7.7 and is 25% unionized at a pH of 7.4. The heptane:buffer partition coefficient is 2.9.

Main action Local anaesthetic.

Mode of action Local anaesthetics diffuse in their uncharged base form through neural sheaths and the axonal membrane to the internal surface of cell membrane Na^+ channels; here they combine with hydrogen ions to form a cationic species which enters the internal opening of the Na^+ channel and combines with a receptor. This produces blockade of the Na^+ channel, thereby decreasing Na^+ conductance and preventing depolarization of the cell membrane.

Routes of administration/doses Lidocaine may be administered topically, by infiltration, intrathecally, or epidurally; the toxic dose of lidocaine is 3 mg/kg (7 mg/kg with adrenaline). The maximum dose is 300 mg (500 mg with adrenaline). The adult intravenous dose for the treatment of acute ventricular dysrhythmias is a bolus injection of 1 mg/kg, administered over 2 minutes. A second dose may be administered according to the response of the patient. This is normally followed by an infusion at a rate of 20–50 micrograms/kg/min. Lidocaine acts in 2–20 minutes (dependent on the rate of administration and the presence of vasoconstrictors and the concentrations used). The speed of onset of lidocaine may be increased by the addition of bicarbonate to increase the pH of the solution, thereby increasing the unionized fraction of drug. The pH of the drug is approximately 6.4.

Effects

CVS In low concentrations, lidocaine decreases the rate of rise of phase 0 of the cardiac action potential by blockade of inactivated sodium channels.

This results in a rise in the threshold potential, with the duration of the action potential and effective refractory period being shortened. It has few haemodynamic effects when used in low doses, except to cause a slight increase in the systemic vascular resistance, leading to a mild increase in the blood pressure. In toxic concentrations, the drug decreases the peripheral vascular resistance and myocardial contractility, producing hypotension and possibly cardiovascular collapse.

RS The drug causes bronchodilatation at subtoxic concentrations. Respiratory depression occurs in the toxic dose range.

CNS The principal effect of lidocaine is reversible neural blockade; this leads to a characteristically biphasic effect in the CNS. Initially, excitation (light-headedness, dizziness, visual and auditory disturbances, and seizure activity) occurs due to inhibition of inhibitory interneurone pathways in the cortex. With increasing doses, depression of both facilitatory and inhibitory pathways occurs, leading to CNS depression (drowsiness, disorientation, and coma). Local anaesthetic agents block neuromuscular transmission when administered intraneurally; it is thought that a complex of neurotransmitter, receptor, and local anaesthetic is formed, which has negligible conductance.

AS Local anaesthetics depress contraction of the intact bowel.

Metabolic/other Lidocaine may have some anticholinergic and antihistaminergic activity.

Toxicity/side effects Lidocaine is intrinsically less toxic than bupivacaine. Allergic reactions to the amide-type local anaesthetic agents are extremely rare. The side effects are predominantly correlated with excessive plasma concentrations of the drug, as described above. Methaemoglobinaemia may occur if doses in excess of 600 mg are used and is caused by the metabolite O-toluidine, although this condition may occur at lower doses in patients suffering from anaemia or a haemoglobinopathy or in patients receiving therapy known to also precipitate methaemoglobinaemia (sulfonamides). Use of lidocaine for paracervical block or pudendal nerve block in obstetric patients is not recommended, as this may give rise to methaemoglobinaemia in the neonate, as the erythrocytes are deficient in methaemoglobin reductase.

Kinetics

Absorption The absorption of local anaesthetic agents is related to:
1. the site of injection (intercostal > caudal > epidural > brachial plexus > subcutaneous)
2. the dose—a linear relationship exists between the total dose and the peak blood concentrations achieved, and
3. the presence of vasoconstrictors which delay absorption.

Distribution Lidocaine is 64–70% protein-bound in the plasma, predominantly to alpha-1 acid glycoprotein; the V_D is 0.7–1.5 l/kg.

Metabolism Lidocaine is metabolized in the liver by N-dealkylation, with subsequent hydrolysis to monoethylglycine and xylidide. Monoethylglycine is further hydrolysed, whilst xylidide undergoes hydroxylation to 4-hydroxy-2,6-xylidine which is the main metabolite and excreted in the urine. Metabolites of lidocaine may lower the fit threshold, thereby potentiating seizure activity, whilst others have some antiarrhythmic properties.

Excretion Less than 10% of the dose is excreted unchanged in the urine. The clearance is 6.8–11.6 ml/min/kg, and the elimination half-life is 90–110 minutes. The clearance is reduced in the presence of cardiac and hepatic failure.

Special points The onset and duration of conduction blockade are related to the pKa, lipid solubility, and the extent of protein binding. A low pKa and high lipid solubility are associated with a rapid onset time; a high degree of protein binding is associated with a long duration of action. Local anaesthetic agents significantly increase the duration of action of both depolarizing and non-depolarizing relaxants.

Due to the narrow therapeutic index of lidocaine, the plasma concentrations of the drug need to be monitored in patients with cardiac and hepatic impairment.

Lidocaine is not removed by haemodialysis.

Intravenous administration of lidocaine decreases N_2O and halothane requirements by 10% and 28%, respectively.

EMLA® (Eutectic Mixture of Local Anaesthetics) is a white cream used to provide topical anaesthesia prior to venepuncture and has also been used to provide anaesthesia for split skin grafting. It contains 2.5% prilocaine and 2.5% lidocaine in an oil–water emulsion. When applied topically under an occlusive dressing, local anaesthesia is achieved after 1–2 hours and lasts for up to 5 hours. The preparation causes temporary blanching and oedema of the skin; detectable methaemoglobinaemia may also occur in the presence of excessive O-toluidine plasma levels as a metabolite of prilocaine.

Lidocaine

Linezolid

Uses Linezolid is used in the treatment of:
1. nosocomial and community-acquired pneumonia
2. complex skin and soft tissue infections, and
3. MRSA infection and vancomycin-resistant *Enterococcus* (VRE).

Chemical An oxazolidinone.

Presentation As 600 mg tablets and a solution for intravenous administration containing 2 mg/ml of linezolid.

Main action Antibacterial active against a wide range of Gram-positive organisms, particularly *Enterococcus*, *Streptococcus*, and staphylococcal spp., and Gram-positive anaerobes, including *Clostridium perfringens*.

Mode of action Linezolid inhibits bacterial protein synthesis by binding specifically to the 50S ribosomal subunit, thereby preventing initiation complex formation.

Routes of administration/doses The adult oral and intravenous dose is 600 mg 12-hourly.

Toxicity/side effects Headache, abnormalities of liver function tests, taste alteration, and gastrointestinal disturbances are common. Fertility may be affected reversibly. Skin and bleeding disorders, phlebitis, and pancreatitis may also occur.

Kinetics

Absorption Linezolid is rapidly absorbed after oral administration and has an oral bioavailability approaching 100%.

Distribution The drug is 31% protein-bound in the plasma; the V_D is 0.64 l/kg.

Metabolism Linezolid is metabolized by oxidation to two inactive carboxylic acid metabolites.

Excretion 30% is excreted unchanged in the urine; the metabolites are excreted in the urine and faeces. The elimination half-life is 5 hours, and the clearance 120 ml/min.

Special points Linezolid is a reversible non-selective MAOI. It enhances the effects of ephedrine on the blood pressure.

Lithium

Uses Lithium is used in the treatment of:
1. mania and hypomania and in the prophylaxis of
2. recurrent bipolar depression
3. recurrent affective disorders, and
4. as an adjunct in the treatment of chronic pain of non-malignant origin.

Chemical An alkali metal.

Presentation As tablets containing 200/250/400/450 mg of lithium carbonate.

Main action Antipsychotic.

Mode of action The precise mode of action of lithium is unknown; it may act by stabilization of membranes or by alteration of central neurotransmitter function.

Routes of administration/doses The adult oral dose is 0.4–1.2 g/day; serum levels should be monitored within 1 week of starting lithium and regularly thereafter, as the drug has a narrow therapeutic index. The therapeutic level is 0.5–1.5 mmol/l.

Effects

CVS Prolonged lithium therapy may lead to reversible ECG changes, especially T-wave depression.

CNS The drug has no effect on CNS function in normal subjects, although an increase in muscle tone occurs commonly. Lithium appears to lower the seizure threshold in epileptics.

GU Over one-third of patients receiving lithium develop polyuria and polydipsia due to antagonism of the effects of ADH.

Metabolic/other With prolonged use of lithium, retention of sodium (secondary to an increase in aldosterone secretion) may occur, as may hypercalcaemia and hypermagnesaemia. The drug has mild insulin-like effects on carbohydrate metabolism.

Toxicity/side effects At therapeutic serum levels, disturbances of thyroid function, weight gain, tremor, pretibial oedema, and allergic phenomena may occur. Excessive serum concentrations may result in nausea and vomiting, abdominal pain, diarrhoea, ataxia, convulsions, coma, dysrhythmias, and death. Nephrogenic diabetes insipidus occurs in 5–20% of patients on long-term lithium treatment.

Kinetics

Absorption The drug is rapidly absorbed when administered orally; the bioavailability is 100%.

Distribution Lithium exhibits no demonstrable protein binding in the plasma; the V_D is 0.45–1.13 l/kg.

Excretion 95% of a dose of lithium is excreted in the urine, the remainder in sweat. The clearance is 0.24–0.46 ml/min/kg, and the elimination half-life is 14–30 hours.

Special points Renal, cardiac, and thyroid function should be monitored regularly during lithium therapy. Co-administration of lithium and diazepam has been reported to lead to hypothermia; the drug may also increase the duration of action of both depolarizing and non-depolarizing relaxants.

The drug is removed by haemodialysis.

Lorazepam

Uses Lorazepam is used:
1. in the short-term treatment of anxiety
2. as a hypnotic
3. in premedication and
4. for the treatment of status epilepticus.

Chemical A hydroxybenzodiazepine.

Presentation As 1/2.5 mg tablets and as a clear, colourless solution for injection containing 4 mg/ml of lorazepam.

Main actions
1. Hypnosis
2. Sedation
3. Anxiolysis
4. Anterograde amnesia
5. Anticonvulsant, and
6. Muscular relaxation.

Mode of action Benzodiazepines are thought to act via specific benzodiazepine receptors found at synapses throughout the CNS, but concentrated especially in the cortex and midbrain. Benzodiazepine receptors are closely linked with GABA receptors and appear to facilitate the activity of the latter. Activated GABA receptors open chloride ion channels which then either hyperpolarize or short-circuit the synaptic membrane.

Routes of administration/doses The adult oral or sublingual dose is 1–4 mg/day in divided doses. The intravenous or intramuscular dose is 0.025–0.05 mg/kg; intramuscular injection is painful.

Effects
CVS Lorazepam appears to have no direct cardiac effects.

RS Mild respiratory depression occurs, following the administration of the drug, which is of clinical significance only in patients with lung disease.

CNS The drug produces sedation, anterograde amnesia, and an anticonvulsant effect.

AS Lorazepam has no effect on basal gastric acid secretion but decreases pentagastrin-stimulated gastric acid secretion by 25%.

Metabolic/other Circulating cortisol and glucose levels fall when lorazepam is used in premedication, probably secondarily to its anxiolytic effect.

Toxicity/side effects Drowsiness, sedation, confusion, and impaired coordination occur in a dose-dependent fashion. Paradoxical stimulation has been reported and occurs more frequently when hyoscine is administered concurrently. Tolerance and dependence may occur with prolonged use of benzodiazepines; acute withdrawal of benzodiazepines in these circumstances may produce insomnia, anxiety, confusion, psychosis, and perceptual disturbances.

Kinetics

Absorption Lorazepam has a bioavailability of 90% when administered by the oral or intramuscular route.

Distribution The drug is 88–92% protein-bound in the plasma; the V_D is 1 l/kg. Lorazepam is less extensively distributed than diazepam and thus has a longer duration of action despite the shorter elimination half-life of lorazepam.

Metabolism Lorazepam is conjugated directly in the liver to glucuronide to form an inactive water-soluble metabolite.

Excretion 80% of an orally administered dose appears in the urine as the glucuronide. The clearance is 1 ml/min/kg, and the elimination half-life is 8–25 hours—this is unaffected by renal disease.

Special points The co-administration of cimetidine does not impair the metabolic clearance of lorazepam.

   The drug is not removed by haemodialysis.

Macrolides

Uses Macrolides are used in the treatment of:
1. respiratory tract infections
2. skin, soft tissue, and bone infections
3. ocular, ear, and oral infections
4. gastrointestinal infections
5. GU infections
6. as surgical prophylaxis and
7. for the prophylaxis of subacute bacterial endocarditis
8. and have been used as a prokinetic in intensive care.

Chemical A macrocyclic lactone ring to which deoxy sugars are attached.

Presentation Macrolides in clinical use include erythromycin, clarithromycin, and azithromycin. Erythromycin is available in a form for topical use as a treatment for acne vulgaris, as a powder for oral suspension, in tablet and capsule formulations, and as an intravenous formulation. Clarithromycin is available as an oral preparation or for intravenous use. The drug is also available in combination with other agents for *Helicobacter pylori* eradication therapy. Azithromycin is available in tablet, oral suspension, or intravenous formulations.

Main action Macrolides are bactericidal/bacteriostatic antibiotics that are active predominantly against:
1. Gram-positive bacteria
2. some Gram-negative bacteria (particularly with azithromycin)
3. Gram-positive and negative anaerobes
4. obligate intracellular parasites (*Legionella, Mycoplasma*).

Mode of action Macrolides bind to specific bacterial ribosomal proteins (50S subunit) and inhibit peptide translocase, thereby preventing the formation of polymerized peptides.

Routes of administration/doses Macrolides may be administered topically as creams or ointments, orally or intravenously, or via the intrathecal/intraventricular route. The specific dose, route, and frequency of an agent administered are dependent on the clinical indication, age of the patient, and particular agent being used. Doses should be reduced in patients with renal impairment.

Effects

AS Erythromycin has a prokinetic effect on gut motility.

Toxicity/side effects Common side effects include nausea, vomiting, and diarrhoea. Hepatic dysfunction, allergic phenomena, and ototoxicity have also been reported.

Kinetics

Absorption Macrolides are absorbed to varying degrees, depending on the specific agent: erythromycin (10–60%), clarithromycin (50%), azithromycin (37%). Erythromycin undergoes first-pass metabolism.

Distribution The V_D for erythromycin is 0.34–1.22 l/kg, and for azithromycin 0.44 l/kg. The percentage of drug bound to plasma proteins is 81–87% for erythromycin, 8% for clarithromycin, and 12–50% for azithromycin. High concentrations are found within the lung tissue. The CSF is poorly penetrated by these agents.

Metabolism Macrolides undergo hepatic metabolism in man. Erythromycin undergoes demethylation; clarithromycin is converted to 14-hydroxyclarithromycin as part of first-pass metabolism. This metabolite is microbiologically active. Clarithromycin is also metabolized in the liver via N-dealkylation. Azithromycin is metabolized via hepatic N- and O-demethylation to inactive metabolites.

Excretion Erythromycin and clarithromycin are excreted renally. The clearance of erythromycin is 5–13.2 ml/min/kg; the half-life is 1.6 hours, with 2–15% of the drug being excreted unchanged in the urine. The clearance of clarithromycin is unknown, as it exhibits non-linear kinetics; the half-life is 5–6 hours, with 33% of the drug being excreted unchanged in the urine and 11% as the 14-hydroxyclarithromycin metabolite. Ten percent of an administered dose of clarithromycin is excreted via the bile. Azithromycin has a clearance of 10.18 ml/kg/min, a prolonged half-life of 68 hours, with 12% of the drug being excreted unchanged in the urine. The major excretion pathway for azithromycin is via the bile.

Special points Erythromycin and clarithromycin may cause QT prolongation in the critically ill. All macrolides inhibit CYP450 3A4, which may lead to increased drug levels of the following agents if administered concurrently to a patient: methylprednisolone, warfarin, phenytoin, ciclosporin, theophylline, sodium valproate, tacrolimus, midazolam, digoxin.

Erythromycin and clarithromycin are not removed by haemofiltration or dialysis, and, therefore, the dose should be halved in patients receiving renal replacement therapy. No dose adjustment is necessary for azithromycin.

Erythromycin should be avoided in patients with suspected or confirmed porphyria.

Antimicrobial agents should always be administered, following consideration of local pharmacy and microbiological policies.

Magnesium

Uses Magnesium has been used in the management of:
1. pre-eclampsia and eclampsia
2. hypomagnesaemia associated with malabsorption syndromes (especially chronic alcoholism), diuretics, and critical illness
3. premature labour (as a tocolytic)
4. acute myocardial infarction
5. torsades de pointes and other ventricular dysrhythmias
6. barium poisoning
7. asthma
8. cerebral oedema
9. spasms occurring with tetanus
10. autonomic hyperreflexia secondary to chronic spinal cord injury and is
11. a component of cardioplegic solutions.

Chemical An inorganic sulfate.

Presentation A clear, colourless solution of magnesium sulfate containing 2.03 mmol/ml of ionic magnesium 50%.

Main actions Magnesium is an essential cofactor in over 300 enzyme systems. It is also essential for the production of ATP, DNA, RNA, and protein function.

Mode of action The precise mechanism of the anticonvulsant activity of magnesium remains unknown; it produces a dose-dependent pre-synaptic inhibition of acetylcholine release at the neuromuscular junction.

Routes of administration/doses Magnesium sulfate may be administered intravenously or intramuscularly. A number of dose regimes have been described for the use of magnesium sulfate in the management of pre-eclampsia, e.g. 16 mmol administered intravenously over 20 minutes followed by an infusion of 4–8 mmol/hour. Serum concentrations should be monitored repeatedly, and the dose adjusted correspondingly. Loss of deep tendon reflexes is a useful clinical sign of impending toxicity.

Effects

CVS Magnesium acts peripherally to cause vasodilation and may cause hypotension when used in high doses. The drug slows the rate of sinoatrial node impulse formation and prolongs sinoatrial conduction time, the PR interval, and AV nodal effective refractory period. Magnesium attenuates both the vasoconstrictor and arrhythmogenic actions of adrenaline.

RS Magnesium is an effective bronchodilator and attenuates hypoxic pulmonary vasoconstriction.

CNS The drug is a CNS depressant and exhibits anticonvulsant properties. High concentrations inhibit catecholamine release from adrenergic nerve terminals and the adrenal medulla.

AS Magnesium sulfate acts as an osmotic laxative when administered orally.

GU The drug exerts a renal vasodilator and diuretic effect. It decreases uterine tone and contractility; placental perfusion may increase, secondary to a decrease in uterine vascular resistance. Magnesium crosses the placenta and may cause neonatal hypotonia and neonatal depression.

Metabolic/other Magnesium prolongs the clotting time of whole blood, decreases thromboxane B2 synthesis, and inhibits thrombin-induced platelet aggregation.

Toxicity/side effects Minor side effects include warmth, flushing, nausea, headache, and dizziness. Dose-related side effects include somnolence, areflexia, AV and intraventricular conduction disorders, progressive muscular weakness, and cardiac arrest. The toxic effects can be reversed by the administration of calcium. Intramuscular injection of magnesium sulfate is painful.

Kinetics

Absorption 25–65% of ingested magnesium is absorbed.

Distribution Magnesium is 30% protein-bound in the plasma.

Excretion More than 50% of an exogenous magnesium load is excreted in the urine, even in the presence of significant magnesium deficiency.

Special points Magnesium enhances the effects of other CNS depressants and NMB agents; 30–50% of the normal dose of non-depolarizing relaxants should be used to maintain neuromuscular blockade in the presence of magnesium sulfate. Acute administration of magnesium sulfate prior to the use of suxamethonium appears to prevent potassium release and may reduce the incidence and severity of muscle pains.

Magnesium deficiency is present in 20–65% of patients receiving intensive care.

Mannitol

Uses Mannitol is used:
1. to reduce the pressure and volume of CSF
2. to preserve renal function during the perioperative period in jaundiced patients and in those undergoing major vascular surgery
3. in the short-term management of patients with acute glaucoma
4. for bowel preparation prior to colorectal procedures
5. to initiate a diuresis in transplanted kidneys, and
6. in the treatment of rhabdomyolysis.

Chemical An alcohol, derived from *Dahlia* tubers.

Presentation As sterile, pyrogen-free solutions of 10% and 20% mannitol in water; crystallization may occur at low temperatures.

Main actions Osmotic diuresis and antioxidant.

Mode of action Mannitol is a low-molecular-weight (182 daltons) compound and is thus freely filtered at the glomerulus and not reabsorbed, nor does it cross the intact blood–brain barrier. Its action as a diuretic rests upon the fact that it increases the osmolality of the glomerular filtrate and tubular fluid, increasing urinary volume by an osmotic effect. Mannitol decreases CSF volume and pressure by:
1. decreasing the rate of CSF formation and
2. by withdrawing brain extracellular water across the blood–brain barrier into the plasma; if the barrier is disrupted, mannitol passes into the brain extravascular space and is ineffective.

Mannitol also acts as a hydroxyl radical scavenger.

Routes of administration/doses For the reduction of elevated intracranial pressure, a dose of 1 g/kg is infused intravenously over 15 minutes prior to operative treatment. Subsequently, intermittent doses of 0.25–0.5 g/kg may be used for the treatment of persistently elevated intracranial pressure. The diuretic dose is 0.5–1 g/kg. Mannitol acts within a few minutes and lasts 1–4 hours.

The oral dose for bowel preparation is 100 ml of the 20% solution—care should be taken to maintain adequate hydration.

Effects

CVS The acute administration of mannitol increases the cardiac output; blood pressure increases by 5–10 mmHg.

CNS Mannitol induces a significant reduction in intracranial pressure with preservation of cerebral blood flow in patients with intact autoregulation; in patients with defective autoregulation, a minimal reduction in intracranial pressure with an increase in cerebral blood flow occurs.

GU Renal blood flow is increased, and the rate of renin secretion decreases; mannitol washes out the medullary interstitial gradient, leading to a decreased ability to produce concentrated urine. Diuresis occurs 1–3 hours after administration.

Metabolic/other The plasma sodium and potassium concentrations may fall and that of urea increase with the use of high doses of mannitol.

Toxicity/side effects Circulatory overload and rebound increases in intracranial pressure may occur, following the use of mannitol. Allergic responses are rare; the drug is irritant to tissues and veins. Mannitol may have toxic effects on the distal convoluted tubule and collecting duct cells, causing vacuolization.

Kinetics

Absorption After oral administration, approximately 17.5% is absorbed in the small bowel.

Distribution The drug shows a biphasic distribution to plasma and extracellular water; complex fluid shifts occur in response to this. The V_D is 0.47 l/kg.

Metabolism Mannitol is not metabolized in man.

Excretion The drug is excreted unchanged in the urine; the clearance is 7 ml/min/kg, and the elimination half-life is 72 minutes.

Special points Blood should not be co-administered with mannitol. A total dose exceeding 3 g/kg/day may produce a serum osmolality >320 mOsm/l. Rebound increases in intracranial pressure may occur after the cessation of mannitol therapy.

Metaraminol

Uses Metaraminol is used as an adjunct in the treatment of hypotension occurring during general or neuroaxial anaesthesia.

Chemical A synthetic sympathomimetic amine.

Presentation As a clear solution containing 10 mg/ml of metaraminol tartrate.

Main action Peripheral vasoconstriction.

Mode of action Metaraminol is a direct- and indirect-acting sympathomimetic agent that has agonist effects mainly at alpha-1 adrenoceptors, but also has some beta-adrenoceptor activity. The drug also causes noradrenaline to be released from intracytoplasmic stores, in addition to causing adrenaline release.

Routes of administration/doses The adult dose by intravenous infusion of metaraminol diluted in saline or glucose should be titrated according to response; bolus doses of 0.5–5 mg may be administered intravenously with extreme caution. The corresponding intramuscular or subcutaneous dose for the prevention of hypotension is 2–10 mg. The onset of effect after intravenous administration occurs within 1–2 minutes, with maximum effect at 10 minutes, and lasts 20–60 minutes. The onset of effect after intramuscular or subcutaneous administration occurs within 10 minutes and lasts 1–1.5 hours.

Effects

CVS Metaraminol causes a sustained increase in the systolic and diastolic blood pressures due to an increase in the systemic vascular resistance; it also increases PVR. A reflex bradycardia occurs. The drug has positive inotropic properties, although the cardiac output may fall due to the increase in systemic vascular resistance. Coronary blood flow is increased by metaraminol by an indirect mechanism.

RS The drug causes a slight decrease in the respiratory rate and an increase in the tidal volume.

CNS The cerebral blood flow is decreased by the administration of metaraminol.

GU The renal blood flow is decreased by metaraminol, and the drug causes contraction of the pregnant uterus and reduces uterine artery blood flow via its effect at alpha-adrenoceptors.

Metabolic/other Metaraminol increases glycogenolysis and inhibits insulin release, leading to hyperglycaemia. Lipolysis is increased, and the concentration of free fatty acids may become elevated. The drug may increase oxygen consumption and elevate body temperature.

Toxicity/side effects Headaches, dizziness, tremor, nausea, and vomiting may occur with the use of the drug. Rapid and large increases in blood pressure resulting in left ventricular failure and cardiac arrest have been reported after the administration of metaraminol. Extravascular injection of the drug may lead to tissue necrosis and abscess formation at the injection site.

Excessive hypertension may occur when metaraminol is administered to patients with hyperthyroidism or those receiving MAOIs.

Kinetics There are limited quantitative data available. The effect starts 1–2 minutes after intravenous injection, 10 minutes after intramuscular injection, and 5–20 minutes after subcutaneous injection. It is reportedly 45% protein-bound.

The drug does not cross the blood–brain barrier.

Metformin

Uses Metformin is used in the treatment of non-insulin-dependent (type II) diabetes mellitus.

Chemical A biguanide.

Presentation As 500/850 mg tablets of metformin hydrochloride.

Main action Hypoglycaemia.

Mode of action Biguanides have no effect in the absence of circulating insulin; they do not alter insulin concentration but do enhance its peripheral action. They appear to act by inhibiting the intestinal absorption of glucose and decreasing the peripheral utilization of glucose, both by increasing the rate of anaerobic glycolysis and by decreasing the rate of gluconeogenesis.

Routes of administration/doses The adult oral dose is 1.5–3 g daily in divided doses. Metformin has a duration of action of 8–12 hours.

Effects

CVS Metformin reduces the intestinal absorption of glucose, folate, and vitamin B12; it has no effects on gastric motility. The drug may also increase the intestinal utilization of glucose and cause weight loss.

Metabolic/other Metformin increases the sensitivity to the peripheral actions of insulin by increasing the number of low-affinity binding sites for insulin in red blood cells, adipocytes, hepatocytes, and skeletal muscle cells. The drug does not cause hypoglycaemia in diabetic subjects receiving metformin monotherapy. Metformin inhibits the metabolism of lactate and causes a decrease in the plasma triglyceride, cholesterol, and pre-beta lipoprotein concentrations.

Toxicity/side effects Metformin is normally well tolerated; gastrointestinal disturbances may occur. Lactic acidosis may complicate the use of the drug rarely.

Kinetics

Absorption The drug is slowly absorbed from the small intestine; the oral bioavailability is 50–60%.

Distribution Metformin is not protein-bound in the plasma.

Metabolism No metabolites of the drug have been detected in man.

Excretion The drug is excreted essentially unchanged in the urine. The clearance exceeds the glomerular filtration rate, implying active tubular secretion. The elimination half-life is 1.7–4.5 hours. The drug is not recommended for use in patients with renal impairment.

Methohexital

Uses Methohexital is used for the induction and maintenance of anaesthesia.

Chemical A methylated oxybarbiturate.

Presentation As a white, crystalline powder in vials containing 0.1/ 0.5 g of methohexital sodium mixed with sodium carbonate; this is dissolved in water before administration to yield a clear, colourless solution with a pH of 11 and a pKa of 7.9, which is stable in solution for 6 weeks.

Main action Hypnotic.

Mode of action Barbiturates are thought to act primarily at synapses by depressing post-synaptic sensitivity to neurotransmitters and by impairing pre-synaptic neurotransmitter release. Multi-synaptic pathways are depressed preferentially; the reticular activating system is particularly sensitive to the depressant effects of barbiturates. The action of barbiturates at the molecular level is unknown. They may act in a manner analogous to that of local anaesthetic agents by entering cell membranes in the unionized form, subsequently becoming ionized and exerting a membrane-stabilizing effect by decreasing Na^+ and K^+ conductance, decreasing the amplitude of the action potential, and slowing the rate of conduction in excitable tissue. In high concentrations, barbiturates depress the enzymes involved in glucose oxidation, inhibit the formation of ATP, and depress calcium-dependent action potentials. They also inhibit calcium-dependent neurotransmitter release and enhance chloride ion conductance in the absence of GABA.

Routes of administration/doses The drug is usually administered intravenously in a dose of 1–1.5 mg/kg; it acts in one arm–brain circulation time, and awakening occurs in 2–3 minutes. The drug may also be administered intramuscularly in a dose of 6.6 mg/kg or rectally in a dose of 15–20 mg/kg.

Effects

CVS Methohexital has negatively inotropic effects and decreases the systemic vascular resistance; it may also depress transmission in autonomic ganglia and thus lead to hypotension.

RS Methohexital is a more powerful respiratory depressant than thiopental and obtunds the ventilatory response to both hypoxia and hypercarbia. The drug may cause pronounced coughing and hiccuping.

CNS At low doses, methohexital may cause paradoxical excitement. Induction of anaesthesia with the drug is associated with an increased incidence of excitatory phenomena when compared to thiopental. Methohexital decreases both the cerebral blood flow and intracranial pressure. The drug may cause epileptiform EEG patterns; abnormal muscle movements may also occur due to neurotransmitter release.

AS The drug causes some depression of intestinal activity and constriction of the splanchnic vasculature.

GU Methohexital decreases renal plasma flow and increases ADH secretion, leading to a decrease in the urine output. It has no effect on the tone of the gravid uterus.

Metabolic/other The drug decreases the production of superoxide anions by polymorphonuclear leucocytes.

Toxicity/side effects Methohexital causes pain on injection in up to 80% of patients. It is less irritant than thiopental when extravasation occurs but, when administered intra-arterially, may lead to arterial constriction and thrombosis. Anaphylactoid reactions occur with a frequency similar to that observed with thiopental. Nausea and vomiting may complicate the use of methohexital.

Kinetics

Distribution The drug is 51–65% protein-bound in the plasma, predominantly to albumin; 20% is sequestered in red blood cells; the V_D is 1.13 l/kg. The rapid onset of action of the drug is due to:
1. the high blood flow to the brain
2. the lipophilicity of the drug and
3. its low degree of ionization—only the non-ionized fraction crosses the blood–brain barrier (methohexital is 75% non-ionized at pH 7.4; hyperventilation increases the non-bound fraction and increases the anaesthetic effect). The relatively brief duration of anaesthesia following a bolus of methohexital is due to redistribution to muscle and later to fat. Methohexital has a shorter duration of action than thiopental due to its very short distribution half-life and a high clearance which is four times greater than that of thiopental.

Metabolism Occurs in the liver, primarily to a 4-hydroxy metabolite.

Excretion The metabolites are excreted in the urine; 1% of the dose is excreted unchanged. The clearance is 7.9–13.9 ml/min/kg, and the elimination half-life is 1.8–6 hours.

Special points The drug may induce acute clinical and biochemical manifestations in patients with porphyria and is also not recommended for use in epileptics. Methohexital should be used with caution in patients with fixed cardiac output states, hepatic or renal dysfunction, myxoedema, dystrophia myotonica, myasthenia gravis, familial periodic paralysis, and in the elderly or in patients who are hypovolaemic.

Methoxamine

Uses Methoxamine is used for:
1. the correction or prevention of hypotension during spinal or general anaesthesia and cardiopulmonary bypass and
2. the treatment of supraventricular tachycardias.

Chemical A synthetic sympathomimetic amine.

Presentation As a clear solution containing 20 mg/ml of methoxamine hydrochloride.

Main actions Peripheral vasoconstriction and bradycardia.

Mode of action Methoxamine is a selective alpha-1 adrenergic agonist.

Routes of administration/doses Methoxamine is administered intravenously at a rate of 1 mg/min to a total dose of 5–10 mg in an adult; it acts within 1–2 minutes and has a duration of action of 1 hour. The corresponding intramuscular dose is 5–20 mg when the onset of action is 15–20 minutes, and the duration of effect is 90 minutes.

Effects

CVS Methoxamine commonly produces a reflex and intrinsic bradycardia, accompanied by an increase in the systolic and diastolic blood pressures and central venous pressure. The drug has no effect on the cardiac output but prolongs the effective refractory period and slows AV conduction.

RS The drug has no effect on respiratory function.

AS Contraction of gastrointestinal sphincters follows the administration of methoxamine.

GU The drug produces renal arterial vasoconstriction, leading to a fall in the glomerular filtration rate. Contraction of the pregnant uterus and a decrease in uterine blood flow may occur.

Metabolic/other Mydriasis, piloerection, and diaphoresis are produced by the drug. Glycogenolysis and gluconeogenesis are stimulated; this is accompanied by a decrease in insulin secretion.

Toxicity/side effects Headaches, projectile vomiting, sensations of coldness, and the desire to urinate have been reported in association with the use of methoxamine.

Kinetics There are no data available.

Special points The drug may precipitate severe hypertension in patients with uncontrolled hyperthyroidism or who are receiving MAOIs or tricyclic antidepressants.

Methyldopa

Uses Methyldopa is used in the treatment of:
1. hypertension and
2. pre-eclampsia.

Chemical A phenylalanine derivative.

Presentation As 125/250/500 mg tablets and a suspension containing 50 mg/ml of methyldopa. A solution for intravenous administration containing 50 mg/ml of methyldopa hydrochloride is also available.

Main actions Antihypertensive.

Mode of action Methyldopa is metabolized to alpha-methyl noradrenaline which is stored in adrenergic nerve terminals within the CNS; the latter is a potent agonist at alpha-2 (pre-synaptic) nerve terminals and reduces central sympathetic discharge, thereby lowering the blood pressure (cf. clonidine).

Routes of administration/doses The adult oral dose is 0.5–3 g/day in 2–3 divided doses.

Effects

CVS Methyldopa decreases the systemic vascular resistance, with little accompanying change in either the cardiac output or heart rate. Postural hypotension occurs uncommonly with the use of the drug.

GU Methyldopa has little effect on the renal or uteroplacental blood flow, the glomerular filtration rate, or filtration fraction.

Metabolic/other Plasma renin activity and noradrenaline concentrations decrease after administration of the drug.

Toxicity/side effects The reported side effects after the administration of methyldopa are numerous. CVS disturbances that may result from the use of the drug include orthostatic hypotension, bradycardia, and peripheral oedema. CNS disturbances may also occur, including sedation, depression, weakness, paraesthesiae, and dizziness. Gastrointestinal, dermatological, and haematological disturbances, including thrombocytopenia, a positive Coombs' test (in 10–20%), and haemolytic anaemia, have also been reported. Methyldopa may also cause hepatic damage.

Kinetics

Absorption Methyldopa has a variable absorption when administered orally; the bioavailability is 8–62% by this route due to a significant first-pass metabolism.

Distribution The drug is 50% protein-bound in the plasma; the V_D is 0.21–0.37 l/kg.

Metabolic/other Methyldopa is conjugated to sulfate, as it traverses the intestinal mucosa and is metabolized in the liver to a variety of poorly characterized metabolites.

Excretion 20–40% of an administered dose is excreted in the urine, two-thirds of this unchanged. The clearance is 2.2–4 ml/min/kg, and the elimination half-life is 2.1–2.8 hours.

Special points The hypotension effects of the drug are additive with those produced by volatile anaesthetic agents; methyldopa also decreases the apparent MAC of the latter.

The action of the drug is prolonged in the presence of renal failure; it is removed by haemodialysis.

Methyldopa commonly produces nasal congestion; care should be exercised during nasal intubation in patients receiving the drug.

Methylphenidate

Uses Methylphenidate is used for the treatment of:
1. attention-deficit/hyperactivity disorder (ADHD)
2. narcolepsy and has been used for the treatment of
3. post-anaesthetic shivering
4. hiccuping during general anaesthesia
5. depression and
6. brain injury.

Chemical A piperidine derivative.

Presentation As 5/10/20 mg tablets of methylphenidate hydrochloride and a range of extended-release formulations.

Main actions Central nervous stimulation.

Mode of action Methylphenidate binds to the dopamine transporter in pre-synaptic cell membranes, blocking its reuptake, thereby increasing extracellular dopamine levels. It also affects noradrenaline reuptake and binds weakly to 5-hydroxytryptamine (5HT) receptors.

Routes of administration/doses The drug is administered orally to a maximum of 60 mg/day in divided doses.

Effects

CVS The drug causes dose-dependent hypertension and tachycardia.

CNS Methylphenidate causes generalized CNS stimulation.

Metabolic/other Methylphenidate decreases growth velocity.

Toxicity/side effects Insomnia, nervousness, anorexia, hypertension, and tachycardia occur relatively frequently. The drug has significant potential for abuse.

Kinetics

Absorption Methylphenidate is almost completely absorbed after oral administration.

Distribution The drug exhibits a low degree of protein binding.

Metabolism Occurs primarily by de-esterification to ritalinic acid.

Excretion 60–80% of the dose is administered in the urine. The elimination half-life is 2.5 hours.

Metoclopramide

Uses Metoclopramide is used in the treatment of:
1. digestive disorders, e.g. hiatus hernia, reflux oesophagitis, and gastritis
2. nausea and vomiting due to a variety of causes, e.g. drugs (general anaesthetic agents, opiates, and cytotoxic gents), radiotherapy, hepatic and biliary disorders
3. diagnostic radiology of the gastrointestinal tract
4. migraine, and
5. post-operative gastric hypotonia.

Chemical A chlorinated procainamide derivative.

Presentation As 10 mg tablets, a syrup containing 1 mg/ml, and as a clear, colourless solution for injection containing 5 mg/ml of metoclopramide hydrochloride.

Main actions Increased gastrointestinal motility and antiemetic.

Mode of action The effects of metoclopramide on gastrointestinal motility appear to be mediated by:
1. antagonism of peripheral dopaminergic (D2) receptors
2. augmentation of peripheral cholinergic responses, and
3. direct action on smooth muscle to increase tone.

The antiemetic effects of the drug appear to be mediated by:
1. central dopaminergic (D2) blockade, leading to an increased threshold for vomiting at the chemoreceptor trigger zone and
2. decrease in the sensitivity of visceral nerves supplying afferent information to the vomiting centre.

Routes of administration/doses Metoclopramide may be administered orally, intravenously, or intramuscularly; the adult dose by all routes is 10 mg 8-hourly. A dose of 1–2 mg/kg is recommended for the treatment of nausea and vomiting associated with cisplatin treatment.

Effects

CVS There have been occasional reports of hypotension during general anaesthesia and cardiac arrest, dysrhythmias, and hypertension in patients with phaeochromocytoma following the administration of metoclopramide.

CNS Metoclopramide raises the threshold for vomiting at the chemoreceptor trigger zone and prevents apomorphine-induced vomiting in man. The drug has neuroleptic effects (including an antipsychotic action), as would be expected of a centrally acting dopamine antagonist.

AS Metoclopramide increases the tone of the lower oesophageal sphincter by about 17 mmHg, accelerates gastric emptying and the amplitude of gastric contractions, and accelerates small intestinal transit time. Its effects on large bowel motility are variable. The drug has no effect on gastric secretion.

GU The drug may increase ureteric peristaltic activity.

Metabolic/other Metoclopramide stimulates prolactin release and also causes a transient increase in aldosterone secretion.

Toxicity/side effects Occur in 11% of patients receiving the drug; drowsiness, dizziness, faintness, and bowel disturbances are the most frequently reported side effects. Extrapyramidal side effects occur; the commonest manifestations are akathisia and oculogyric crises; extrapyramidal effects occur more frequently with higher doses, and in patients with renal impairment and the elderly. The neuroleptic malignant syndrome has been reported in association with metoclopramide.

Kinetics

Absorption The drug is rapidly absorbed after oral administration and has a bioavailability by this route of 32–97%. This wide variability is due primarily to first-pass conjugation to sulfate.

Distribution Metoclopramide is 13–22% protein-bound in the plasma; the V_D is 2.2–3.4 l/kg.

Metabolism Occurs primarily in the liver; the major metabolite is a sulfate derivative. Two other metabolites have been identified in man.

Excretion 80% of an oral dose is excreted in the urine within 24 hours; 20% of this is unchanged, and the remainder appears as non-metabolized drug conjugated to a sulfate or glucuronide and as the sulfated metabolite. The clearance is 8.8–11.6 ml/min/kg, and the elimination half-life is 2.6–5 hours.

Metoclopramide is not significantly removed by haemodialysis.

Metronidazole

Uses Metronidazole is used for:
1. the treatment and prophylaxis of infections due to anaerobic bacteria, especially *Bacteroides fragilis* and *Clostridia* spp., and the treatment of
2. protozoal infections such as amoebiasis, giardiasis, and trichomoniasis
3. acute dental infections, and
4. pseudomembranous colitis.

Chemical A synthetic imidazole derivative.

Presentation As 200/400/500 mg tablets; 500 mg or 1 g suppositories; as an oral suspension of 200 mg/5 ml; and as a clear, colourless 0.5% solution for intravenous injection of metronidazole.

Main actions Metronidazole is an antimicrobial agent with a high degree of activity against anaerobes and protozoa.

Mode of action The drug acts via a reactive intermediate which reacts with bacterial DNA, so that the resultant DNA complex can no longer function as an effective primer for DNA and RNA polymerases—all nucleic acid synthesis is thus effectively terminated.

Routes of administration/doses The adult oral dose is 200–800 mg, and the corresponding rectal dose is 1 g 8-hourly. The intravenous dose is 500 mg 8-hourly, administered at a rate of 5 ml/min.

Effects

Metabolic/other Metronidazole decreases the cholesterol content of bile.

Toxicity/side effects Unpleasant taste, nausea and vomiting, gastrointestinal disturbances, rashes, and darkening of urine have been reported. Peripheral neuropathy and leucopenia may occur with chronic use of the drug.

Kinetics

Absorption The bioavailability of oral metronidazole is 80% and by the rectal route is 75%.

Distribution Metronidazole is distributed in virtually all tissues and body fluids in concentrations that do not differ markedly from their serum levels. Approximately 10% is protein-bound in the plasma. The V_D is 0.75 l/kg.

Metabolism Occurs by oxidation and glucuronidation in the liver.

Excretion 60% of the dose is excreted unchanged in the urine; the drug does not usually accumulate in renal failure. The clearance is 1.22 ml/kg/min, and the elimination half-life is 6–10 hours.

Special points Metronidazole increases the anticoagulant effect of warfarin and exhibits a disulfiram-like interaction with alcohol, producing an acute confusional state and vomiting.

Prolongation of the action of vecuronium by the co-administration of the drug has been demonstrated in animals.

Metronidazole may cause reddish brown discoloration of the urine.

Metronidazole is removed by haemodialysis.

Midazolam

Uses Midazolam is used:
1. for induction of anaesthesia
2. for sedation during endoscopy and procedures performed under local anaesthesia and during intensive care
3. as a hypnotic
4. for premedication prior to general anaesthesia and may be of use
5. in the treatment of chronic pain, including deafferentation syndromes.

Chemical A water-soluble imidazobenzodiazepine.

Presentation As a clear, colourless solution of midazolam hydrochloride containing 1/2/5 mg/ml.

Main actions
1. Hypnosis
2. Sedation
3. Anxiolysis
4. Anterograde amnesia
5. Anticonvulsant and
6. Muscular relaxation.

Mode of action Benzodiazepines are thought to act via specific benzodiazepine receptors found at synapses throughout the CNS, but concentrated especially in the cortex and midbrain. Benzodiazepine receptors are closely linked with GABA receptors and appear to facilitate the activity of the latter. Activated GABA receptors open chloride ion channels which then either hyperpolarize or short-circuit the synaptic membrane. Midazolam has kappa-opioid agonist activity *in vitro*, which may explain the mechanism of benzodiazepine-induced spinal analgesia.

Routes of administration/doses The intramuscular dose (used for premedication) is 0.07–0.08 mg/kg; the intravenous dose for sedation is 0.07–0.1 mg/kg, titrated according to response. The end point for sedation is drowsiness and slurring of speech; response to commands is, however, maintained. The drug may also be administered intrathecally in an adult dose of 0.3–2 mg or epidurally in a dose of 0.1–0.2 mg/kg.

Effects

CVS Systolic blood pressure decreases by 5% and diastolic pressure by 10%, and the systemic vascular resistance falls by 15–33%, following the administration of the drug; the heart rate increases by 18%. Midazolam in combination with fentanyl obtunds the pressor response to intubation to a greater extent than thiopental in combination with fentanyl.

RS Midazolam decreases the tidal volume, but this is offset by an increase in the respiratory rate; the minute volume is thus little changed. Apnoea occurs in 10–77% of patients when midazolam is used as an induction agent. The drug impairs the ventilatory response to hypercapnia.

CNS The drug produces hypnosis, sedation, and anterograde amnesia. There have been no studies of the anticonvulsant activity of midazolam in man. The cerebral oxygen consumption and cerebral blood flow are decreased in a dose-related manner, but a normal relationship is maintained between the two. When administered intrathecally or epidurally, the drug has anti-nociceptive effects.

AS A midazolam–fentanyl induction sequence is associated with a lower incidence of post-operative vomiting than with a thiopental–fentanyl sequence. The drug reduces hepatic blood flow.

GU Midazolam decreases renal blood flow.

Metabolic/other Midazolam decreases the adrenergic, but not the cortisol and renin, response to stress. The drug causes significant inhibition of phagocytosis and leucocyte bactericidal activity.

Toxicity/side effects Side effects are confined to occasional discomfort at the site of injection. Withdrawal phenomena may occur in children after prolonged infusion.

Kinetics

Absorption The bioavailability when administered by the oral route is 44% and by the intramuscular route is 80–100%.

Distribution The drug is 96% protein-bound in the plasma; the V_D is 0.8–1.5 l/kg. The V_D may increase to 3.1 l/kg in the critically ill.

Metabolism Midazolam is virtually completely metabolized in the liver to hydroxylated derivatives which are then conjugated to a glucuronide. Metabolites bind to CNS benzodiazepine receptors and are pharmacologically active.

Excretion Occurs in the urine, predominantly as the hydroxylated derivatives; renal impairment thus has little effect. The clearance is 5.8–9 ml/min/kg, and the elimination half-life is 1.5–3.5 hours. The elimination half-life may increase to 5.4 hours in the critically ill.

Special points The short duration of action of midazolam is due to its high lipophilicity, high metabolic clearance, and rapid rate of elimination. However, this may not be the case after prolonged dosing on intensive care.

The use of midazolam in premedication decreases the MAC of volatile agents by approximately 15%.

The clinical effects of the drug can be reversed by physostigmine, glycopyrronium bromide, and flumazenil.

Milrinone

Uses Milrinone is used in the acute management of:
1. severe treatment-resistant congestive cardiac failure and in
2. low cardiac output states following cardiac surgery.

Chemical Milrinone is a bipyridine molecule.

Presentation As a clear, colourless to pale yellow solution for injection in 10 and 20 ml glass ampoules containing 1 mg/ml of milrinone lactate. The pKa of milrone is 9.67, and the pH is 6.35.

Main actions Positive inotropism and vasodilatation.

Mode of action Milrinone acts by selective inhibition of type III cAMP phosphodiesterase in cardiac and vascular muscle. This causes an increase in intracellular ionized calcium and contractile force in cardiac muscle. It also causes cAMP-dependent protein phosphorylation and subsequent vascular muscle relaxation. It does not have beta-adrenergic agonist activity. The drug improves left ventricular diastolic relaxation.

Routes of administration/doses Milrinone is administered intravenously. In adult patients, a loading dose of 50 micrograms/kg administered over 10 minutes is recommended, followed by a continuous infusion of between 0.375 micrograms/kg/min and 0.75 micrograms/kg/min, titrated to haemodynamic response. In paediatric patients, a loading dose of between 50 and 75 microgram/kg is administered over 30–60 minutes, followed by a continuous infusion of between 0.25 and 0.75 micrograms/kg/min.

Effects

CVS Milrinone has a positive inotropic action and leads to an increase in the cardiac output. The cardiac index increases by 25–30%. Pulmonary capillary wedge pressure decreases by 20%, together with a decrease in the systemic vascular resistance and mean arterial pressure. The drug may increase AV nodal conductance which may lead to an increase in ventricular response in patients with atrial fibrillation or atrial flutter.

GU The urine output and glomerular filtration rate may increase, secondary to an increase in the cardiac output and renal perfusion.

Toxicity/side effects Commonly reported side effects include ventricular ectopics, arrhythmias, and hypotension. Arrhythmias are often associated with an underlying cause (e.g. pre-existing arrhythmia, electrolyte abnormality).

Kinetics

Distribution Milrinone is 70–80% protein-bound. The V_D is 0.38 l/kg following a loading dose, and 0.45 l/kg following a continuous intravenous infusion.

Metabolism 12% of an administered dose undergoes hepatic metabolism to an O-glucuronide metabolite.

Excretion 83% of milrinone is excreted renally. Following a loading dose, the half-life is 2.3 hours, with a clearance of 0.13 l/kg/hour. Following a continuous infusion, the half-life is 2.4 hours, with a clearance of 0.14 l/kg/hour.

Special points The infusion rate should be decreased in patients with severe renal impairment, as the half-life is prolonged in the presence of a reduced glomerular filtration rate.

Mivacurium

Uses Mivacurium is used to facilitate intubation and controlled ventilation.

Chemical A benzylisoquinolinium which is a mixture of three stereoisomers: trans–trans (57%), cis–trans (36%), cis–cis (4–8%). The cis–cis isomer is estimated to have <5% of the neuromuscular-blocking potency of the other two stereoisomers.

Presentation As a clear, pale yellow aqueous solution in 5 and 10 ml ampoules containing 2.14 mg/ml of mivacurium hydrochloride. It has a pH of approximately 4.5.

Main action Competitive, non-depolarizing neuromuscular blockade.

Mode of action Mivacurium acts by competitive antagonism of acetylcholine at nicotinic (N2) receptors at the post-synaptic membrane of the neuromuscular junction.

Routes of administration/doses Mivacurium is administered by intravenous injection; in adults, the mean dose to reach the ED95 is 0.07 mg/kg. The recommended intubating dose in adults is 0.2 mg/kg administered over 30 seconds or a dose of 0.25 mg/kg administered as a divided dose (0.15 mg/kg, followed 30 seconds later by 0.1 mg/kg), which provides good to excellent intubating conditions within 2–2.5 minutes and 1.5–2 minutes (following completion of the first divided dose), respectively. Maintenance doses of 0.1 mg/kg are required at approximately 15-minute intervals in adults and children. Continuous infusion of mivacurium in adults may also be administered at a rate of 8–10 micrograms/kg/min (0.5–0.6 mg/kg/hour). The ED95 in infants and children is 0.07 mg/kg and 0.1 mg/kg, respectively. The corresponding recommended doses for tracheal intubation are 0.15 mg/kg for infants and 0.2 mg/kg for children, with times to maximal neuromuscular block of 1.4 and 1.7 minutes, respectively. Average infusion rates to maintain 89–99% neuromuscular block are 11–14 micrograms/kg/min for children aged 2 months to 12 years old (0.7–0.9 mg/kg/hour). The duration of neuromuscular blockade is related to the bolus dose; doses in adults of 0.07, 0.15, 0.2, and 0.25 mg/kg produce clinically effective block for approximately 13, 16, 20, and 25 minutes, respectively. Spontaneous recovery after a continuous infusion is independent of the duration of infusion and is similar to recovery reported for single doses. Tachyphylaxis or cumulative neuromuscular blockade is not associated with continuous infusion of mivacurium. Significant train-of-four fade is not seen during the onset of block with mivacurium, and intubation of the trachea may be possible before the train-of-four count has been abolished.

Effects

CVS Mivacurium has minimal CVS effects; a slight (7%) transient decrease in the blood pressure and a slight (7%) increase in the heart rate may occur after rapid intravenous injection. The drug has no significant vagal or ganglion-blocking properties in the normal dosage range.

RS Neuromuscular blockade leads to apnoea; bronchospasm may occur, secondary to histamine release.

Toxicity/side effects Transient cutaneous flushing occurs in approximately 16% of patients and is the commonest side effect. Hypotension, tachycardia, bronchospasm, erythema, and urticaria may all occur, with an incidence of <1%, and are attributed to histamine release. There have been rare reports of fatal anaphylactoid reactions with the administration of mivacurium. Cross-sensitivity may occur with vecuronium, rocuronium, and pancuronium.

Kinetics

Distribution The V_D of the *trans–trans* isomer is 147 ml/kg, that of the *cis–trans* isomer is 276 ml/kg, and that of the *cis–cis* isomer is 335 ml/kg.

Metabolism The primary mechanism of metabolism of the *trans–trans* and *cis–trans* stereoisomers is enzymatic hydrolysis by plasma cholinesterases to yield a quaternary alcohol and a quaternary monoester metabolite which appear to be inactive. Some hydrolysis by liver esterases also occurs. The clearance of the *cis–cis* isomer is independent of plasma cholinesterase.

Excretion The metabolites are excreted in the bile and urine, together with some unchanged drug. The clearance of the *trans–trans* isomer is 53 ml/kg/min, that of the *cis–trans* isomer is 99 ml/kg/min, and that of the *cis–cis* isomer is 4.6 ml/kg/min. The elimination half-life of the *trans–trans* isomer is 2.0 minutes, that of the *cis–trans* isomer is 1.8 minutes, and that of the *cis–cis* isomer is 53 minutes. The clearance of the *trans–trans* and *cis–trans* stereoisomers in elderly patients may decrease to 32 and 47 ml/kg/min, respectively, resulting in prolongation of action by approximately 20–30%. Renal impairment increases the clinical duration of action of mivacurium by a factor of 1.5, and hepatic impairment increases it by a factor of 3.

Special points The duration of action of mivacurium is prolonged by isoflurane and enflurane, and it is recommended that the initial dose be reduced by 25%. Concomitant use of halothane causes minimal prolongation of action of the drug, and dosage reduction is not required. Data suggest that sevoflurane may reduce the mivacurium infusion rate requirement in children by up to 70%. Mivacurium is metabolized by plasma cholinesterase and, as such, its duration of activity prolonged in individuals possessing a genetic abnormality of plasma cholinesterase or an acquired reduction in its activity. The following drugs may reduce plasma cholinesterase activity: oral contraceptives, glucocorticoids, MAOIs, ketamine, lithium, ester local anaesthetic agents, metoclopramide, ecothiopate, trimetaphan, and edrophonium. Acquired conditions associated with a reduced activity of plasma cholinesterase include: malignancy, renal impairment, hepatic impairment, cardiac failure, pregnancy, thyrotoxicosis. The following drugs enhance the neuromuscular effects of mivacurium: aminoglycoside antibiotics, propranolol, calcium channel blockers, diuretics, and magnesium and lithium salts.

In patients who are obese, the ideal body weight should be used for dose calculation.

Mivacurium can be reversed using neostigmine (together with an inhibitor of vagal activity). Administration of between 0.03 and 0.06 mg/kg of neostigmine at 10% recovery from neuromuscular block produces 95% recovery of muscle twitch response and a T4:T1 ratio of >75% in approximately 10 minutes.

Mivacurium does not act as a trigger agent for malignant hyperpyrexia in animal models.

The drug is physically incompatible with alkaline solutions (e.g. barbiturates).

Morphine

Uses Morphine is used:
1. for premedication
2. as an analgesic in the management of moderate to severe pain
3. in the treatment of left ventricular failure
4. to provide analgesia during terminal care, and
5. in combination with kaolin in the symptomatic treatment of diarrhoea.

Chemical A phenanthrene derivative.

Presentation As 5/10/30/60/100/200 mg tablets, as a syrup containing 2/10/20 mg/ml, as 15/30 mg suppositories, and as a clear, colourless solution for injection containing 10/15/30 mg/ml of morphine sulfate; preservative-free morphine must be used for epidural/spinal use.

Main actions Analgesia and respiratory depression.

Mode of action Morphine is an agonist at mu- and kappa-opioid receptors. Opioids appear to exert their effects by increasing intracellular calcium concentration which, in turn, increases potassium conductance and hyperpolarization of excitable cell membranes. The decrease in membrane excitability that results may decrease both pre- and post-synaptic responses.

Routes of administration/doses The initial adult oral dose is 5–20 mg 4-hourly, increased as required. The dose by the rectal route is 15–30 mg 4-hourly. The corresponding intramuscular or subcutaneous dose is 0.1–0.2 mg/kg, and the intravenous dose is 0.05–0.1 mg/kg 3- to 4-hourly. Morphine may also be administered intrathecally; an adult dose of 0.2–1 mg has been recommended. The drug has a peak analgesic effect 30–60 minutes after intramuscular injection and has a duration of effect of 3–4 hours.

Effects

CVS Morphine has minimal effects on the CVS; the predominant effect is that of orthostatic hypotension, secondary to a decrease in the systemic vascular resistance, at least part of which is mediated by histamine release. The drug may also cause bradycardia when administered in high doses.

RS The principal effect of the drug is respiratory depression with a decreased ventilatory response to hypoxia and hypercapnia. Morphine also has a potent antitussive action. Bronchoconstriction may occur with the use of high doses of the drug.

CNS Morphine is a potent analgesic agent and may also cause drowsiness, relief of anxiety, and euphoria. Miosis is produced by the drug as a result of stimulation of the Edinger–Westphal nucleus. Seizures and muscular rigidity may occur with the use of high doses of morphine.

AS Morphine decreases gastrointestinal motility and decreases gastric acid, biliary, and pancreatic secretions; it also increases the common bile duct pressure by causing spasm of the sphincter of Oddi. The drug may also cause nausea, vomiting, and constipation.

GU The drug increases the tone of the ureters, bladder detrusor muscle, and sphincter, and may precipitate urinary retention.

Metabolic/other Mild diaphoresis and pruritus may result from histamine release. Morphine increases the secretion of ADH and may therefore lead to impaired water excretion and hyponatraemia. The drug causes a transient decrease in adrenal steroid secretion.

Toxicity/side effects Respiratory depression, nausea and vomiting, hallucinations, and dependence may complicate the use of morphine. Pruritus may occur after epidural or spinal administration of the drug.

Kinetics

Absorption Morphine is well absorbed when administered orally; the bioavailability by this route is 15–50% due to an extensive first-pass metabolism.

Distribution The drug is 20–40% protein-bound in the plasma, predominantly to albumin; the V_D is 3.4–4.7 l/kg. Morphine equilibrates slowly between the plasma and CSF; there is no clear correlation between the degree of analgesia and the plasma concentration of the drug.

Metabolism Occurs in the liver to morphine-3-glucuronide, morphine-6-glucuronide, and normorphine. In animal models, morphine-6-glucuronide has analgesic effects, and morphine-3-glucuronide has effects on arousal. Enterohepatic cycling of the metabolites probably does not occur.

Excretion Occurs predominantly in the urine as the glucuronide conjugates; 7–10% appears in the faeces as conjugated morphine. The clearance is 12–23 ml/min/kg, and the elimination half-life is 1.7–4.5 hours. Cumulation of morphine-6-glucuronide occurs in the presence of renal failure; a reduction in the dose of the drug is necessary under these circumstances.

Special points Morphine should be used with caution in the presence of hepatic failure, as the drug may precipitate encephalopathy. Similarly, the use of the drug in patients with hypopituitarism may precipitate coma. In common with other opioids, morphine decreases the apparent MAC of co-administered volatile agents. The actions of the drug are all reversed by naloxone, although the analgesia afforded by the epidural administration of morphine is well preserved after the administration of naloxone.

Morphine is not removed by haemodialysis or by peritoneal dialysis.

Nalbuphine

Uses Nalbuphine is used:
1. for premedication and
2. as an analgesic in the treatment of moderate to severe pain.

Chemical A semi-synthetic phenanthrene derivative.

Presentation As a clear, colourless solution for injection containing 10 mg/ml of nalbuphine hydrochloride.

Main action Analgesia.

Mode of action Nalbuphine is an agonist at kappa-opioid receptors and an antagonist at MOP receptors; it thus produces analgesia (a kappa effect), whilst antagonizing both the respiratory depressant effects and the potential for dependency that are associated with the mu-receptor.

Routes of administration/doses The drug may be administered intravenously, intramuscularly, or subcutaneously in an adult dose of 10–20 mg. Nalbuphine acts within 2–3 minutes when administered intravenously and within 15 minutes when administered intramuscularly. The duration of action is 3–6 hours.

Effects

CVS Nalbuphine has little significant effect on the heart rate, mean arterial pressure, systemic or pulmonary vascular resistance, or cardiac output.

RS The drug has a respiratory depressant effect equal to that of morphine but demonstrates a ceiling effect at a dose of 0.5 mg/kg. It will antagonize the respiratory depressant effects of co-administered pure mu-agonists, whilst adding to the analgesic effect of the latter.

CNS Nalbuphine has an analgesic potency equivalent to that of morphine. It has no euphorian effects.

AS The drug causes less inhibition of gastrointestinal activity than other opioids.

Toxicity/side effects Sedation, dizziness, vertigo, dry mouth, and headache may complicate the use of nalbuphine. The drug causes less nausea and vomiting, psychotomimetic effects, and dependence than does morphine.

Kinetics

Absorption The bioavailability by the oral route is 12–17% due to a significant first-pass hepatic metabolism. The bioavailability is 80% by the intramuscular and subcutaneous routes.

Distribution Nalbuphine is 25–40% protein-bound in the plasma; the V_D is 162–498 l.

Metabolic/other Occurs predominantly in the liver to two inactive conjugates which are secreted into the bile.

Excretion The metabolites are predominantly excreted (with some unchanged nalbuphine) via the faeces. A small fraction is excreted unchanged in the urine. The clearance is 0.8–2.3 l/min, and the elimination half-life is 110–160 minutes. Care should be exercised during the use of the drug in patients with renal or hepatic impairment.

Special points Nalbuphine is ineffective in obtunding the cardiovascular responses to laryngoscopy and intubation. The drug will precipitate withdrawal symptoms in opiate addicts; its effects are reversed by naloxone.

Nalbuphine has been used in the management of post-operative shivering.

Naloxone

Uses Naloxone is used for:
1. the reversal of respiratory depression due to opioids
2. the diagnosis of suspected opioid overdose and has been used in the treatment of
3. clonidine overdose.

Chemical A substituted oxymorphone derivative.

Presentation As a clear solution for injection containing 0.02/0.4 mg/ml of naloxone hydrochloride.

Main actions Reversal of MOP receptor effects such as sedation, hypotension, respiratory depression, and the dysphoric effects of partial agonists. The drug will precipitate acute withdrawal symptoms in opiate addicts.

Mode of action Naloxone is a competitive antagonist at mu-, delta-, kappa-, and sigma-opioid receptors.

Routes of administration/doses For the reversal of opioid-induced respiratory depression, the drug should be administered intravenously in small incremental doses, until the desired end point of reversal of respiratory depression without reversal of analgesia is reached; in adults, 0.1–0.2 mg will normally achieve this effect. In the treatment of known or suspected opioid overdose, 0.4–2.0 mg may be administered intravenously, intramuscularly, or subcutaneously. The drug acts within 2 minutes when administered intravenously and has a duration of effect (approximately 20 minutes) that may be shorter than the opioid whose effects it is desired to counteract. It may therefore be necessary to administer additional doses of naloxone intravenously or intramuscularly.

Effects

CVS The drug has no effect at normal doses. In doses of 0.3 mg/kg, the blood pressure may increase. Naloxone has been shown to reverse the hypotension associated with endotoxic and hypovolaemic shock in some animal studies.

CNS Naloxone causes slight drowsiness at very high doses. Some forms of stress-induced analgesia are obtunded by naloxone; the drug also decreases the tolerance to pain in subjects with high pain thresholds.

AS Naloxone reverses opioid-induced spasm of the sphincter of Oddi.

Toxicity/side effects Serious ventricular dysrhythmias occurring in patients with irritable myocardia after the administration of naloxone have been reported.

Kinetics

Absorption The drug is 91% absorbed when administered orally but has a bioavailability by this route of 2% due to an extensive first-pass metabolism.

Distribution The drug is 46% protein-bound in adult plasma. The V_D is 2 l/kg.

Metabolism The drug is metabolized in the liver, primarily by conjugation to glucuronide.

Excretion The clearance is 25 ml/min/kg, and the plasma half-life is 1.2 hours.

Special points Naloxone is effective in alleviating the pruritus, nausea, and respiratory depression associated with the epidural or spinal administration of opioids.

Neostigmine

Uses Neostigmine is used:
1. for the reversal of non-depolarizing neuromuscular blockade and in the treatment of
2. myasthenia gravis
3. paralytic ileus and
4. urinary retention.

Chemical A quaternary amine which is an ester of an alkyl carbamic acid.

Presentation As 15 mg tablets of neostigmine bromide and as a clear, colourless solution for injection containing 2.5 mg/ml of neostigmine metilsulfate. A fixed-dose combination containing 0.5 mg of glycopyrronium bromide and 2.5 mg of neostigmine metilsulfate per ml is also available.

Main actions Cholinergic.

Mode of action Neostigmine is a reversible, acid-transferring cholinesterase inhibitor which binds to the esteratic site of acetylcholinesterase and is hydrolysed by the latter, but at a much slower rate than is acetylcholine. The accumulation of acetylcholine at the neuromuscular junction allows the competitive antagonism of any non-depolarizing relaxant that may be present.

Routes of administration/doses The adult oral dose is 15–50 mg 2- to 4-hourly. The intravenous dose for the reversal of non-depolarizing neuromuscular blockade is 0.05–0.07 mg/kg, administered slowly and in combination with an appropriate dose of an anticholinergic agent. The peak effect of the drug when administered intravenously occurs at 7–11 minutes; a single dose of neostigmine has a duration of action of 40–60 minutes.

Effects

CVS The effects of neostigmine on the CVS are variable and depend upon the prevailing autonomic tone. The drug may cause bradycardia, leading to a fall in cardiac output; it decreases the effective refractory period of cardiac muscle and increases conduction time in conducting tissue. In high doses, neostigmine may cause hypotension, secondary to a central effect.

RS Neostigmine increases bronchial secretion and may cause bronchoconstriction.

CNS In small doses, the drug has a direct action on skeletal muscle, leading to muscular contraction. In high doses, neostigmine may block neuromuscular transmission by the combination of a direct effect and by allowing the accumulation of acetylcholine. Miosis and failure of accommodation may be precipitated by the administration of the drug.

AS The drug increases salivation, lower oesophageal and gastric tone, gastric acid output, and lower gastrointestinal tract motility. Nausea and vomiting may occur.

GU Neostigmine increases ureteric peristalsis and may lead to involuntary micturition.

Metabolic/other Sweating and lacrimation are increased.

Toxicity/side effects The side effects are manifestations of its pharmacological actions, as described above. Cardiac arrest has been reported after the use of neostigmine.

Kinetics Data are incomplete.

Absorption Neostigmine is poorly absorbed when administered orally; the bioavailability by this route is 1–2%.

Distribution The drug is highly ionized and therefore does not cross the blood–brain barrier to any significant extent. Neostigmine is 6–10% protein-bound in the plasma; the V_D is 0.4–1 l/kg.

Metabolism Neostigmine is predominantly metabolized by plasma esterases to a quaternary alcohol; some hepatic metabolism with subsequent biliary excretion may also occur.

Excretion 50–67% of an administered dose is excreted in the urine. The clearance is 5.7–11.1 ml/min/kg, and the elimination half-life is 15–80 minutes; the clearance is decreased, and the elimination half-life is increased in the presence of renal impairment.

Special points Neostigmine prolongs the duration of action of suxamethonium. There is some evidence that the use of neostigmine to reverse neuromuscular blockade is associated with an increased incidence of gastrointestinal anastomotic breakdown.

Nifedipine

Uses Nifedipine is used in the treatment of:
1. angina
2. mild to severe hypertension (including pregnancy-induced hypertension)
3. Raynaud's phenomenon and
4. coronary artery spasm occurring during coronary angiography or angioplasty.

Chemical A dihydropyridine derivative.

Presentation As 5/10 mg capsules and a slow-release preparation containing 10/20/30/60 mg per tablet. A fixed-dose combination with atenolol is also available.

Main actions Relaxation of arterial smooth muscle in both the coronary and peripheral circulations.

Mode of action Nifedipine causes competitive blockade of cell membrane slow calcium channels, leading to decreased influx of Ca^{2+} into cells. This produces electromechanical decoupling, inhibition of contraction, and relaxation of cardiac and smooth muscle fibres, and leads to a negative inotropic effect and vasodilatation. It may also act by increasing red cell deformability and preventing platelet clumping and thromboxane release.

Routes of administration/doses The adult oral dose of nifedipine is 10–20 mg 8-hourly (20–40 mg 12-hourly for the slow-release preparation); 100–200 micrograms may be infused via a coronary catheter over 2 minutes.

Effects

CVS The mean arterial pressure decreases by 20–33%; this effect is more pronounced in hypertensive patients. This is accompanied by a reflex increase in the heart rate by up to 28%. The systemic and pulmonary vascular resistance and left ventricular end-diastolic and pulmonary artery pressures all decrease. Cardiac output is increased; nifedipine also causes a sustained relaxation of epicardial conductance vessels, leading to increased coronary blood flow in patients with ischaemic heart disease. Nifedipine is 3–10 times more effective in inhibiting contraction in coronary artery smooth muscle than in myocardial contractile cells. The drug may also protect the myocardium during reperfusion after cardiac bypass.

RS Nifedipine demonstrates no intrinsic bronchodilator effect in most studies. The drug appears to inhibit hypoxic pulmonary vasoconstriction.

CNS The drug causes a marginal increase in the cerebral blood flow due to vasodilatation of large cerebral vessels.

AS Contractility throughout the gut and lower oesophageal pressure are decreased by nifedipine. The hepatic blood flow is increased.

GU Nifedipine has no marked effect on the renal blood flow or glomerular filtration rate. Uterine activity is decreased by the drug.

Metabolic/other Plasma renin activity and catecholamines are increased; short-term use may decrease glucose tolerance. Platelet aggregation is impaired by the drug; thromboxane synthesis is inhibited, and nifedipine may thus decrease thromboxane-induced coronary artery spasm.

Toxicity/side effects Occur in 20% of patients; headache, flushing, and dizziness (secondary to vasodilatation) are common; oedema of the legs, eye pain, and gum hyperplasia have been reported.

Kinetics

Absorption Nifedipine is completely absorbed when administered orally; the bioavailability by this route is 45–68%.

Distribution The drug is 92–98% protein-bound in the plasma, the V_D is 0.62–1.12 l/kg.

Metabolism 95% of the dose is metabolized in the liver to three inactive metabolites.

Excretion 90% of the metabolites are excreted in the urine, the rest in the faeces. The clearance is 27–66 l/hour, and the elimination half-life is 1.3–11 hours, dependent upon the route of administration.

Special points Nifedipine is a safe and effective drug for the treatment of post-surgical hypertension; the reduction in mean arterial pressure is associated with an increase in the cardiac index and systemic oxygen transport.

All volatile agents in current use decrease Ca^{2+} release from the sarcoplasmic reticulum and decrease Ca^{2+} flux into cardiac cells; the negatively inotropic effects of nifedipine are thus additive with those of the volatile agents. When used in combination with isoflurane, the negative inotropic effects of the drugs are additive and may result in a profound decrease in cardiac output.

Experiments in animals have demonstrated an increased risk of sinus arrest if volatile agents and calcium antagonists are used concurrently. If withdrawn acutely (especially in the post-operative period) after chronic oral use, severe rebound hypertension may result.

Calcium channel antagonists may also:
1. reduce the MAC of volatile agents by up to 20% and
2. increase the efficacy of NMB agents.

Administration of nifedipine immediately prior to induction appears to aggravate redistribution hypothermia. The drug is not removed by dialysis.

Nimodipine

Uses Nimodipine is used:
1. in the prevention and treatment of cerebral vasospasm secondary to subarachnoid haemorrhage and may be of use in the management of
2. migraine
3. acute cerebrovascular accidents and
4. drug-resistant epilepsy.

Chemical A dihydropyridine.

Presentation As an intravenous infusion containing 200 micrograms/ml of nimodipine containing ethanol 20% and macrogol '400' 17%, and as 30 mg tablets.

Main action Dilation of cerebral vessels, leading to improved cerebral perfusion.

Mode of action Nimodipine is a calcium antagonist that binds to specific sites in the cell membranes of vascular smooth muscle and prevents Ca^{2+} influx through 'slow' Ca^{2+} channels, leading to vasodilatation; the drug has a relatively specific action on cerebral arterioles.

Routes of administration/doses The drug should be administered into a running crystalloid infusion via a central vein at the rate of 1 mg/hour for the first 2 hours and thereafter at the rate of 2 mg/hour for 5–14 days. The oral dose is 60 mg every 4 hours, starting within 4 days of subarachnoid haemorrhage.

Effects

CVS In normal subjects, doses of 2 mg/hour decrease the systolic and diastolic blood pressures. In the anaesthetized patient, an infusion of 1 microgram/kg/min decreases the systemic vascular resistance by 10–40% and increases the cardiac output by 25–45%.

CNS Nimodipine increases the cerebral blood flow by up to 18%, with no demonstrable 'steal' effect in patients who have had a subarachnoid haemorrhage. The use of nimodipine in such patients leads to a significant reduction in mortality and morbidity.

Toxicity/side effects Side effects occur infrequently, although flushing, headache, nausea, hypotension, and reversible abnormalities of liver function tests may complicate the use of the drug.

Kinetics

Absorption Nimodipine is rapidly and well absorbed when administered orally but has a bioavailability by this route of only 3–28% due to a significant first-pass metabolism.

Distribution The drug is 98% protein-bound in the plasma; the V_D is 0.94–2.3 l/kg.

Metabolism Nimodipine is initially demethylated and dehydrogenated to an inactive pyridine analogue which subsequently undergoes further degradation.

Excretion Half of the dose appears as metabolites in the urine, and a third in the faeces. The clearance is 420–520 l/hour, and the elimination half-life is 0.9–7.2 hours (dependent upon the route of administration). The clearance is decreased by hepatic impairment; the effect of renal impairment is unclear.

Special points Nimodipine has some effect in obtunding the cardiovascular responses to intubation and surgical stimulation; the peak blood pressures post-intubation and post-incision are consistently 10–15% lower in patients receiving the drug than those recorded in untreated patients.

The drug is adsorbed onto polyvinyl chloride tubing and is also light-sensitive; however, it remains stable in diffuse daylight for up to 10 hours.

Nitric oxide

Uses Nitric oxide (NO) is used as a selective pulmonary vasodilator in pulmonary hypertension.

Chemical An inorganic gas.

Presentation In aluminium cylinders containing 100/800 ppm of NO and nitrogen; the cylinders may contain either 353 l at standard temperature and pressure (STP) of NO in nitrogen or 1963 l at STP. Pure NO is toxic and corrosive. NO can also be supplied via stainless steel medical gas piping.

Main actions Vasodilatation.

Mode of action NO is produced *in vivo* by NO synthase which uses the substrate L-arginine. NO diffuses to the vascular smooth muscle layer and stimulates guanylate cyclase; the cyclic guanosine monophosphate (cGMP) produced activates a phosphorylation cascade which leads to smooth muscle relaxation and vasodilatation.

Routes of administration/doses NO is administered by inhalation in a dose of 5–20 ppm; the drug can either be injected into the patient limb of the inspiratory circuit of a ventilator during inspiration only or administered using a continuous-flow system which delivers NO throughout the respiratory cycle. The former technique reduces a 'bolus' effect seen with a continuous-flow technique, in addition to reducing nitrogen dioxide formation. This latter effect is achieved by decreasing the time allowed for oxygen and NO to mix. The delivery system is designed to minimize the oxidation of NO to nitrogen dioxide. Monitoring of NO concentrations can be achieved by a chemiluminescence monitor or electrochemical detector.

Effects

CVS NO is a potent vasodilator that mediates the hypotension and significant vascular leak characteristic of septic shock. Inhaled NO is a selective pulmonary vasodilator, since it is avidly bound to haemoglobin and thereby inactivated before reaching the systemic circulation. NO released from the vascular endothelium inhibits platelet aggregation and attenuates platelet and white cell adhesion.

RS NO inhibits hypoxic pulmonary vasoconstriction and preferentially increases blood flow through well-ventilated areas of the lung, thereby improving ventilation:perfusion relationships.

CNS NO increases the cerebral blood flow and appears to have a physiological role as a neurotransmitter within the autonomic and central nervous systems.

GU NO may play a role in the regulation of renin production and sodium homeostasis in the kidney. It is the physiological mediator of penile erection.

Metabolic/other NO released from macrophages reacts with superoxide ion to form the free radical peroxynitrite which is toxic to bacteria. Insulin release appears to be modulated by NO.

Toxicity/side effects Exposure to 500–2000 ppm of NO results in methaemoglobinaemia and pulmonary oedema. Contamination by nitrogen dioxide can similarly lead to pneumonitis and pulmonary oedema.

Kinetics

Absorption NO is highly lipid-soluble and diffuses freely across cell membranes.

Metabolism Following inhalation, NO combines with oxyhaemoglobin that is 60–100% saturated, producing methaemoglobin and nitrate. NO has a half-life of <5 seconds. During the first 8 hours of NO exposure, methaemoglobin concentrations increase.

Excretion The main metabolite is nitrate (70%) which is excreted by the kidneys.

Special points Prolonged inhalation (up to 27 days) of the gas appears safe and is not associated with tachyphylaxis.

Abrupt cessation of NO can cause a profound decrease in PaO_2 and increase in pulmonary artery pressure, possibly via downregulation of endogenous NO production or guanylate cyclase activity. The dose should be reduced slowly to avoid this from occurring, even in patients who may not have clinically responded to NO therapy. During treatment, concentrations of nitrogen dioxide must be monitored.

NO therapy is contraindicated in neonates known to have circulations dependent on a right-to-left shunt or significant left-to-right shunts.

Development of methaemoglobinaemia usually rapidly resolves on discontinuation of treatment over several hours. Persistent methaemoglobinaemia can be treated using methylthioninium chloride.

Mortality does not appear to be affected by the administration of NO in ARDS.

The occupational exposure limits are 25 ppm for NO and 3 ppm for nitrogen dioxide.

Nitrous oxide

Uses N_2O is used:
1. as an adjuvant to the induction and maintenance of general anaesthesia
2. as an analgesic during labour and other painful procedures
3. in cryosurgery as a refrigerant
4. as a gas of recreational use.

Chemical An inorganic gas.

Presentation As a liquid in cylinders at a pressure of 44 bar at 15°C; the cylinders are French blue and are available in six sizes (C–J, containing 450–18 000 l, respectively), following manufacture by heating ammonium nitrate to 250°C. The gauge pressure does not correlate with the cylinder content, until all N_2O is in the gaseous phase. It is a sweet-smelling, colourless gas; it is non-flammable but supports combustion. It has a molecular weight of 44, specific gravity of the gas of 1.53, a boiling point of −88.5°C, a critical temperature of 36.5°C, and a critical pressure of 71.7 atmospheres. Due to the critical temperature being close to the ambient temperature, the filling ratio of the cylinder is 0.75 in temperate regions, but reduced to 0.67 in tropical regions. The MAC of N_2O is 105, the oil:water partition coefficient 3.2, and the blood:gas partition coefficient 0.47 (compared to 0.015 for nitrogen). There are trace amounts of CO_2, carbon monoxide, and NO/nitrogen dioxide present in cylinders of N_2O at the following maximum amounts: 300 vpm, 10 vpm, 2 vpm, respectively.

Entonox® is the trade name given to a 50/50 mixture of oxygen and N_2O and is produced by bubbling oxygen through liquid N_2O. It is available in cylinders which are French blue, with white and blue shoulders in the following four sizes: SD, D, F, G, containing 440–5000 l, respectively. The cylinder pressure is 137 bar at 15°C. At normal temperatures, both of the components of Entonox® are present in pressurized cylinders in the gaseous phase (due to the Poynting effect); below its pseudocritical temperature of −7°C, liquefaction of N_2O occurs, resulting in the separation of the two components.

N_2O is also available commercially as small cannisters.

Main actions Analgesia and depression of the CNS.

Mode of action The mode of action of the anaesthetic action of N_2O is via non-competitive inhibition of the NMDA-subtype of glutamate receptors (N-methyl-D-aspartate)—this provides the predominant analgesic component of N_2O. It may also act via the two-pore domain potassium channels (e.g. TREK-1) which increase potassium conductance and subsequent neurone hyperpolarization. It appears to have minimal effect at $GABA_A$ receptors. The analgesic action of N_2O occurs via supraspinal activation of opioid receptors and GABA-ergic interneurones in the periaqueductal grey matter, and noradrenergic neurones in the locus coeruleus. The latter activation pathway appears to be triggered by the hypothalamic release of corticotrophin-releasing factor, mediated by N_2O antagonism at the NMDA receptor.

Routes of administration/dose N_2O is administered by inhalation; a concentration of 70% in oxygen is conventionally used as an adjunct to general anaesthesia. Entonox® is used to provide analgesia for a range of painful procedures.

Effects

CVS N_2O decreases myocardial contractility *in vitro*; *in vivo*, the mean arterial pressure is usually well maintained by a reflex increase in the peripheral vascular resistance. Deterioration in left ventricular function occurs when N_2O is added to a high-dose opioid–oxygen anaesthetic sequence, volatile agents, or a propofol infusion.

RS The gas causes a slight depression in respiration, with a decrease in the tidal volume and an increase in the respiratory rate. N_2O is non-irritant and does not cause bronchospasm.

CNS N_2O is a CNS depressant and, when administered in a concentration of 80%, will cause loss of consciousness in most subjects. The gas is a powerful analgesic in concentrations of >20%. Its administration causes a rise in the intracranial pressure.

GU N_2O has no effect on the uterine tone.

Toxicity/side effects 15% of patients receiving N_2O will experience nausea and vomiting. The gas is 35 times more soluble than nitrogen in the blood; N_2O will therefore cause an increase in the size of air-filled spaces (e.g. pneumothorax, intestines, air cysts in the middle ear) in the body. A further manifestation of this physical property of the gas is the Fink effect (diffusion hypoxia); when N_2O is discontinued, the ingress of the gas into the alveoli lowers the alveolar oxygen concentration. The prolonged use of high concentrations of N_2O (>6 hours) leads to oxidation of the cobalt ion of cobalamin (vitamin B12). The resulting cobalt cation prevents cobalamin from acting as a coenzyme for methionine synthetase. This cytosolic enzyme is involved in the synthesis of DNA, RNA, myelin, and catecholamines. The resultant clinical syndrome is akin to pernicious anaemia, megaloblastic anaemia, and pancytopenia. Twenty percent of elderly patients are deficient in cobalamin. N_2O may decrease the proliferation of human peripheral blood mononuclear cells and alter neutrophil chemotaxis. Prolonged use/abuse of the gas may lead to altered mental state, paraesthesiae, ataxia, lower limb weakness, and spasticity. Subacute combined degeneration of the cord may occur and may be irreversible. In neonatal rats, N_2O exacerbates isoflurane-induced apoptotic neuronal death. N_2O is teratogenic in animals when administered during early pregnancy. The maximum exposure to N_2O in the UK is 100 ppm.

Kinetics

Absorption N_2O diffuses freely across the normal alveolar epithelium. The rate of uptake of the gas is increased by a decreased cardiac output, an increased concentration, and increased alveolar ventilation. Due to its relative insolubility, the alveolar concentration of the gas approaches the inspired concentration rapidly; 90% equilibration occurs within 15 minutes, and 100% equilibration within 5 hours.

Metabolism Little, if any, metabolism occurs in man.

Excretion N_2O is excreted unchanged through the lungs and skin.

Special points N_2O exhibits the following two effects. The 'concentration effect' implies that the greater the inspired anaesthetic concentration, the more rapid the rise in the alveolar concentration. The 'second gas effect' refers to the ability of one gas administered in a high concentration (e.g. N_2O) to accelerate the uptake of another gas (e.g. halothane) that is co-administered. Sixty-six percent of N_2O in oxygen decreases the MAC of halothane to 0.29, of enflurane to 0.6, of isoflurane to 0.5, of sevoflurane to 0.66, and of desflurane to 2.8. The use of N_2O is safe in patients susceptible to malignant hyperpyrexia.

Noradrenaline

Uses Noradrenaline is used in the treatment of refractory hypotension.

Chemical A catecholamine.

Presentation As a clear, colourless solution containing 2 mg/ml of noradrenaline acid tartrate for dilution prior to infusion.

Main action Increased systemic vascular resistance.

Mode of action Noradrenaline is a directly and indirectly acting sympathomimetic amine that exerts its action predominantly at alpha-adrenergic receptors, with a minor action at beta-receptors.

Routes of administration/doses Noradrenaline is administered through a central vein as an infusion in glucose or saline in a concentration of 40 micrograms/ml (expressed as the base) at a rate titrated according to the response desired. The drug has a duration of action of 30–40 minutes; tachyphylaxis occurs with prolonged administration.

Effects

CVS Noradrenaline increases the peripheral vascular resistance, leading to an increase in the systolic and diastolic blood pressures; the cardiac output remains unchanged or decreases slightly. Reflex vagal stimulation leads to a compensatory bradycardia. The drug produces coronary vasodilatation, leading to a marked increase in coronary blood flow. The circulating blood volume is reduced by noradrenaline due to loss of protein-free fluid to the extracellular fluid. Noradrenaline may also cause nodal rhythm, AV dissociation, and ventricular dysrhythmias.

RS The drug causes a slight increase in the minute volume, accompanied by a degree of bronchodilatation.

CNS The cerebral blood flow and oxygen consumption are decreased by the administration of noradrenaline; mydriasis also occurs.

AS The hepatic and splanchnic blood flow are decreased by the drug.

GU Noradrenaline decreases the renal blood flow; the glomerular filtration rate is usually well maintained. The tone of the bladder neck is increased. Noradrenaline increases the contractility of the pregnant uterus; this may lead to fetal bradycardia and asphyxia.

Metabolic/other Noradrenaline may decrease insulin secretion, leading to hyperglycaemia; the concentration of free fatty acids and the plasma renin activity may increase.

Toxicity/side effects Anxiety, headache, photophobia, pallor, sweating, gangrene, and chest pain may occur with the use of the drug. Extravasation of noradrenaline may lead to sloughing and tissue necrosis.

Kinetics

Absorption Noradrenaline undergoes significant first-pass metabolism and is inactive when administered orally.

Distribution The V_D is 0.09–0.4 l/kg.

Metabolism Exogenous noradrenaline is metabolized by two pathways: by oxidative deamination to the aldehyde by mitochondrial monoamine oxidase (in the liver, brain, and kidney) and by methylation by cytoplasmic catechol-O-methyl transferase to normetanephrine. The predominant metabolite appearing in the urine is 3-methoxy, 4-hydroxymandelic acid (vanillylmandelic acid, VMA).

Excretion 5% of an administered dose of noradrenaline is excreted unchanged; the clearance is 27.9–100 ml/min/kg, and the half-life is 0.57–2.4 minutes.

Special points The use of noradrenaline during halothane anaesthesia may lead to the appearance of serious cardiac dysrhythmias; if co-administered with MAOIs or tricyclic antidepressants, serious hypertensive episodes may be precipitated.

The drug is pharmaceutically incompatible with barbiturates and sodium bicarbonate.

Omeprazole

Uses Omeprazole is used in the treatment of:
1. peptic ulcer disease
2. peptic oesophagitis
3. the Zollinger–Ellison syndrome
4. prevention of NSAID-associated ulcers and
5. following endoscopic treatment of peptic ulcer bleeding.

Chemical A substituted benzimidazole derivative.

Presentation As capsules containing 10/20/40 mg of omeprazole and in 40 mg vials as a powder of the sodium salt of omeprazole.

Main actions Inhibition of basal and stimulated gastric acid secretion.

Mode of action Omeprazole acts via a derivative which binds irreversibly to parietal cell H-K-ATPase and non-competitively inhibits it. The activity of the parietal cell 'proton pump', which represents the final common pathway of hydrogen ion secretion, is thus inhibited.

Routes of administration/doses The adult oral dose for the treatment of peptic ulcer disease is 20–40 mg daily for a period of 4–8 weeks; the corresponding dose for the treatment of the Zollinger–Ellison syndrome is 20–120 mg daily. The intravenous dose is administered over 5 minutes.

Effects

AS Omeprazole significantly reduces the volume of gastric juice but has no effect on the rate of gastric emptying. A single 20 mg dose will effectively control acid secretion for 24 hours. In animals, orally administered omeprazole appears to confer protection against stress-induced gastric ulceration.

Metabolic/other The drug has no demonstrable effect on endocrine function.

Toxicity/side effects Omeprazole is usually well tolerated; rashes, nausea, headache, gastrointestinal disturbances, liver dysfunction, and arrhythmia may occur.

Kinetics

Absorption Oral omeprazole is rapidly absorbed and has a bioavailability of 40–97%, dependent upon the formulation and dose. The drug may increase its own bioavailability, since degradation occurs under acidic conditions.

Distribution The drug is 95–96% protein-bound in the plasma, predominantly to albumin and alpha-1-acid glycoprotein. The V_D is 0.3–0.4 l/kg.

Metabolism Omperazole is rapidly and completely metabolized by oxidation to a sulfone, reduction to a sulfide, and hydroxylation.

Excretion 80% of an oral dose is excreted in the urine, the remainder in the faeces. The clearance is 533–666 ml/min, and the elimination half-life is 0.5–1.5 hours.

Special points Omeprazole is 2–10 times as potent as cimetidine; furthermore, it heals ulcers significantly more rapidly than conventional H2 antagonist regimes and may be effective in patients resistant to conventional therapy. Proton pump inhibitors reduce the risk of rebleeding from peptic ulcer disease and the need for surgery.

The pharmacokinetics of the drug are unaltered by renal impairment, and it is not removed by haemodialysis; no dose reduction is required in patients with renal or hepatic impairment. Omeprazole decreases the clearance of co-administered diazepam, phenytoin, and warfarin.

Administration of omeprazole (as with other proton pump inhibitors) is associated with ventilator-associated pneumonia in critically ill patients.

Ondansetron

Uses Ondansetron is used:
1. in the management of nausea and vomiting induced by chemotherapy and radiotherapy and
2. in the prevention and treatment of PONV.

Chemical A synthetic carbazole.

Presentation As a clear, colourless aqueous solution in 2/4 ml ampoules containing 2 mg/ml ondansetron hydrochloride dihydrate. It is also available as 4/8 mg tablets, as a strawberry-flavoured lyophilizate (4/8 mg), and as a suppository containing 16 mg of ondansetron.

Main action Antiemetic.

Mode of action Ondansetron is a highly selective antagonist at $5HT_3$ receptors and acts both centrally and peripherally. Emetogenic stimuli appear to cause release of 5HT in the small intestine and initiate a vomiting reflex by activating vagal afferents via $5HT_3$ receptors; ondansetron blocks the initiation of this reflex. Activation of vagal afferents may also result in the release of 5HT in the area postrema, promoting emesis via a central mechanism.

Routes of administration/doses For prevention of chemotherapy- or radiotherapy-induced nausea and vomiting, the route of administration and dose of ondansetron should be flexible in the range of 8–32 mg/day. For prophylaxis against PONV, the drug may be administered as a single dose of 4 mg by intramuscular or slow intravenous injection. The paediatric dose is 0.1 mg/kg. Identical doses are recommended for treatment of established PONV.

Effects

CVS Ondansetron has no demonstrable effects on the CVS.

RS The drug has no effect on the ventilatory response to CO_2.

CNS Ondansetron has no sedative effects and does not impair performance in psychomotor tests.

AS Ondansetron has no effect on gastric motility but does increase large bowel transit time.

Metabolic/other Ondansetron has no effect on serum prolactin concentration or haemostatic function.

Toxicity/side effects Constipation, headache, and flushing may occur. Bradycardia may occur, following rapid intravenous administration. Rare cases of anaphylaxis have been reported.

Kinetics

Absorption Ondansetron is passively and completely absorbed, following oral administration, and undergoes first-pass metabolism. Oral bioavailability of the drug is 60–65%. Peak plasma concentrations of approximately 30 ng/ml are achieved in about 1.5 hours, following an 8 mg oral dose. Following intramuscular injection, peak plasma levels of 25 ng/ml are reached within 10 minutes, and, following a 4 mg intravenous dose, peak plasma levels of 65 ng/ml are achieved.

Distribution The drug is 70–76% protein bound in the plasma; the V_D is 2 l/kg.

Metabolism Ondansetron is extensively metabolized in the liver by multiple hepatic cytochrome P450 enzymes (CYP3A4, CYP2D6, and CYP1A2). The drug is metabolized by hydroxylation or N-demethylation of the indole nucleus, followed by conjugation with glucuronic acid or sulfate. Due to the number of enzyme systems involved, inhibition or deficiency of one (e.g. CYP2D6 deficiency/debrisoquine polymorphism) is normally compensated by other enzymes, resulting in little or no significant change in ondansetron clearance or dose requirement. Patients receiving CYP3A4 inducers (e.g. carbamazepine, phenytoin, rifampicin) may have increased clearance of ondansetron, although this does not require dosage adjustment.

Excretion Less than 5% of the drug is excreted unchanged in the urine. The clearance is 6.3 ml/kg/min, and the elimination half-life is 3 hours.

Special points In patients with renal impairment, both the systemic clearance and V_D are reduced, following intravenous administration of ondansetron, resulting in an increase in the elimination half-life (>4 hours). This increase is not clinically significant, and no alteration of dose is required in patients with renal impairment. Hepatic impairment significantly reduces the clearance of the drug, with prolonged elimination half-lives (15–32 hours) and an oral bioavailability approaching 100% due to reduced pre-systemic metabolism. As a result of these effects, the dose of ondansetron should be limited to 8 mg/day in patients with hepatic impairment.

The drug may reduce the analgesic effect of tramadol.

Ondansetron contains <23 mg of sodium per dose.

Ondansetron may reduce the incidence of post-anaesthetic shivering.

Ondansetron may be used in combination with dexamethasone in the treatment of PONV.

Oseltamivir

Uses Oseltamivir is used in the treatment of:
1. influenza virus infections and
2. for the prophylaxis of influenza virus infections.

Chemical A synthetic ethyl ester.

Presentation As 30/45/75 mg capsules and as a granulate powder for oral suspension at a concentration of 12 mg/ml of oseltamivir phosphate.

Main action Oseltamivir is an antiviral agent active against influenza virus.

Mode of action Oseltamivir phosphate is a pro-drug and requires ester hydrolysis to convert it into the active component oseltamivir carboxylate. Oseltamivir carboxylate selectively inhibits influenza A and B neuramini-dases *in vitro*, leading to inhibition of virus infection and replication.

Routes of administration/doses The adult oral dose for treatment of influenza infection is 150 mg in divided doses for 5 days. The dose in children aged between 1 and 12 years old is dependent on the patient's weight as follows: ≤15 kg (30 mg twice daily), >15–23 kg (45 mg twice daily), >23–40 kg (60 mg twice daily), >40 kg (75 mg twice daily), for 5 days. The dose for infants <12 months of age is 3 mg/kg (3–12 month olds), 2.5 mg/kg (1–3 month olds), 2 mg/kg (0–1 month old), twice daily for 5 days. The recommended dose for post-exposure prophylaxis is 75 mg once daily for 10 days in adults. The dose in children aged between 1 and 12 years old is dependent on the patient's weight as follows: ≤15 kg (30 mg once daily), >15–23 kg (45 mg once daily), >23–40 kg (60 mg once daily), >40 kg (75 mg once daily), for 10 days. The dose for infants <12 months of age is 3 mg/kg (3–12 month olds), 2.5 mg/kg (1–3 month olds), 2 mg/kg (0–1 month old), once daily for 10 days. Efficacy has been demonstrated when treatment initiation occurs within 2 days of first onset of symptoms (for treatment) or within 2 days of exposure to an infected individual (for prophylaxis).

Toxicity/side effects The most commonly reported side effects are nausea (11%) and vomiting (8%), following use of the drug in adults. The incidence of these effects is higher in paediatric patients.

Kinetics

Absorption The drug is readily absorbed from the gastrointestinal tract. Oseltamivir phosphate is converted by hepatic esterases to oseltamivir carboxylate. At least 75% of an oral dose reaches the systemic circulation as oseltamivir carboxylate.

Distribution The drug is 3% protein-bound in the plasma; the V_D at steady state is approximately 23 l.

Metabolic/other Oseltamivir phosphate is extensively converted to oseltamivir carboxylate by hepatic esterases. It undergoes no further metabolism prior to elimination. Neither the pro-drug nor its active metab-olite interacts with the hepatic cytochrome P450 system.

Excretion Oseltamivir carboxylate is eliminated by renal excretion (>99%) via tubular secretion.

Special points Dose reduction is recommended in patients with severe renal impairment. No dose adjustment is required in patients with hepatic impairment.

In vitro studies have demonstrated that virus isolates with reduced susceptibility to oseltamivir carboxylate can be recovered. Resistance to the drug is associated with mutations, resulting in amino acid substitutions in viral neuraminidase, haemagglutinin, or both. Resistant mutations are usually viral subtype-specific and may be naturally occurring (i.e. no prior exposure to oseltamivir required to cause resistance).

Oxycodone

Uses Oxycodone is used for:
1. the treatment of moderate to severe pain in patients with cancer and post-operative pain and
2. in the treatment of severe pain requiring a strong opioid.

Chemical A semi-synthetic opium alkaloid derivative.

Presentation Oxycodone is available in immediate- and controlled-release preparations. The drug is available in 10 mg/ml and 50 mg/ml preparations for intravenous use; 5/10/20 mg capsules for oral use; and 1 mg/ml and 10 mg/ml as liquid formulations for oral use. The controlled-release preparation is available in 5/10/15/20/30/40/60/80/120 mg tablets.

Main actions The drug has opioid agonist activity, producing analgesia and anxiolysis, together with antitussive and sedative effects.

Mode of action Oxycodone has an affinity for mu-, kappa-, and delta-opioid receptors. The MOP receptor appears to be specifically involved in the mediation of analgesia. Opioids appear to exert their effects by interacting with pre-synaptic Gi-protein receptors, leading to hyperpolarization of the cell membrane by increasing K^+ conductance. Inhibition of adenylate cyclase, leading to reduced production of cAMP and closure of voltage-sensitive calcium channels, also occurs. The decrease in membrane excitability that results may decrease both pre- and post-synaptic responses.

Routes of administration/doses The drug may be administered orally, intravenously, or subcutaneously. The initial adult intravenous dose is 1–10 mg, administered slowly over 1–2 minutes and titrated to effect. The initial adult oral dose is 5 mg 4- to 6-hourly, titrated to effect. Ten mg of oral oxycodone is equivalent to 20 mg of oral morphine; 2 mg of oral oxycodone is equivalent to 1 mg of parenteral oxycodone. There are no data available on the use of oxycodone in children. Dose reductions are required in elderly patients and those with renal and hepatic impairment.

Effects

CVS Oxycodone has minimal effects on the CVS; the predominant effect is that of orthostatic hypotension, secondary to a decrease in the systemic vascular resistance, partly mediated by histamine release.

RS The principal effect of the drug is respiratory depression with a decreased ventilatory response to hypoxia and hypercapnia. Oxycodone also has an antitussive action. Bronchoconstriction may occur with high doses of the drug.

CNS Oxycodone is a powerful analgesic agent and may also cause drowsiness, relief of anxiety, and euphoria. Miosis is produced by the drug as a result of stimulation of the Edinger–Westphal nucleus. Increased muscle tone and seizure activity may occur with the use of high doses of oxycodone.

AS Oxycodone decreases gastrointestinal motility. The drug may also cause nausea, vomiting, and constipation.

GU The drug increases the tone of the ureters, bladder detrusor muscle, and sphincter, and may precipitate urinary retention.

Metabolic/other The drug may cause histamine release, resulting in pruritus.

Toxicity/side effects Respiratory depression, nausea and vomiting, hallucinations, and dependence may complicate the use of oxycodone.

Kinetics

Absorption The oral bioavailability of oxycodone is 60–87%. The time to P_{max} is 1–1.5 hours, following administration of immediate-release oxycodone. The controlled-release preparation has the same bioavailability, but, due to a biphasic release pattern, the time to reach P_{max} is 3 hours.

Distribution The V_D of oxycodone is 2.6 l/kg at steady state. Approximately 45% of the drug is bound to plasma proteins. The drug penetrates the placenta and is found in breast milk.

Metabolism The drug undergoes extensive hepatic metabolism via CYP450 3A to noroxycodone and CYP450 2D6 to oxymorphone and various other conjugated glucuronides.

Excretion Oxycodone and its metabolites undergo renal elimination. Up to 19% of free drug, up to 50% of conjugated oxycodone, and up to 14% of conjugated oxymorphone may be found in the urine. The elimination half-life of immediate-release oxycodone is 3 hours, and that of controlled release preparations 4.5 hours. Steady state is reached in approximately 24 hours. The clearance is 800 ml/min.

Special points Oxycodone should be used with caution in the presence of hepatic failure, as the drug may precipitate encephalopathy. In common with other opioids, oxycodone decreases the apparent MAC of co-administered volatile agents. The actions of the drug are all reversed by naloxone.

Prochlorperazine is chemically incompatible with oxycodone. The drug is compatible with hyoscine, dexamethasone, haloperidol, midazolam, and metoclopramide.

There is no evidence to suggest that blockade of CYP450 2D6 and CYP450 3A4 results in clinically significant effects.

Oxygen

Uses Oxygen is used:
1. in the management of all forms of hypoxia (other than histotoxic)
2. as an adjunct in the management of shock and in the treatment of
3. carbon monoxide poisoning
4. pneumatosis coli
5. decompression sickness and
6. anaerobic infections.

Chemical A gaseous inorganic element.

Presentation As a compressed gas in cylinders at a pressure of 137 bar (13 700 kPa) at 15°C; the cylinders are black with white shoulders and are available in several different sizes. Those cylinders commonly used in hospital are C–J containing 170–6800 l, respectively. Size J cylinders are used for cylinder manifolds. The AZ cylinder is MRI-compatible and contains 170 l. Oxygen is also available commercially in liquid form, one volume of liquid oxygen yielding 840 volumes of gaseous oxygen at 15°C and 1013 mb. Liquid oxygen is stored in a vacuum-insulated evaporator (VIE) which ranges in liquid capacity from 1600 to 18 675 l, depending on its size.

Oxygen is a colourless, odourless, tasteless gas which supports combustion and is explosive in the presence of grease. It has a molecular weight of 32, a specific gravity of 1.105, a critical temperature of −118.4°C, and a critical pressure of 50.8 atmospheres.

It is supplied at 99.5% purity with maximum amounts of carbon monoxide and CO_2 of 5.0 vpm and 300.0 vpm, respectively. Liquid oxygen appears pale blue.

Main action The essential role of oxygen is in the process of oxidative phosphorylation.

Mode of action Elemental oxygen is combined with hydrogen ions via mitochondrial cytochrome oxidase; the energy released is used for the synthesis of ATP.

Routes of administration Oxygen is administered by inhalation via fixed-performance or variable-performance devices. Depending on the device used, inspired concentrations of up to 100% may be achieved. Fixed-performance devices include anaesthetic breathing systems with a suitably large reservoir and Venturi-operated devices (also known as high airflow oxygen enrichment, or HAFOE, devices). Variable-performance devices include Hudson face masks, partial rebreathing masks, nasal cannulae, and nasal catheters. A number of factors determine the FiO_2 delivered by a variable-performance device: gas flow rate, peak inspiratory flow rate, respiratory rate, and how tightly fitting the face mask is.

Effects

CVS The administration of 100% oxygen causes a slight decrease in the heart rate (due to an effect on chemoreceptors), a slight increase in the diastolic blood pressure, and a decrease of 8–20% in the cardiac output due to myocardial depression. The coronary blood flow decreases, secondary to coronary arterial vasoconstriction. In contrast, the PVR and mean arterial pressure decrease.

RS Mild respiratory depression (due to a decrease in sensitivity of the respiratory centre to CO_2) results from the administration of 100% oxygen. Nitrogen is eliminated from the lungs within 2–3 minutes (leading to atelectasis subsequent to the loss of the 'splinting' effect of nitrogen), from the blood within 5 minutes, and from the body within 2 hours. The binding of oxygen with haemoglobin tends to displace CO_2 from the blood (the Haldane effect).

CNS The administration of 100% oxygen causes cerebrovascular constriction (due to an increased sensitivity to adrenergic agonists), resulting in a decrease in the cerebral blood flow.

Toxicity/side effects The following toxic effects are associated with the use of high concentrations of oxygen:
1. CO_2 retention in patients with respiratory failure who are predominantly dependent upon a hypoxic drive to respiration
2. retrolental fibroplasia in neonates
3. acute oxygen toxicity (the Paul–Bert effect) may occur if hyperbaric 100% oxygen is used; the symptoms are altered mood, vertigo, loss of consciousness, and convulsions
4. chronic oxygen toxicity may occur when concentrations >60% are used for prolonged periods at atmospheric pressure; the symptoms of this are tracheobronchial irritation, sore throat, and substernal pain, and the signs are pulmonary congestion, atelectasis, and a decreased vital capacity
5. prolonged administration of 100% oxygen may interfere with red blood cell formation.

Kinetics

Absorption The gas is freely permeable through normal alveolar tissue.

Distribution Oxygen is transported in the blood predominantly combined to haemoglobin; in addition, each 100 ml of plasma contains 0.3 ml of dissolved oxygen at normal atmospheric pressure and an FiO_2 of 0.21. When 100% oxygen is administered at atmospheric pressure, each 100 ml of plasma contains approximately 1.7 ml of dissolved oxygen. If 100% oxygen is administered at 3 atmospheres, approximately 6 ml of dissolved oxygen is contained within each 100 ml of plasma.

Metabolism Occurs within mitochondria to produce CO_2 and water.

Excretion As exhaled CO_2 and metabolic water.

Oxytocin

Uses Oxytocin is used:
1. for the induction and acceleration of labour
2. to promote lactation and in the management of
3. missed and incomplete abortion and
4. post-partum haemorrhage.

Chemical A naturally occurring polypeptide from the posterior lobe of the pituitary gland.

Presentation As a clear solution for injection containing 5/10 units/ml of synthetic oxytocin (which is free from vasopressin and extraneous animal protein) and in a fixed-dose combination for injection containing 5 units/ml of oxytocin and 500 micrograms of ergometrine maleate (which has a more sustained effect on the uterus than does oxytocin).

Main actions Stimulation of uterine contraction.

Mode of action Oxytocin is thought to act by binding to specific receptors on smooth muscle cells and increasing the permeability of the myometrial cell membrane to K^+, thereby decreasing the membrane potential and increasing the excitability of the uterine smooth muscle.

Routes of administration/doses Oxytocin is administered by intravenous infusion at a rate of 1.5–12 milliunits/min, titrated against the frequency and duration of uterine contractions. The intramuscular dose of the oxytocin–ergometrine preparation is 1 ml.

Effects

CVS Bolus intravenous administration of oxytocin causes a decrease in the blood pressure that occurs within 30 seconds and lasts up to 10 minutes—this response is exaggerated in the anaesthetized subject. A reflex tachycardia and an increase in the cardiac output by up to 1.5 l/min occur. ECG changes, such as prolongation of the QT interval and T-wave flattening, may reflect poor coronary artery filling.

AS Oxytocin has no effect on the lower oesophageal sphincter pressure during pregnancy.

GU Infusions of oxytocin increase the renal blood flow in animal models.

Metabolic/other Oxytocin has an antidiuretic effect (exerted by a direct action on the renal tubules) which may, when it is administered in high doses with large volumes of electrolyte-free fluid, lead to water intoxication. Oxytocin also causes milk ejection by causing contraction of modified smooth muscle within the mammary gland, forcing milk from alveolar channels into large sinuses.

Toxicity/side effects Oxytocin may cause uterine spasm and rupture, leading to fetal asphyxia when infused too rapidly. Anaphylactoid reactions to the drug have also been reported. Water intoxication has been described above.

Kinetics Data are incomplete.

Absorption Oxytocin is active when administered by any parenteral route but is inactivated by chymotrypsin when administered orally.

Metabolism Oxytocin is rapidly removed from the plasma by hydrolysis in the liver and kidney (by the action of oxytocinase).

Excretion The elimination half-life is 1–7 minutes.

Special points Oxytocin should not be infused through the same intravenous line as blood and plasma, as rapid inactivation of the polypeptide by plasma oxytocinase occurs. Infusions of oxytocin may alter the action of co-administered suxamethonium, leading to a decrease in the fasciculations caused by the latter and an increased dose requirement for suxamethonium.

Pancuronium

Uses Pancuronium is used to facilitate intubation and controlled ventilation.

Chemical A bis-quaternary aminosteroid.

Presentation As a clear colourless solution for injection containing 2 mg/ml of pancuronium bromide. The solution has a pH of 4.

Main action Pancuronium acts by competitive antagonism of acetylcholine at nicotinic (N2) receptors at the post-synaptic membrane of the neuromuscular junction. The drug also has some pre-junctional action.

Routes of administration/doses The drug is administered intravenously. The ED95 of pancuronium is estimated to be 0.05 mg/kg. An initial dose of 0.05–0.1 mg/kg is recommended in adults, providing muscle relaxation for between 65 and 100 minutes. Endotracheal intubation can be achieved within 90–150 seconds of an intravenous dose, with maximal resultant neuromuscular blockade achieved within 4 minutes following administration. Maintenance of neuromuscular blockade may be achieved with bolus doses of 0.01–0.02 mg/kg. An initial dose of 0.06–0.1 mg/kg is recommended in children. If pancuronium is administered after suxamethonium, then the initial intravenous dose of the former should be reduced to 0.02–0.06 mg/kg in both adults and children. The initial recommended dose in neonates is 0.03–0.04 mg/kg. The drug should not be given by infusion.

Effects

CVS Pancuronium causes an increase in the heart rate, blood pressure, and cardiac output, secondary to a vagolytic action. The systemic vascular resistance remains unchanged after the administration of the drug. A slight fall in central venous pressure may occur.

RS Neuromuscular blockade results in apnoea. Pancuronium has a very low potential for histamine release; bronchospasm is extremely uncommon.

AS Reports of salivation have been noted.

Metabolic/other Pancuronium may decrease the partial thromboplastin time and prothrombin time.

Toxicity/side effects There have been rare reports of fatal anaphylactoid reactions with the administration of pancuronium. Cross-sensitivity may exist with vecuronium and rocuronium. A transient rash may occur, following the administration of pancuronium.

Kinetics

Distribution Pancuronium is 15–30% protein-bound in the plasma, predominantly to albumin and gamma globulin; the V_D is 0.241–0.280 l/kg, which is increased by approximately 50% in patients with cirrhosis. The drug does not cross the blood–brain barrier. Pancuronium has been shown to cross the placenta in small doses.

Metabolism 30–45% of an administered dose undergoes hepatic metabolism by deacetylation to 3-hydroxy-, 17-hydroxy-, and 3,17-hydroxy derivatives, with subsequent biliary excretion. The 3-hydroxy derivative (up to 25% of an injected dose) has half the NMB activity of the parent drug, compared to the other metabolites (<5% of an injected dose) which have approximately 50 times less potency than pancuronium.

Excretion Pancuronium drug levels appear to decrease in a triphasic manner. Forty to 50% of the dose is excreted in the urine (80% as unchanged drug), with 5–11% appearing in the bile. The clearance is 1.10–2.22 ml/kg/min, and the elimination half-life is 69–161 minutes (decreased by 22% and doubled, respectively, in patients with cirrhosis).

Special points The duration of action of pancuronium, in common with other non-depolarizing relaxants, is prolonged by hypokalaemia, hypocalcaemia, hypermagnesaemia, hypoproteinaemia, dehydration, acidosis, and hypercapnia. The following drugs, when co-administered with pancuronium, increase the effect of the latter: volatile anaesthetic agents, induction agents, fentanyl, suxamethonium, diuretics, calcium channel blockers, alpha- and beta-adrenergic antagonists, protamine, lidocaine, metronidazole, and the aminoglycoside antibiotics. Pancuronium appears to decrease the MAC of halothane; it also tends to counteract the depressant effect of halothane on the blood pressure.

Due to the increased V_D seen in patients with cirrhosis, the initial dose to achieve adequate muscle relaxation may be higher. However, the duration of action of the drug may be prolonged in patients with cirrhosis, biliary dysfunction, and renal impairment. The dose should be reduced in the presence of renal impairment.

The use of pancuronium appears to be safe in patients susceptible to malignant hyperpyrexia.

Paracetamol

Uses Paracetamol is used:
1. as an analgesic for the relief of pain of mild to moderate severity and
2. as an antipyretic agent.

Chemical As acetanilide derivative.

Presentation As tablets and suppositories containing 60/125/250/500 mg of paracetamol and a syrup containing 24/50 mg/ml. A number of fixed-dose combinations with codeine, dihydrocodeine, pentazocine, and metoclopramide are also available. The drug is often a component of proprietary cold cures. A dispersible tablet form is available but has a high sodium content due to the presence of sodium bicarbonate. An intravenous preparation for infusion containing 10 mg/ml of paracetamol is available in 50 ml and 100 ml vials. The intravenous preparation also contains cysteine hydrochloride monohydrate, disodium phosphate dihydrate, sodium hydroxide, and mannitol. The sodium content is <23 mg per 100 ml. The preparation is sealed in a glass vial also containing argon, as the drug is unstable in an oxygen-rich environment. The drug should be infused over a 15-minute period. An intravenous preparation containing the pro-drug propacetamol, 1 g of which is equivalent to 500 mg of paracetamol, is also available.

Main action Analgesic and antipyretic.

Mode of action The mode of action of paracetamol is poorly understood, although there is evidence of activity involving prostaglandin synthesis inhibition, and serotonergic and cannabinoid pathways. The drug inhibits COX isoenzymes COX-1 and COX-2, particularly in areas of low inflammation (cf. non-steroidal anti-inflammatory drugs). Prostaglandin synthesis within the CNS is inhibited which accounts for the antipyretic effect of the drug; specifically, it inhibits the synthesis of the E series of prostaglandins that are normally produced in the anterior hypothalamus in response to pyrogens. There is evidence that paracetamol enhances inhibitory serotonergic pain pathways, as well as inhibits the uptake of anandamide, an endocannabinoid, involved in nociception. The drug also acts peripherally by blocking impulse generation within the bradykinin-sensitive chemoreceptors responsible for the generation of afferent nociceptive impulses.

Routes of administration/doses The dose for adolescents and adults weighing >50 kg is 500 mg to 1 g 4- to 6-hourly (maximum daily dose 4 g) for the oral, rectal, and intravenous routes. Analgesic doses in children range from 60 to 90 mg/kg/day in divided doses, depending on the age and route of administration. Analgesic doses in neonates range from 30 to 60 mg/kg/day in divided doses, depending on the post-conceptual age and route of administration. A loading dose may be given.

Effects

CNS The maximum analgesic effect of paracetamol appears to be greater than that of any other non-opioid analgesic.

AS Paracetamol is occasionally used as a model for drug absorption, as its rate of absorption is proportional to the gastric emptying rate. Drugs which alter gastric emptying alter the rate of paracetamol absorption. The drug has no effect on the liver, unless taken in overdose, and does not cause gastric ulceration.

Metabolic/other The drug potentiates the effect of ADH. It has a dose-dependent effect on platelets, causing reduced aggregation via platelet COX-1 inhibition and a subsequent decrease in thromboxane A2 synthesis. This degree of inhibition is unlikely to cause clinically significant bleeding.

Toxicity/side effects Gastrointestinal disturbances, skin reactions, and idiosyncratic haemopoietic disorders (thrombocytopenia, neutropenia) may occur with therapeutic doses. Approximately 5% of patients who are allergic to aspirin show cross-sensitivity to paracetamol.

Kinetics

Absorption The drug is rapidly absorbed from the upper gastrointestinal tract; the bioavailability when administered by the oral route is 63–89% due to first-pass metabolism. Absorption is variable when administered rectally, and the bioavailability by this route is 24–98% of that observed after oral administration.

Distribution At therapeutic levels, paracetamol is 0–5% protein-bound in the plasma; the V_D is 0.7–1 l/kg. Being a non-ionized, lipid-soluble substance, paracetamol penetrates tissues and the blood–brain barrier well. The drug crosses the placenta.

Metabolism Occurs predominantly in the liver, 80–90% being metabolized to glucuronide (60–80%) and sulfate (20–30%) and 10% by cytochrome P450 (CYP2E1) to a highly reactive intermediate metabolite (N-acetyl-p-benzo-quinoneimine (NAPQI)) which, in turn, is inactivated by conjugation with glutathione. In the CNS, paracetamol is metabolized to P-aminophenol and then to N-arachidonoylphenolamine.

Excretion 1–5% is excreted unchanged in the urine; the glucuronide and sulfate metabolites are actively secreted in the renal tubules at low concentrations and actively reabsorbed at high concentrations. The clearance is 5 ml/kg/min, and the elimination half-life is 2–4 hours in normal adults, 4–5 hours in neonates, and 11 hours in premature neonates.

Special points Paracetamol should be used with caution in patients with renal or hepatic impairment. The dose interval should be increased in patients with severe renal impairment. Paracetamol is removed by haemodialysis. The drug may lead to an increase in the INR of patients taking warfarin, possibly due to reduced synthesis of vitamin K-dependent clotting factors.

Hepatic damage occurs readily with doses exceeding 15 g of the drug; with toxic doses, the supply of glutathione becomes depleted, and the highly reactive intermediate metabolite (NAPQI) combines with hepatic cell membranes, leading eventually to centrilobular necrosis. N-acetylcysteine (NAC) and methionine act as alternative supplies of glutathione and can protect against paracetamol-induced liver damage if administered within

10–12 hours of ingestion of paracetamol. A treatment intervention graph is widely available. The major complication is fulminant hepatic failure (with or without acute renal failure), usually occurring at 2–7 days. Liver function tests are a poor prognostic indicator under these circumstances. Criteria for referral to a specialist liver centre are: encephalopathy, INR >3 on day 2 (>4.5 on day 3 or any increase thereafter), creatinine >200 micromoles/l or oliguria, arterial pH <7.3, hypoglycaemia. Patients may be considered for transplantation if arterial pH is <7.3 (or <7.25 if NAC administered) or the combination of prothrombin time >100 seconds, creatinine >300 micromoles/l, and grade III encephalopathy. The following are associated with a poor outcome: bilirubin levels >4 mg/100 ml, INR >2.2, lactate >3.5 mmol/l at 4 and 12 hours, low factor V levels.

Methionine has been added to paracetamol preparations to decrease the risk of hepatotoxicity in overdosage.

Penicillin

Uses Penicillin is used in the treatment of infections of:
1. the respiratory tract
2. ear, nose, and throat
3. skin, bone, soft tissues, and wounds, and in the treatment of
4. gonorrhoea
5. meningitis and
6. subacute bacterial endocarditis.

Chemical The prototype penicillin.

Presentation The preparation for oral use is phenoxymethylpenicillin (penicillin V) which is presented as 125/250 mg tablets and in an elixir as the potassium salt. The parenteral preparation is benzylpenicillin (penicillin G) which is a white crystalline powder presented in vials containing 0.3/0.6/3/6 g of sodium benzylpenicillin.

Main actions Penicillin is a bactericidal antibiotic with a narrow spectrum of activity, which includes *Streptococcus, Neisseria, Haemophilus, Corynebacterium, Bacillus, Clostridium, Listeria*, and *Treponema* spp., some sensitive staphylococcal strains, and oral anaerobes. Penicillin is destroyed by beta-lactamases produced by some strains of *Pseudomonas, Enterobacteriaceae*, and *Bacteroides*.

Mode of action Penicillin binds specifically to PBPs (transpeptidases and carboxypeptidases) in the bacterial cell wall and prevents peptidoglycan cross-linking, thereby decreasing the mechanical stability of the bacterial cell wall.

Routes of administration/doses The adult oral dose is 125–250 mg 4- to 6-hourly; the corresponding intravenous and intramuscular dose is 0.6–4.8 g/day in 2–4 divided doses. One mega unit is 600 mg. Penicillin may also be administered intrathecally.

Effects
Metabolic/other High doses of benzylpenicillin may produce hypernatraemia and hypokalaemia.

Toxicity/side effects Gastrointestinal disturbances, allergic phenomena (including anaphylaxis), rashes, and haemolytic anaemia may occur with the use of the drug. High parenteral doses of penicillin may cause neuropathy and nephropathy.

Kinetics
Absorption 15–30% of an oral dose of benzylpenicillin (the drug is unstable under acid conditions) and 60% of an oral dose of phenoxymethylpenicillin is absorbed. The pharmacokinetics after absorption is similar for both preparations.

Distribution Penicillin is 59–67% protein-bound in the plasma, predominantly to albumin; the V_D is 0.32–0.81 l/kg.

Metabolism Penicillin is metabolized to penicilloic acid which is inactive with subsequent transformation to penamaldic and penicillenic acid.

Excretion 60–90% of a dose is excreted in the urine by active tubular secretion; up to 25% is excreted unchanged. The elimination half-life is 0.7 hours.

Special points Penicillin is removed by haemodialysis.

Pethidine

Uses Pethidine is used:
1. for premedication
2. as an analgesic in the management of moderate to severe pain and
3. as an antispasmodic agent in the treatment of renal and biliary colic.

Chemical A synthetic phenylpiperidine derivative.

Presentation As 50 mg tablets and a clear, colourless solution for injection containing 10/50 mg/ml of pethidine hydrochloride.

Main actions Analgesia and respiratory depression.

Mode of action Pethidine is an agonist at mu- and kappa-opioid receptors. Opioids appear to exert their effects by increasing intracellular calcium concentration which, in turn, increases potassium conductance and hyperpolarization of excitable cell membranes. The decrease in membrane excitability that results may decrease both pre- and post-synaptic responses.

Routes of administration/doses The adult oral dose is 50–150 mg 4-hourly; the corresponding dose by the intramuscular route is 25–150 mg and by the intravenous route 25–100 mg. Pethidine may also be administered via the epidural route; a dose of 25 mg is usually employed. The drug acts within 15 minutes when administered orally and within 10 minutes when administered intramuscularly; the duration of action is 2–3 hours.

Effects

CVS Pethidine causes orthostatic hypotension due to the combination of histamine release and alpha-adrenergic blockade that it produces. The drug also has a mild quinidine-like effect and anticholinergic properties, which may lead to the development of tachycardia.

RS The drug is a potent respiratory depressant, having a greater effect on the tidal volume than on the respiratory rate. Pethidine obtunds the ventilatory response to both hypoxia and hypercapnia. Chest wall rigidity may occur with the use of the drug. It has little antitussive activity.

CNS Pethidine is one-tenth as potent an analgesic as morphine. It appears to cause more euphoria and less nausea and vomiting than an equipotent dose of morphine. Miosis and corneal anaesthesia follow the use of the drug.

AS In common with other opioids, pethidine decreases the rate of gastric emptying. The drug appears to cause a less marked increase in bile duct pressure and less depression of intestinal activity (and therefore constipation) than equipotent doses of morphine.

GU The drug decreases the ureteric tone; it may increase the amplitude of contractions of the pregnant uterus.

Metabolic/other Pethidine increases ADH secretion and decreases adrenal steroid secretion.

Toxicity/side effects Respiratory depression, nausea and vomiting, hallucinations, and dependence may complicate the use of pethidine. The drug evokes less histamine release than morphine.

Kinetics

Absorption The bioavailability, when administered orally, is 45–75% due to a significant first-pass effect. The drug has a bioavailability of 100% when administered intramuscularly (into the deltoid muscle).

Distribution Pethidine is 49–67% protein-bound in the plasma; the V_D is 3.5–5.3 l/kg. The drug crosses the placenta; the mean cord blood concentration at delivery is 75–90% of the maternal venous concentration.

Metabolism Occurs in the liver by N-demethylation to norpethidine and by hydrolysis to pethidinic acid; norpethidine is further hydrolysed to norpethidinic acid. The acid metabolites are further conjugated prior to excretion. Norpethidine may accumulate in the presence of renal failure and has 50% the analgesic potency of the parent compound and marked convulsant properties.

Excretion 1–25% of the administered dose is excreted unchanged in the urine, dependent upon the urinary pH. Norpethidine is excreted in the urine; accumulation may occur in the presence of renal or hepatic impairment. The clearance is 12–22 ml/min/kg, and the elimination half-life is 2.4–7 hours. The clearance is reduced by the co-administration of halothane.

Special points Pethidine may precipitate a severe hypertensive episode in patients receiving MAOIs. The drug reduces the apparent MAC of co-administered volatile agents. By convention, pethidine is used in asthmatic patients, although there is no published evidence that the drug causes bronchospasm less frequently than morphine in this group of patients.

Pethidine effectively inhibits post-anaesthetic shivering.

Phenelzine

Uses Phenelzine is used in the treatment of:
1. non-endogenous depression and
2. phobic disorders.

Chemical A substituted hydrazine.

Presentation As tablets containing 15 mg of phenelzine sulfate.

Main action Antidepressant.

Mode of action Phenelzine is an irreversible inhibitor of mitochondrial monoamine oxidase, an enzyme involved in the metabolism of catecholamines and 5HT. It is assumed that the antidepressant activity of the drug is related to the increased concentration of monoamines in the CNS that results from the use of the drug.

Routes of administration/doses The adult oral dose is 15 mg 6- to 8-hourly; this is reduced once a satisfactory response has been obtained. The maximum inhibition of enzyme activity is achieved within a few days, but the antidepressant effect of the drug may take 3–4 weeks to become established.

Effects
CVS The predominant effect of the drug is orthostatic hypotension; MAOIs were formerly used as antihypertensive agents.

CNS Phenelzine is an effective antidepressant which may also produce stimulation of the CNS, resulting in tremor and insomnia. The MAOIs suppress REM sleep very effectively.

AS Constipation occurs commonly with the use of the drug; the mechanism of this effect is unknown.

Metabolic/other Inappropriate secretion of ADH has been reported in association with the use of phenelzine.

Toxicity/side effects Disturbances of the CNS (including convulsions and peripheral neuropathy), anticholinergic side effects, and hepatotoxicity may complicate the use of the drug. More importantly, a host of serious and potentially fatal interactions may occur between MAOIs and tyramine-containing substances, sympathomimetic agents, and CNS depressants (v.i.).

Kinetics Data are incomplete.
Absorption Phenelzine is readily absorbed when administered orally.

Metabolism 80% of the dose is metabolized by oxidation and hydroxylation to phenylacetic acid and parahydroxyphenylacetic acid. The drug may inhibit its own metabolism.

Excretion Occurs predominantly in the urine as free and unconjugated aromatic forms of the drug.

Special points MAOIs demonstrate several important drug interactions:

1. drugs, such as pethidine, fentanyl, morphine, and barbiturates, whose action is terminated by oxidation, have a more profound and prolonged effect in the presence of MAOIs; this is particularly marked in the case of pethidine. Marked hyperpyrexia, possibly due to 5HT release, may also occur when pethidine is administered to a patient who is already receiving MAOIs

2. indirectly acting sympathomimetic agents (e.g. ephedrine) produce an exaggerated pressor response in the presence of co-administered MAOIs; severe hypertensive episodes (which are best treated with phentolamine) may result from this interaction

3. MAOIs markedly exaggerate the depressant effects of volatile anaesthetic agents on the blood pressure and CNS

4. MAOIs inhibit plasma cholinesterase and may therefore prolong the duration of action of co-administered suxamethonium

5. MAOIs may also potentiate the effects of antihypertensive and hypoglycaemic agents, anti-parkinsonian drugs, and local anaesthetics.

A period of 2 weeks is required to restore amine metabolism to normal after the cessation of administration of phenelzine. This is the recommended period that should elapse between discontinuation of MAOI therapy and elective surgery. Post-operative analgesia for patients who are still receiving MAOI therapy has been safely provided using chlorpromazine and codeine.

Phenoxybenzamine

Uses Phenoxybenzamine is used in the treatment of:
1. hypertensive crises
2. Raynaud's phenomenon and
3. in the preoperative preparation of patients due for the removal of a phaeochromocytoma.

Chemical A tertiary amine which is a haloalkylamine.

Presentation As 10 mg tablets and a clear, colourless solution for injection containing 50 mg/ml of phenoxybenzamine hydrochloride.

Main actions Vasodilatation (predominantly arterial).

Mode of action Phenoxybenzamine acts via a highly reactive carbonium ion derivative which binds covalently to alpha-adrenergic receptors to produce irreversible competitive alpha-blockade. The drug increases the rate of peripheral turnover of noradrenaline and the amount of noradrenaline released per impulse by blockade of pre-synaptic alpha-2 receptors. Haloalkylamines also inhibit the response to serotonergic, histaminergic, and cholinergic stimulation.

Routes of administration/doses The adult dose by the oral route is 10–60 mg/day in divided doses. The corresponding dose by intravenous infusion (diluted in glucose or saline) over 1 hour is 10–40 mg. After intravenous administration, the drug acts in 1 hour and has a duration of action of 3–4 days.

Effects

CVS Phenoxybenzamine produces a decrease in the peripheral vascular resistance, which leads to a decrease in the diastolic blood pressure and pronounced orthostatic hypotension. A reflex tachycardia and an increase in cardiac output follow the administration of the drug. Phenoxybenzamine inhibits catecholamine-induced cardiac dysrhythmias. The drug causes a shift of fluid from the interstitial to the vascular compartment due to vasodilatation of pre- and post-capillary resistance vessels.

CNS The drug decreases cerebral blood flow only if marked hypotension occurs. Motor excitability may follow the administration of phenoxybenzamine; however, sedation is the usual effect observed. Miosis occurs commonly.

AS Phenoxybenzamine produces little change in gastrointestinal tone or splanchnic blood flow.

GU The drug causes little alteration of renal blood flow; it decreases the motility of the non-pregnant uterus.

Toxicity/side effects Dizziness, sedation, a dry mouth, paralytic ileus, and impotence may result from the use of phenoxybenzamine. The drug is irritant if extravasation occurs.

Kinetics Data are incomplete.

Absorption Phenoxybenzamine is incompletely absorbed after oral administration; the bioavailability by this route is 20–30%.

Distribution The drug is highly lipophilic.

Metabolism Phenoxybenzamine is predominantly metabolized in the liver by deacetylation.

Excretion Occurs via the urine and bile; the half-life is 24 hours.

Special points Systemic administration of the drug may lead to an increase in the systemic absorption of co-administered local anaesthetic agents. Phenoxybenzamine causes marked congestion of the nasal mucosa, and this may make nasal instrumentation more traumatic if topical vasoconstrictors are not used.

Phentolamine

Uses Phentolamine is used for:
1. the diagnosis and perioperative management of patients with phaeochromocytoma
2. the acute treatment of hypertension occurring during anaesthesia and
3. the treatment of left ventricular failure complicating myocardial infarction.

Chemical An imidazoline.

Presentation As a clear solution for injection containing 10 mg/ml of phentolamine mesilate.

Main actions Hypotension, positive inotropism, and chronotropism.

Mode of action Phentolamine acts by transient, competitive alpha-adrenergic blockade (it is 3–5 times as active at alpha-1 as at alpha-2 receptors); it also has some beta-adrenergic agonist and anti-serotonergic activity.

Routes of administration/doses The adult intramuscular dose for the control of paroxysmal hypertension is 5–10 mg; the drug may also be administered by intravenous infusion (diluted in glucose or saline) at the rate of 0.1–0.2 mg/min.

Effects

CVS Phentolamine causes a marked reduction in the systemic vascular resistance, producing a decrease in blood pressure and a reflex tachycardia. The drug has a positive inotropic action, which is probably an indirect effect due to alpha-2 blockade leading to noradrenaline release. The coronary blood flow increases; the drug also has class I antiarrhythmic effects. In patients with heart failure, phentolamine causes an increase in the heart rate and cardiac output, with a concomitant decrease in the pulmonary arterial pressure, systemic vascular resistance, and left ventricular end-diastolic pressure.

RS The drug increases the vital capacity, FEV_1, and maximum breathing capacity in normal subjects, and prevents histamine-induced bronchoconstriction. Respiratory tract secretions are increased by the drug. Phentolamine is a pulmonary arterial vasodilator.

AS The drug increases salivation, gastric acid, pepsin secretion, and gastrointestinal motility.

Metabolic/other The drug increases insulin secretion.

Toxicity/side effects Phentolamine is generally well tolerated but may cause orthostatic hypotension, dizziness, abdominal discomfort, and diarrhoea. Cardiovascular collapse and death have followed the administration of phentolamine when it is used as a diagnostic test for phaeochromocytoma.

Kinetics Data are incomplete.

Absorption The bioavailability is 20% when administered orally.

Metabolism The drug is extensively metabolized.

Excretion 10% of the dose is excreted in the urine unchanged. The plasma half-life is 10–15 minutes.

Special points Phentolamine causes marked congestion of the nasal mucosa, and this may make nasal instrumentation more traumatic if topical vasoconstrictors are not used.

Phenylephrine

Uses Phenylephrine is used as an adjunct in the treatment of:
1. hypotension occurring during general or spinal anaesthesia
2. as a nasal decongestant and
3. as a mydriatic agent.

Chemical A synthetic sympathomimetic amine.

Presentation As a clear solution containing 10 mg/ml of phenylephrine hydrochloride.

Main action Peripheral vasoconstriction.

Mode of action Phenylephrine is a direct-acting sympathomimetic agent that has agonist effects at alpha-1 adrenoceptors. The drug does not affect beta-adrenoceptors.

Routes of administration/doses Phenylephrine may be administered subcutaneously or intramuscularly in a dosage of 2–5 mg, with further doses titrated to response. The drug may be administered intravenously, following dilution in 0.9% sodium chloride (e.g. 10 mg of phenylephrine diluted in 100 ml of 0.9% sodium chloride yields a 100 micrograms/ml solution which can be diluted further, producing a 25 micrograms/ml solution) in 50–100 micrograms boluses. When administered intravenously, it has a duration of action of 5–10 minutes. When administered intramuscularly or subcutaneously, it has a duration of action of up to 1 hour.

Effects

CVS Phenylephrine causes a rapid increase in the systolic and diastolic blood pressures due to an increase in the systemic vascular resistance. A reflex bradycardia occurs, which may cause a decrease in cardiac output.

RS The drug is not known to cause bronchodilatation or act as a respiratory stimulant.

CNS Phenylephrine has no stimulatory effects on the CNS. Phenylephrine causes mydriasis.

GU The drug reduces uterine artery blood flow via its effect at alpha-adrenoceptors. Renal blood flow is decreased.

Metabolic/other The drug may cause alterations in glucose metabolism.

Toxicity/side effects Headaches, sweating, hypersalivation, tremor, and urinary retention may complicate the use of the drug. Extravascular injection of the drug may lead to tissue necrosis at the injection site.

Kinetics There are no quantitative data available.

Metabolism The drug is metabolized in the gastrointestinal tract and liver by monoamine oxidase.

Special points Excessive hypertension may occur when phenylephrine is administered to patients with hyperthyroidism or those receiving MAOIs. Patients receiving cardiac glycosides, tricyclic antidepressants, or quinidine are at an increased risk of developing dysrhythmias when phenylephrine is administered.

Phenytoin

Uses Phenytoin is used:
1. in the prophylaxis and treatment of generalized tonic–clonic and partial epilepsies and in the treatment of
2. fast atrial and ventricular dysrhythmias resulting from digoxin toxicity and
3. trigeminal neuralgia.

Chemical A hydantoin derivative.

Presentation As 25/50/100/300 mg capsules, a syrup containing 6 mg/ml, and as a clear, colourless solution for injection containing 50 mg/ml of phenytoin sodium.

Main actions Anticonvulsant and antiarrhythmic.

Mode of action Phenytoin has membrane-stabilizing activity and slows inward Na^+ and Ca^{2+} flux during depolarization in excitable tissue; it also delays outward K^+ flux. There appears to be a high-affinity binding site within the CNS for phenytoin, which suggests the existence of an endogenous ligand.

Routes of administration/doses The adult oral dose is 200–600 mg/day; a small dose should be used initially and gradually increased thereafter. The corresponding intramuscular dose is 100–200 mg 4-hourly for 48–72 hours, decreasing to 300 mg daily. The intravenous loading dose for the management of epilepsy is 10–15 mg/kg (administered slowly), followed by a maintenance dose of 100 mg 6- to 8-hourly. When used in the treatment of cardiac dysrhythmias, the corresponding intravenous dose is 3.5 mg/kg. The therapeutic range is 10–20 mg/l.

Effects

CVS Phenytoin exhibits class I antiarrhythmic properties and enhances AV nodal conduction. Hypotension may complicate rapid intravenous administration of the drug; complete heart block, ventricular fibrillation, and asystole have also been reported under these circumstances.

CNS 80% of newly diagnosed epileptics can be controlled with phenytoin monotherapy. The drug acts as an anticonvulsant by stabilizing, rather than raising, the seizure threshold and by preventing the spread of seizure activity, rather than by abolishing a primary discharging focus.

Metabolic/other Hyperglycaemia, hypocalcaemia, and alterations in liver function tests have been described consequent to phenytoin therapy. The drug suppresses ADH secretion.

Toxicity/side effects Phenytoin has both idiosyncratic and concentration-dependent side effects. The idiosyncratic side effects include acne, gingival hyperplasia, hirsutism, coarsened facies, folate-dependent megaloblastic anaemia and other blood dyscrasias, osteomalacia, erythroderma, lymphadenopathy, systemic lupus erythematosus, hepatotoxicity, and allergic phenomena. The concentration-dependent side effects include nausea and vomiting, drowsiness, behavioural disturbances, tremor, ataxia, nystagmus, paradoxical seizures, peripheral neuropathy, and cerebellar damage. The drug is irritant if extravasation occurs when given intravenously and may cause muscular damage when administered intramuscularly.

Kinetics

Absorption Absorption is very slow by both the intramuscular and oral routes. The oral bioavailability is 85–95%.

Distribution Phenytoin is 90–93% protein-bound in the plasma; the V_D is 0.5–0.7 l/kg.

Metabolism There is a large genetic variation in the rate of metabolism of phenytoin, which occurs in the liver predominantly to a hydroxylated derivative which is subsequently conjugated to glucuronide. Phenytoin exhibits zero-order elimination kinetics just above the therapeutic range; the implication of this is that the dose required to produce a plasma concentration within the therapeutic range is close to that which will produce toxicity.

Excretion 70–80% of the dose is excreted in the urine by active tubular secretion as the major metabolite; 5% is excreted unchanged. The clearance is 5.5–9.5 ml/kg/day, and the elimination half-life is 9–22 hours in the first-order kinetics range; the latter increases at higher dose ranges when the capacity of the hepatic mono-oxygenase system becomes saturated. The dose of phenytoin should be reduced in the presence of hepatic impairment, but renal impairment requires little alteration of dosage (despite the fact that the free fraction of the drug increases in the presence of uraemia, an increase in the clearance and V_D tends to offset this).

Special points Phenytoin is a potent enzyme inducer and demonstrates a plethora of drug interactions, among which the most important are the precipitation of phenytoin toxicity by metronidazole and isoniazid and a reduced effectiveness of benzodiazepines, pethidine, and warfarin caused by the co-administration of phenytoin. The drug may also decrease the MAC of volatile agents and enhance the CNS toxicity of local anaesthetics; it appears to increase the dose requirements of all the non-depolarizing relaxants (with the exception of atracurium) by 60–80%.

The parenteral preparation of phenytoin precipitates in the presence of most crystalloid solutions.

The drug is not removed by dialysis.

Piperacillin

Uses Piperacillin is used in the treatment of:
1. urinary and respiratory tract infections
2. intra-abdominal and biliary tract sepsis
3. gynaecological and obstetric infections
4. infections of skin, soft tissue, bone, and joints
5. septicaemia
6. meningitis and for
7. perioperative prophylaxis.

Chemical A semi-synthetic penicillin.

Presentation In vials containing 1/2 g and infusion bottles containing 4 g of piperacillin sodium. A fixed-dose combination with tazobactam is also available.

Main actions Piperacillin is a bactericidal broad-spectrum antibiotic that is effective against many beta-lactamase-producing organisms. In vitro, it shows activity against the Gram-negative organisms Escherichia coli, Haemophilus influenzae, and Klebsiella, Neisseria, Proteus, Shigella, and Serratia spp.; anaerobes, including Bacteroides and Clostridium spp.; and the Gram-positive enterococci Staphylococcus, and Streptococcus spp. It is particularly effective against Pseudomonas, indole-positive Proteus, Streptococcus faecalis, and Serratia marcescens.

Mode of action Piperacillin binds to cell wall PBPs and inhibits their activity; specifically, it affects PBP 1A/B which are involved in the cross-linking of cell wall peptidoglycans, PBP 2 which is involved in the maintenance of the rod shape, and PBP 3 which is involved in septal synthesis.

Routes of administration/doses The adult intravenous dose is 4 g 6 to 8 hourly (each gram should be infused over 3–5 minutes), and the intramuscular dose 2 g 6 to 8 hourly.

Effects

Metabolic/other Piperacillin has a lower sodium content than other disodium penicillins and causes less fluid and electrolyte derangements; serum potassium levels may decrease after the administration of the drug.

Toxicity/side effects Gastrointestinal upsets, abnormalities of liver function tests, allergic reactions, and transient leucopenia and neutropenia may complicate the use of the drug. Deterioration in renal function has been reported in patients with pre-existent severe renal impairment treated with piperacillin.

Kinetics

Absorption Piperacillin is poorly absorbed when administered orally and is hydrolysed by gastric acids.

Distribution The drug is 16% protein-bound in the plasma; the V_D is 0.32 l/kg. High concentrations are found in most tissues and body fluids.

Metabolism Piperacillin is not metabolized in man.

Excretion 20% is excreted in the bile; the remainder is excreted in the urine by glomerular filtration and tubular secretion. The elimination half-life is 36–72 minutes.

Special points The dose of piperacillin should be reduced in the presence of renal impairment; the drug is 30–50% removed by haemodialysis.

Prednisolone

Uses Prednisolone is used:
1. as replacement therapy in adrenocortical deficiency states and in the treatment of
2. allergy and anaphylaxis
3. hypercalcaemia
4. asthma
5. panoply of autoimmune disorders
6. some forms of red eye and
7. in leukaemia chemotherapy regimes and
8. for immunosuppression after organ transplantation.

Chemical A synthetic glucocorticosteroid.

Presentation As 1/2.5/5/20 mg tablets of prednisolone, a solution for injection containing 25 mg/ml of prednisolone acetate, and as eye/ear drops and retention enemas.

Main actions Anti-inflammatory.

Mode of action Corticosteroids act by controlling the rate of protein synthesis; they react with cytoplasmic receptors to form a complex which directly influences the rate of RNA transcription. This directs the synthesis of lipocortins.

Routes of administration/doses The adult oral dose is 5–60 mg/day in divided doses, using the lowest dose that is effective and on alternate days, if possible, to limit the development of side effects. The intramuscular or intra-articular dose is 25–100 mg once or twice weekly.

Effects

CVS In the absence of corticosteroids, vascular permeability increases; small blood vessels demonstrate an inadequate motor response, and the cardiac output decreases. Steroids have a positive effect on myocardial contractility and cause vasoconstriction by increasing the number of alpha-1 adrenoreceptors and beta-adrenoreceptors and stimulating their function.

CNS Corticosteroids increase the excitability of the CNS; the absence of glucocorticoid leads to apathy, depression, and irritability.

AS Prednisolone increases the likelihood of peptic ulcer disease. It decreases the gastrointestinal absorption of calcium.

GU Prednisolone has weak mineralocorticoid effects and produces sodium retention and increased potassium excretion; the urinary excretion of calcium is also increased by the drug. The drug increases the glomerular filtration rate and stimulates tubular secretory activity.

Metabolic/other Prednisolone exerts profound effects on carbohydrate, protein, and lipid metabolism. Glucocorticoids stimulate gluconeogenesis and inhibit the peripheral utilization of glucose; they cause a redistribution of body fat, enhance lipolysis, and also reduce the conversion of amino acids to protein. Prednisolone is a potent anti-inflammatory agent which inhibits all stages of the inflammatory process by inhibiting neutrophil and macrophage recruitment, blocking the effect of lymphokines, and inhibiting the formation of plasminogen activator. Corticosteroids increase red blood cell, neutrophil, and haemoglobin concentrations, whilst depressing other white cell lines and the activity of lymphoid tissue.

Toxicity/side effects Consist of an acute withdrawal syndrome and a syndrome (Cushing's) produced by prolonged use of excessive quantities of the drug. Cushing's syndrome is characterized by growth arrest, a characteristic appearance consisting of central obesity, a moon face, and buffalo hump, striae, acne, hirsutism, skin and capillary fragility, together with the following metabolic derangements—altered glucose tolerance, fluid retention, a hypokalaemic alkalosis, and osteoporosis. A proximal myopathy, cataracts, mania, and an increased susceptibility to peptic ulcer disease may also complicate the use of the drug.

Kinetics

Absorption Prednisolone is rapidly and completely absorbed when administered orally or rectally; the bioavailability by either route is 80–100%.

Distribution The drug is reversibly bound in the plasma to albumin and a specific corticosteroid-binding globulin; the drug is 80–90% protein-bound at low concentrations, but only 60–70% protein-bound at higher concentrations. The V_D is 0.35–0.7 l/kg, according to the dose.

Metabolism Occurs in the liver by hydroxylation with subsequent conjugation.

Excretion 11–14% of the dose is excreted unchanged in the urine. The clearance is dose-dependent and ranges from 170 to 200 ml/min; the elimination half-life is 2.6–5 hours.

Special points Prednisone and prednisolone are metabolically interchangeable; only the latter is active. The conversion of prednisone to prednisolone is rapid and extensive and occurs as a first-pass effect in the liver. Prednisolone is four times as potent as hydrocortisone and six times less potent than dexamethasone. It has been recommended that perioperative steroid cover be given:

1. to patients who have received steroid replacement therapy for 2 weeks prior to surgery or for 1 month in the year prior to surgery and
2. to patients undergoing pituitary or adrenal surgery.

Glucocorticoids antagonize the effects of anticholinesterase drugs.

Pregabalin

Uses Pregabalin is used in the treatment of:
1. peripheral and central neuropathic pain
2. partial seizures with or without secondary generalization and
3. generalized anxiety disorder.

Chemical The drug is a GABA analogue ((S)-3-(aminomethyl)-5-methylhexanoic acid).

Presentation As 25/50/75/100/150/200/225/300 mg capsules. Each capsule contains 35/70/8.25/11/16.5/22/24.75/33 mg of lactose monohydrate, respectively.

Main actions Anticonvulsant, analgesic, and anxiolytic.

Mode of action Pregabalin is structurally related to GABA but does not interact with GABA receptors. The binding site for the drug is the alpha-2 delta subunit of voltage-gated calcium channels.

Routes of administration/doses The dose range is 150–600 mg/day in two or three divided doses. The initial dose is 150 mg/day, increased to 300 mg/day after 1 week, with subsequent increases achieved on a weekly basis, based on individual response and tolerability. Discontinuation of treatment should be performed over at least a week. The dose needs to be reduced in patients with renal impairment.

Effects

CNS Pregabalin has analgesic, anticonvulsant, and anxiolytic properties.

Toxicity/side effects Weight gain may occur in diabetic patients during treatment with pregabalin, requiring dose modification of hypoglycaemic therapies. Pregabalin treatment has been associated with dizziness and somnolence. Data from controlled studies demonstrate an increased incidence of blurred vision, reduced visual acuity, and diplopia.

Kinetics

Absorption Pregabalin is rapidly absorbed orally in the fasted state, has a bioavailability of >90%, and is independent of the dose administered. The rate of absorption is decreased when the drug is given with food.

Distribution The drug is not bound to plasma proteins; the V_D is 0.56 l/kg. Animal studies demonstrate that pregabalin crosses the placenta and is present in breast milk.

Metabolism Pregabalin undergoes minimal metabolism in man; 0.9% of an administered dose is excreted as the major metabolite N-methylated pregabalin.

Excretion Approximately 98% of an administered dose is excreted unchanged in the urine. The elimination half-life is 6.3 hours. Pregabalin plasma and renal clearances are directly proportional to creatinine clearance.

Special points Due to the lactose content of pregabalin preparations, the drug should be avoided in patients with galactose intolerance, lactase deficiency, or glucose–galactose malabsorption.

The drug is removed by haemodialysis, with plasma pregabalin concentrations reduced by approximately 50% following 4 hours of haemodialysis.

Prilocaine

Uses Prilocaine is used as a local anaesthetic.

Chemical A secondary amide which is an amide derivative of toluidine.

Presentation As a clear, colourless solution containing racemic prilocaine hydrochloride (S- and R-enantiomers) in concentrations of 0.5/1/2/4%. A 3% solution with 0.03 IU of felypressin per ml is also available. The pKa of prilocaine is 7.7–7.9 and is 33% unionized at a pH of 7.4. The heptane:buffer partition coefficient is 0.9.

Main action Local anaesthetic.

Mode of action Local anaesthetics diffuse in their uncharged base form through neural sheaths and the axonal membrane to the internal surface of cell membrane Na^+ channels; here they combine with hydrogen ions to form a cationic species which enters the internal opening of the Na^+ channel and combines with a receptor. This produces blockade of the Na^+ channel, thereby decreasing Na^+ conductance and preventing depolarization of the cell membrane.

Routes of administration/doses Prilocaine may be administered topically, by infiltration, or epidurally. The toxic dose of prilocaine is 6 mg/kg (8 mg/kg with felypressin). The maximum dose is 400 mg. The drug has a rapid onset of action and has a duration of action 1.5 times that of lidocaine.

Effects

CVS Prilocaine has few haemodynamic effects when used in low doses, except to cause a slight increase in the systemic vascular resistance, leading to a mild increase in the blood pressure. In toxic concentrations, the drug decreases the peripheral vascular resistance and myocardial contractility, producing hypotension and possibly cardiovascular collapse.

RS The drug causes bronchodilatation at subtoxic concentrations. Respiratory depression occurs in the toxic dose range.

CNS The principal effect of prilocaine is reversible neural blockade; this leads to a characteristically biphasic effect in the CNS. Initially, excitation (light-headedness, dizziness, visual and auditory disturbances, and seizure activity) occurs due to inhibition of inhibitory interneurone pathways in the cortex. With increasing doses, depression of both facilitatory and inhibitory pathways occurs, leading to CNS depression (drowsiness, disorientation, and coma). Local anaesthetic agents block neuromuscular transmission when administered intraneurally; it is thought that a complex of neurotransmitter, receptor, and local anaesthetic is formed, which has negligible conductance.

AS Local anaesthetics depress contraction of the intact bowel.

Toxicity/side effects Prilocaine is intrinsically less toxic than lidocaine. Allergic reactions to the amide-type local anaesthetic agents are extremely rare. The side effects are predominantly correlated with excessive plasma concentrations of the drug, as described above. Methaemoglobinaemia may occur if doses in excess of 600 mg are used and is caused by the metabolite O-toluidine, although this condition may occur at lower doses in patients suffering from anaemia or a haemoglobinopathy, or in patients receiving therapy known to also precipitate methaemoglobinaemia (sulfonamides). Use of prilocaine for paracervical block or pudendal nerve block in obstetric patients is not recommended, as this may give rise to methaemoglobinaemia in the neonate, as the erythrocytes are deficient in methaemoglobin reductase.

Kinetics Data are incomplete.

Absorption The absorption of local anaesthetic agents is related to:
1. the site of injection (intercostal > caudal > epidural > brachial plexus > subcutaneous)
2. the dose—a linear relationship exists between the total dose and the peak blood concentrations achieved and
3. the presence of vasoconstrictors which delay absorption.

The addition of adrenaline to prilocaine solutions does not influence the rate of systemic absorption, as:
1. the drug is highly lipid-soluble, and therefore uptake into fat is rapid and
2. the drug has a direct vasodilatory effect.

Distribution Prilocaine is 55% protein-bound in the plasma, predominantly to alpha-1 acid glycoprotein; the V_D is 190–260 l.

Metabolism Prilocaine is rapidly metabolized in the liver by amide hydrolysis, initially to O-toluidine which is, in turn, metabolized by hydroxylation to 4- and 6-hydroxytoluidine. Some metabolism also occurs in the lungs and kidneys. Excessive plasma concentrations of O-toluidine may lead to the development of methaemoglobinaemia, which responds to the administration of 1–2 mg/kg of methylene blue.

Excretion <5% of the dose is excreted unchanged in the urine. The terminal elimination half-life is 1.6 hours.

Special points The onset and duration of conduction blockade is related to the pKa, lipid solubility, and the extent of protein binding. A low pKa and high lipid solubility are associated with a rapid onset time; a high degree of protein binding is associated with a long duration of action. Local anaesthetic agents significantly increase the duration of action of both depolarizing and non-depolarizing relaxants.

EMLA® is a white cream used to provide topical anaesthesia prior to venepuncture and has also been used to provide anaesthesia for split skin grafting. It contains 2.5% lidocaine and 2.5% prilocaine in an oil–water emulsion. When applied topically under an occlusive dressing, local anaesthesia is achieved after 1–2 hours and lasts for up to 5 hours. The preparation causes temporary blanching and oedema of the skin; detectable methaemoglobinaemia may also occur.

Prochlorperazine

Uses Prochlorperazine is used in the treatment of:
1. nausea and vomiting
2. vertigo
3. psychotic states, including mania and schizophrenia, and
4. in premedication.

Chemical A phenothiazine of the piperazine subclass.

Presentation As tablets containing 3/5/25 mg, suppositories containing 5/25 mg, as a clear, colourless solution for injection containing 12.5 mg/ml of prochlorperazine maleate, and as a syrup containing 1 mg/ml of prochlorperazine mesilate.

Main actions Antiemetic.

Mode of action The antiemetic and neuroleptic effects of the drug appear to be mediated by central dopaminergic (D2) blockade, leading to an increased threshold for vomiting at the chemoreceptor trigger zone; in higher doses, prochlorperazine appears to have an inhibitory effect at the vomiting centre.

Routes of administration/doses The adult dose is 5–20 mg 8 to 12 hourly, and the corresponding intramuscular dose is 12.5 mg 6-hourly.

Effects

CVS Prochlorperazine may cause orthostatic hypotension secondary to alpha-adrenergic blockade. ECG changes, including an increased QT interval, ST depression, and T and U wave changes, may also occur.

RS The drug may cause mild respiratory depression.

CNS Prochlorperazine has neuroleptic properties but appears to be less soporific than perphenazine.

AS Lower oesophageal tone is increased by the drug.

Metabolic/other In common with other phenothiazines, prochlorperazine has anti-adrenergic, anti-inflammatory, antipruritic, anticholinergic, and antihistaminergic effects. The drug may also cause hyperprolactinaemia.

Toxicity/side effects Prochlorperazine may cause extrapyramidal reactions, jaundice, leucopenia, and rashes. The neuroleptic malignant syndrome (a complex of symptoms that include catatonia, cardiovascular lability, hyperthermia, and myoglobinaemia), which has a mortality in excess of 10%, has been reported in association with the use of the drug.

Kinetics Data are incomplete.

Absorption The drug is slowly absorbed when administered orally; the bioavailability is 0–16% by this route.

Distribution The drug is highly protein-bound (91–99%); the V_D is 20–22 l/kg.

Metabolism Prochlorperazine undergoes significant first-pass metabolism in the liver; its metabolic pathways include CYP3A4 and CYP2D6. Metabolism may occur by S-oxidation to a sulfoxide.

Excretion The half-life of prochlorperazine is 6–8 hours.

Special points Prochlorperazine is not removed by haemodialysis.

Promethazine

Uses Promethazine is used in the treatment of:
1. nausea and vomiting (including motion sickness)
2. allergic reactions
3. pruritus and for
4. sedation in children.

Chemical A phenothiazine.

Presentation As 10/25 mg tablets, an elixir containing 1 mg/ml, and a clear, colourless solution for injection containing 25 mg/ml of promethazine hydrochloride.

Main actions Antihistaminergic, sedative, and antiemetic.

Mode of action Promethazine acts primarily as a reversible competitive antagonist at H1 histaminergic receptors; it also has some anticholinergic, anti-serotonergic, and anti-dopaminergic activity.

Routes of administration/doses The adult oral dose is 20–75 mg daily in divided doses; the corresponding intramuscular and intravenous dose is 25–50 mg. The drug acts within 15 minutes and has a duration of action of 8–20 hours.

Effects

CVS When normal therapeutic doses are used, promethazine has no significant cardiovascular effects. Rapid intravenous administration may cause transient hypotension.

RS The drug causes bronchodilatation and a reduction in respiratory tract secretions, and has antitussive properties.

CNS Promethazine is a potent sedative and anxiolytic; it also has a slight antanalgesic effect. It reduces motion sickness by suppression of vestibular end-organ receptors and by an inhibitory action at the chemoreceptor trigger zone. The drug has local anaesthetic properties.

AS Promethazine decreases the tone of the lower oesophageal sphincter.

Toxicity/side effects The drug exhibits predictable anticholinergic side effects and may produce extrapyramidal reactions when used in high doses. Jaundice, photosensitivity, excitatory phenomena, and gastrointestinal and haemopoietic disturbances may complicate the use of promethazine.

Kinetics

Absorption Promethazine is well absorbed when administered orally but undergoes an extensive first-pass metabolism.

Distribution The drug is 93% protein-bound in the plasma; the V_D is 2.5 l/kg.

Metabolism Promethazine is metabolized in the liver by sulfoxidation and N-dealkylation.

Excretion Occurs predominantly in the urine, 2% unchanged. The clearance is 1.41 l/min, and the elimination half-life is 7.5–10 hours.

Special points The depressant effects of the drug on the CNS are additive with those produced by anaesthetic agents.

Promethazine is not removed by haemodialysis.

Propofol

Uses Propofol is used:
1. for the induction and maintenance of general anaesthesia
2. for sedation during intensive care and regional anaesthesia, and has been used
3. in the treatment of refractory nausea and vomiting in patients receiving chemotherapy and
4. in the treatment of status epilepticus.

Chemical Propofol is 2,6-diisopropylphenol; a phenol derivative. The molecular weight is 178.27. It is a weak organic acid with a pKa of 11.

Presentation Being highly lipid-soluble, as a white oil-in-water emulsion containing 1% or 2% w/v of propofol in soybean oil (100 mg/ml), egg lecithin (purified egg phosphatide) (12 mg/ml), benzyl alcohol (1 mg/ml) (to retard the growth of accidental microorganism inoculation), glycerol (22.5 mg/ml), and sodium hydroxide to adjust pH (7–8.5). The drug is also available combined with Lipofundin® containing medium-chain triglycerides.

Main action Hypnotic

Mode of action The mode of action is unclear. It potentiates the inhibitory transmitters glycine and GABA (via different mechanisms to those of thiobarbiturates and benzodiazepines) and may reduce Na^+ channel opening times.

Routes of administration/doses Propofol is administered intravenously in a bolus dose of 1.5–2.5 mg/kg for induction and as an infusion of 4–12 mg/kg/hour for maintenance of anaesthesia in adults. Children require a bolus dose increase of 50% and an increase of maintenance infusion by 25–50%. Patients who are elderly or unstable require dose reductions accordingly (induction 1–1.5 mg/kg, maintenance 3–6 mg/kg/hour). Co-induction of an opioid and/or benzodiazepine, or administration as premedication, will lower the required dose of propofol further. Consciousness is lost in about 30–40 seconds, with emergence occurring approximately after 10 minutes from a single dose. Plasma concentrations of 2–6 micrograms/ml and 0.5–1.5 micrograms/ml are associated with hypnosis and sedation, respectively.

Effects

CVS Propofol produces a 15–25% decrease in the blood pressure and systemic vascular resistance, without a compensatory increase in the heart rate; the cardiac output decreases by 20%. In fit patients, the haemodynamic response to laryngoscopy is attenuated. Vasodilation occurs secondary to propofol-stimulated production and release of NO. Profound bradycardia, possibly through resetting of the baroreceptor reflex, and asystole may complicate the use of the drug.

RS Bolus administration of propofol produces apnoea of variable duration (30 to ≥60 seconds) and suppression of laryngeal reflexes. Infusion of the drug produces a decrease in the tidal volume, tachypnoea, and a depressed ventilatory response to hypercarbia and hypoxia. Propofol causes bronchodilation, possibly via a direct effect on bronchial smooth muscle. The drug does not increase intrapulmonary shunting and may preserve the mechanism of hypoxic pulmonary vasoconstriction.

CNS Propofol produces a smooth, rapid induction, with rapid and clearheaded recovery. Intracranial pressure, cerebral perfusion pressure, and cerebral oxygen consumption all decrease, following drug administration. Up to 10% of patients may manifest excitatory effects in the form of dystonic movements. These may be due to an imbalance between subcortical excitatory and inhibitory centres. Such movements are not accompanied by seizure activity on EEG recordings, and propofol has been used in the treatment of status epilepticus. Animal modules demonstrate that propofol has anticonvulsant properties. There are case reports of vivid dreams, some of a sexual nature, following propofol maintenance.

Intraocular pressure is decreased, following administration of propofol in normal subjects.

AS Propofol appears to possess intrinsic antiemetic properties which may be mediated by antagonism of dopamine D2 receptors.

GU In animals, propofol causes a reduction in the excretion of Na^+.

Metabolic/other Special care should be applied in patients with disorders of fat metabolism or patients receiving total parenteral nutrition as 1 ml of 1%. Propofol contains 0.1 g of fat (medium-chain triglycerides), with a calorific value of 1 cal/ml. Clinically significant impairment of adrenal steroidogenesis does not occur. Propofol is a free-radical scavenger.

Toxicity/side effects Pain on injection occurs in up to 28% of subjects. The incidence may be reduced by the addition of lidocaine (1 ml of 1%), cooling the drug, and the use of large veins. Addition of lidocaine in quantities >20 mg lidocaine per 200 mg propofol results in emulsion instability and increases in globule size, which have been associated with reduced anaesthetic potency in animals. There are case reports of epileptiform movements, facial paraesthesiae, and bradycardia, following the administration of propofol, although the incidence of allergic phenomena is low. The use of propofol appears to be safe in patients susceptible to porphyria (although urinary porphyrin concentrations may increase) and malignant hyperpyrexia. There are reports of neurological sequelae and increased mortality complicating long-term use.

Propofol infusion syndrome has been seen in both children and adults receiving prolonged propofol administration and is characterized by metabolic acidosis, rhabdomyolysis, and multi-organ failure. It is not licensed for sedation on the intensive treatment unit (ITU) for children <16 years of age. The quinol metabolites may occasionally cause green discoloration of the urine and hair. Propofol should not be used in patients allergic to soya or peanuts.

Kinetics

Distribution Propofol is 98% protein-bound in the plasma; the V_D is 4 l/kg. The distribution half-life is 1.3–4.1 minutes, resulting in a brief duration of action following bolus administration of the drug, as it distributes into different compartments (alpha phase). The distribution of propofol is based on a three-compartment pharmacokinetic model which is employed in target-controlled infusion (TCI) programmes.

Metabolism Propofol is rapidly metabolized in the liver, undergoing conjugation to an inactive glucuronide (49–73%), or metabolized to a quinol, which is excreted as sulfate and glucuronide conjugates of the hydroxylated metabolite via cytochrome P450. Inter-patient variability determines the ratio between the glucuronide and hydroxylated pathways. Extrahepatic metabolism probably contributes, since drug clearance exceeds hepatic blood flow. Renal and hepatic disease has no clinically significant effect on the metabolism of propofol.

Excretion The metabolites are excreted in the urine; 0.3% is excreted unchanged. The clearance is 18.8–40.3 ml/kg/min, and the elimination half-life is 9.3–69.3 minutes. The clearance is higher in children and decreased in the presence of renal failure. Following extended administration, its terminal elimination half-life may be prolonged, together with an increasing context-sensitive half-time, although, under normal conditions, propofol is non-cumulative.

Special points Propofol may increase the energy required for successful cardioversion. The drug causes a shortened duration of seizure activity during electroconvulsive therapy, although it does not decrease the efficacy of the treatment. Propofol is physically incompatible with atracurium. Aqueous emulsions of the drug support both bacterial and fungal growth, leading to the development of a formulation of propofol in 0.005% disodium edetate (EDTA) which provides less support for bacterial growth. TCI models can be used for propofol maintenance, such as 'Marsh' or 'Schnider', which use patient covariates to maintain a predetermined plasma or 'effector site' concentration.

There is evidence that preparations containing Lipofundin® produce less discomfort on injection and a shortened ventilation period for patients sedated on the ITU, when compared with other propofol preparations.

In morbidly obese patients, the lean body weight should be used for TCI induction of anaesthesia. The total body weight should be used to calculate TCI maintenance.

Drug structure For the drug structure, please see Fig. 6.

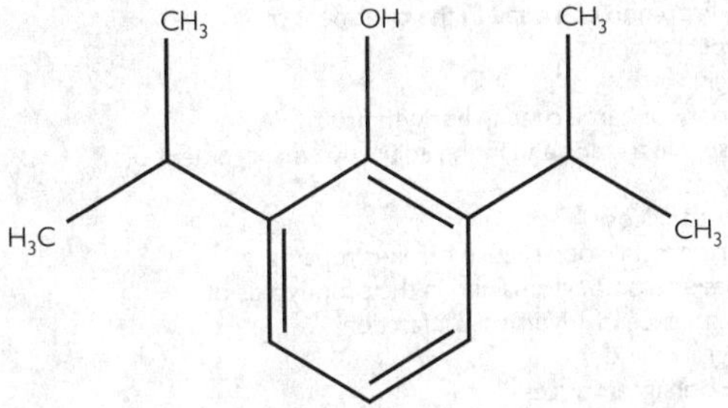

Fig. 6 Drug structure of propofol.

Propranolol

Uses Propranolol is used in the treatment of:
1. hypertension
2. angina
3. variety of cardiac tachydysrhythmias
4. essential tremor and in the adjunctive management of
5. anxiety
6. thyrotoxicosis
7. hypertrophic obstructive cardiomyopathy
8. phaeochromocytoma and in the prophylaxis of
9. recurrence of myocardial infarction
10. migraine and
11. oesophageal varices.

Chemical An aromatic amine.

Presentation As tablets containing 10/40/80/160 mg and as a clear solution for injection containing 1 mg/ml of propranolol hydrochloride.

Main actions Negative inotropism and chronotropism.

Mode of action Propranolol acts by competitive antagonism of beta-1 and beta-2 adrenoceptors; it has no intrinsic sympathomimetic activity. It also exerts a membrane-stabilizing effect when used in very high doses by the inhibition of Na^+ currents.

Routes of administration/doses The adult oral dose is 30–320 mg/day in 2–3 divided doses, according to the condition requiring treatment. The corresponding dose by the intravenous route is 1–10 mg, titrated according to response.

Effects

CVS Propranolol is negatively inotropic and chronotropic, and leads to a decrease in myocardial oxygen consumption; the mechanism of the antihypertensive action of the drug remains poorly defined. Blockade of beta-2 adrenoceptors produces an increase in the peripheral vascular resistance.

RS Propranolol causes a decrease in FEV_1 by increasing airways resistance; it also attenuates the ventilatory response to hypercapnia.

CNS The drug crosses the blood–brain barrier; its central effects may be involved in the mechanism of the antihypertensive action of the drug. Propranolol diminishes physiological tremor and decreases intraocular pressure.

GU Propranolol decreases uterine tone, especially during pregnancy.

Metabolic/other The drug decreases plasma renin activity and suppresses aldosterone release. Propranolol causes a decrease in the plasma free fatty acid concentration and may also cause hypoglycaemia due to blockade of gluconeogenesis. The drug increases total body sodium concentration and thus the extracellular fluid volume. Propranolol prevents the peripheral conversion of levothyroxine to triiodothyronine.

Toxicity/side effects The side effects of propranolol are predictable manifestations of non-specific beta-adrenergic blockade. The drug may thus precipitate heart failure or heart block; exacerbate peripheral vascular disease; lead to bronchospasm, sleep disturbances, and nightmares; mask the symptoms of hypoglycaemia; and cause impaired exercise tolerance.

Kinetics

Absorption 90% of an oral dose of propranolol is absorbed; the bioavailability is 30–35% due to an extensive first-pass metabolism.

Distribution The drug is 90–96% protein-bound in the plasma, predominantly to alpha-1 acid glycoprotein; the V_D is 3.6 l/kg.

Metabolism Propranolol undergoes extensive hepatic metabolism by oxidative deamination and dealkylation, with subsequent glucuronidation; the 4-hydroxy metabolite is active.

Excretion Occurs via the urine; <1% of the dose is excreted unchanged. The clearance is 0.5–1.2 l/min, and the elimination half-life is 2–4 hours. The dose should be reduced in the presence of hepatic failure; no alteration in dose is necessary in the presence of renal impairment.

Special points Beta-adrenergic blockade should be continued throughout the perioperative period; abrupt withdrawal of propranolol may precipitate angina, ventricular dysrhythmias, myocardial infarction, and sudden death. The co-administration of propranolol and non-depolarizing relaxants may lead to a slight potentiation of the latter.

The drug is not removed by dialysis.

Protamine

Uses Protamine is used:
1. to neutralize the anticoagulant effects of heparin and
2. to prolong the effects of insulin.

Chemical A purified mixture of low-molecular-weight cationic proteins prepared from fish sperm.

Presentation As a clear, colourless solution for injection containing 10 mg/ml protamine sulfate.

Main actions Neutralization of the anticoagulant effect of heparin; in high doses, protamine has a weak intrinsic anticoagulant effect.

Mode of action Both *in vitro* and *in vivo*, the strongly basic compound protamine complexes with the strongly acidic compound heparin to form a stable salt—this complex is inactive. The intrinsic anticoagulant effect of the drug appears to be due to the inhibition of the formation and activity of thromboplastin.

Routes of administration/doses Protamine is administered by slow intravenous injection; the dose should be adjusted, according to the amount of heparin that is to be neutralized, the time that has elapsed since the administration of heparin, and the activated coagulation time (ACT). One mg of protamine will neutralize 100 units of heparin. A maximum adult dose of 50 mg of the drug should be administered in any 10-minute period.

Effects

CVS Protamine is a myocardial depressant and may cause bradycardia and hypotension, secondary to complement activation and leukotriene release. The pulmonary artery pressure may increase, leading to an impairment of right ventricular output.

Toxicity/side effects Rapid intravenous administration of protamine may be complicated by acute hypotension, bradycardia, dyspnoea, and flushing. Anaphylactoid reactions may also occur; antibodies to human protamine often develop in vasectomized males and may predispose to hypersensitivity phenomena.

Kinetics Data are incomplete.

Metabolism The metabolic fate of the protamine–heparin complex has not been well elucidated; it may undergo partial degradation, thereby freeing heparin.

Prothrombin complex

Uses Prothrombin complex is used in the treatment and prophylaxis of bleeding resulting from congenital or acquired deficiencies of prothrombin complex coagulation factors.

Chemical Human plasma-derived prothrombin complex coagulation factors (II, VII, IX, and X), together with proteins C and S.

Presentation As a powder in vials containing 250 or 500 IU, together with a solvent for intravenous injection. Following reconstitution, the following approximate concentration of each component is present:
• factor II—20–48 IU/ml
• factor VII—10–25 IU/ml
• factor IX—30–31 IU/ml
• factor X—22–60 IU/ml
• protein C—15–45 IU/ml
• protein S—12–38 IU/ml.

The total protein content following reconstitution is 6–15 mg/ml. The following substances are also present: heparin, human antithrombin III, human albumin, sodium chloride, sodium citrate, and hydrochloric acid or sodium hydroxide for pH adjustment. The sodium content of reconstituted prothrombin complex is up to 343 mg per 100 ml.

Main actions Neutralization of the anticoagulant effect resulting from deficiency in factors II, VII, IX, and X.

Mode of action Increased plasma levels of factors II, VII, IX, and X.

Routes of administration/doses Prothrombin complex is administered intravenously. Advice regarding the dose and administration frequency should be sought from a haematologist prior to administration.

Toxicity/side effects There is a risk of subsequent thrombosis and/or DIC with repeated dosing. There are very rare reports of allergic reactions during or following administration. Development of antibodies to any of the coagulation factors may occur very rarely.

Kinetics Data are incomplete.

Distribution Distribution of prothrombin complex is identical to endogenous coagulation factors.

Metabolism The plasma half-life of each component of prothrombin complex is as follows:
• factor II—60 hours
• factor VII—4 hours
• factor IX—17 hours
• factor X—31 hours

- protein C—47 hours
- protein S—49 hours.

Factors IX and X and proteins C and S exhibit two-compartment model pharmacokinetics. Metabolic pathways involved in prothrombin complex metabolism are identical to those involved in endogenous factor/protein breakdown.

Ranitidine

Uses Ranitidine is used in the treatment of:
1. peptic ulcer disease
2. reflux oesophagitis
3. the Zollinger–Ellison syndrome and
4. for the prevention of stress ulceration in critically ill patients and
5. prior to general anaesthesia in patients at risk of acid aspiration, especially during pregnancy and labour.

Chemical A furan derivative.

Presentation As a clear solution for intravenous or intramuscular injection containing 25 mg/ml, as 150/300 mg tablets, and as a syrup containing 15 mg/ml of ranitidine hydrochloride.

Main actions Inhibition of gastric acid secretion.

Mode of action Ranitidine acts via competitive blockade of histaminergic H2 receptors. Histamine appears to be necessary to potentiate the action of gastrin and acetylcholine on the gastric parietal cell, as well as act directly as a secretagogue.

Routes of administration/doses Ranitidine may be administered by slow intravenous or intramuscular injection, the dose being 50 mg 6- to 8-hourly. The oral dose is 150 mg twice daily.

Effects

CVS No effect is seen with normal clinical dosages.

RS The drug has no effect on respiratory parameters.

AS Ranitidine profoundly inhibits gastric acid secretion, reducing the volume, and hydrogen ion and pepsin content. The drug has a longer duration of anti-secretory activity than cimetidine. Ranitidine has been reported to cause a dose-related increase in lower oesophageal sphincter tone.

Metabolic/other Ranitidine does not show anti-androgenic or anti-dopaminergic effects, nor does it affect cytochrome P450-mediated metabolism that are associated with cimetidine. The drug crosses the placenta, but no adverse effects on fetal well-being have been demonstrated.

Toxicity/side effects Reversible abnormalities of liver function tests, rashes, and anaphylactoid reactions have been reported, following the use of ranitidine. Reversible confusion, thrombocytopenia, and leucopenia occur rarely after administration of the drug.

Kinetics

Absorption Ranitidine has an oral bioavailability of 50–60%.

Distribution The drug is approximately 15% protein-bound in the plasma; the V_D is 1.2–1.8 l/kg.

Metabolism A small fraction of the drug is metabolized by oxidation and methylation.

Excretion Ranitidine is predominantly excreted unchanged by the kidney. The clearance is 10 ml/min/kg, and the elimination half-life is 1.6–2.5 hours.

Special points A reduced dosage of the drug should be used in patients with renal failure; the drug is removed by haemodialysis.

Ranitidine may be associated with an increase in nosocomial pneumonia in ventilated critically ill patients.

Remifentanil

Uses Remifentanil is used:
1. to provide the analgesic component in general anaesthesia
2. to provide analgesia/sedation in intensive care
3. to provide analgesia during labour when regional anaesthesia is not in use
4. to provide analgesia/sedation during 'awake' fibreoptic intubation.

Chemical A synthetic phenylpiperidine derivative of fentanyl.

Presentation As a white lyophilized powder to be reconstituted before use, containing remifentanil hydrochloride in a glycine buffer in 1/2/5 mg vials for dilution prior to infusion. It has a pKa of 7.1 and is 68% unionized at a pH of 7.4.

Main actions Analgesia and respiratory depression.

Mode of action Remifentanil is a pure mu-agonist (or MOP agonist); the mu-opioid receptor (MOP receptor) appears to be specifically involved in the mediation of analgesia. Opioids appear to exert their effects by interacting with pre-synaptic Gi-protein receptors, leading to hyperpolarization of the cell membrane by increasing K^+ conductance. Inhibition of adenylate cyclase, leading to reduced production of cAMP, and closure of voltage-sensitive calcium channels also occur. The decrease in membrane excitability that results may decrease both pre- and post-synaptic responses.

Routes of administration/doses Remifentanil is licensed for intravenous administration only. The drug may be given by slow bolus injection of 1 microgram/kg over at least 30 seconds or by TCI with an approved infusion device incorporating, for example, the 'Minto' pharmacokinetic model with covariates for age and lean body mass. A manual infusion technique may also be used, titrated to response. The drug may be infused at a rate of 0.0125–1 microgram/kg/min, depending on the level of sedation and analgesia required. The peak effect of the drug occurs within 1–3 minutes. The offset is rapid and predictable, even after prolonged infusion, typically occurring within 5–10 minutes of discontinuation of the infusion. Administration of remifentanil reduces the amount of hypnotic/volatile agent required to maintain anaesthesia.

Effects

CVS Remifentanil decreases the mean arterial pressure and heart rate by 20%. Myocardial contractility and cardiac output may also decrease.

RS Remifentanil is a potent respiratory depressant, causing a decrease in both the respiratory rate and tidal volume; it also diminishes the ventilatory response to hypoxia and hypercarbia. Chest wall rigidity (the 'wooden chest' phenomenon) may occur after the administration of remifentanil—this may be an effect of the drug on mu-receptors located on GABA-ergic interneurones. The drug does not cause histamine release.

CNS Remifentanil has a centrally mediated vagal activity. It has an analgesic potency similar to fentanyl and possesses minimal hypnotic or sedative activity. It produces EEG effects similar to those of other opioids—high-amplitude, low-frequency activity. Miosis is produced as a result of stimulation of the Edinger–Westphal nucleus.

AS The drug decreases gastrointestinal motility. There is a relatively low incidence of nausea and vomiting associated with its use.

Toxicity/side effects Respiratory depression, bradycardia, nausea, and vomiting may all complicate the use of remifentanil. Because of its short duration of action, post-operative discomfort may be pronounced if remifentanil is used as a sole analgesic agent perioperatively.

Kinetics

Distribution Remifentanil is 70% bound to plasma proteins, two-thirds to alpha-1 acid glycoprotein. The drug has a low lipid solubility, compared to other mu opioids, with a low V_D of 0.1 l/kg, and distributes into peripheral tissues with a volume of distribution at steady state (VD_{SS}) of 0.25–0.4 l/kg. Remifentanil crosses the placenta and may cause respiratory depression in the neonate. In children aged 1–12 years, the V_D decreases with increasing age. The V_D in neonates is twice that of adults.

Metabolism Remifentanil undergoes rapid ester hydrolysis by non-specific plasma and tissue esterases to a carboxylic acid derivative remifentanil acid, which is 4600-fold less potent than remifentanil. The context-sensitive half-time of remifentanil of 3–5 minutes is fixed, due to the quantity of the above esterases, and does not increase with the duration of the infusion, unlike other opioids. The drug is not metabolized by plasma cholinesterases and is unaffected by its deficiency or by the administration of anticholinesterase drugs.

Excretion The clearance of remifentanil is 4.2–5 l/min and independent of renal and hepatic function. The elimination half-life is 5–14 minutes and is unaltered with renal and hepatic dysfunction. Approximately 95% of an administered dose is excreted in the urine as remifentanil acid which has an elimination half-life of 1.5–2 hours. In children aged 1–12 years, the clearance of remifentanil decreases with increasing age. The clearance in neonates is twice that of adults, although the elimination half-life is approximately the same. The pharmacokinetics of remifentanil acid are similar in children, compared to those seen in adults.

Special points The clearance of the metabolite remifentanil acid is prolonged in patients with renal impairment and may increase to 268 hours. The concentration of the metabolite may increase by 100-fold in intensive care patients with moderate or severe renal impairment at steady state, although there is no evidence that clinically significant mu-opioid effects are seen, even following remifentanil infusions lasting 3 days.

Intravenous lines must be flushed at the end of the infusion due to the risk of respiratory depression by the residual drug in the line dead space.

There is no evidence that remifentanil is extracted during renal replacement therapy.

Remifentanil acid is extracted during haemodialysis by 25–35%.

Patients with hepatic impairment are more sensitive to the respiratory depressant effects of remifentanil.

The lean body weight should be used when using the drug in morbidly obese patients as part of a TCI protocol.

Rivaroxaban

Uses Rivaroxaban is used for the prevention of venous thromboembolism in patients undergoing elective knee and hip replacement surgery.

Chemical An oxazolidinone derivative.

Presentation As 10 mg tablets containing rivaroxaban. Each tablet also contains 27.9 mg lactose monohydrate.

Main actions Direct factor Xa inhibitor.

Mode of action Rivaroxaban directly inhibits factor Xa in a dose-dependent manner, leading to interruption of both the intrinsic and extrinsic coagulation pathways. The drug does not inhibit thrombin and has no effect on platelet function.

Routes of administration/doses The drug is administered orally at a dose of 10 mg. The first dose should be given 6–10 hours after surgery. Treatment should continue for 5 weeks following hip surgery, and 2 weeks following knee surgery. No dose adjustment is required for patients with mild or moderately impaired renal function. The drug should be used with caution in patients with severe renal impairment.

Effects

Metabolic/other The main effect of the drug is its anticoagulation effect. Rivaroxaban does not affect platelet function.

Toxicity/side effects Excessive bleeding is the commonest reported side effect. The use of neuroaxial blocks in patients receiving the drug must be carefully considered, and the timing of block/catheter insertion/removal and commencement/withholding/discontinuation of rivaroxaban must be appropriately timed to minimize the risk of spinal/epidural haematoma formation. It is recommended that, following a dose of rivaroxaban, an epidural catheter should not be removed before 18 hours has elapsed, and any subsequent dose to be delayed by a further 6 hours following catheter removal.

Kinetics

Absorption Rivaroxaban is rapidly absorbed following oral administration, with C_{max} occurring within 2–4 hours of ingestion. The bioavailability of the drug is 80–100%.

Distribution The drug is 92–95% protein-bound; the V_D is approximately 50 l.

Metabolism Two-thirds of an administered dose undergoes oxidative degradation and hydrolysis via CYP450 3A4, CYP450 2J2, and CYP-independent mechanisms. The morpholinone moiety and amide bonds are the main metabolic targets.

Excretion Following hepatic metabolism, 50% of the metabolic products of the drug are renally excreted, whilst the remaining 50% are excreted in the faeces. Unchanged drug is excreted renally. The terminal elimination half-life of a 1 mg dose is 4.5 hours, increasing to 7–11 hours following a 10 mg dose due to absorption rate-limited elimination. The systemic clearance is approximately 10 l/hour.

Special points *In vitro* studies demonstrate that the drug is a substrate of the transporter proteins P-glycoprotein and BCRP (breast cancer resistance protein).

Drug plasma levels may be reduced when rivaroxaban is administered to patients receiving CYP450 3A4 inducers such as rifampicin, phenytoin, carbamazepine, and St John's Wort.

Drug plasma levels may increase when rivaroxaban is administered to patients receiving CYP450 3A4 and P-glycoprotein inhibitors such as ketoconazole, itraconazole, voriconazole, and HIV protease inhibitors.

There is no antidote currently available for rivaroxaban.

The drug is unlikely to be removed by haemodialysis due to high plasma protein binding.

Rocuronium

Uses Rocuronium is used:
1. to facilitate tracheal intubation during routine and modified rapid sequence induction
2. for controlled ventilation.

Chemical An aminosteroid which is structurally related to vecuronium.

Presentation As a clear, colourless solution containing 10 mg/ml of rocuronium bromide. The drug is available in 5 and 10 mg ampoules.

Main action Competitive neuromuscular blockade.

Mode of action Rocuronium acts by competitive antagonism of acetylcholine at nicotinic (N2) receptors at the post-synaptic membrane of the neuromuscular junction; it also has some pre-junctional activity.

Routes of administration/doses Rocuronium is administered intravenously; the normal intubating dose is 0.6 mg/kg, with subsequent doses of 0.15 mg/kg. This intubating dose equates to twice the ED90 for rocuronium (ED90 0.3 mg/kg) and results in 'excellent' intubating conditions in 80% of cases within 60 seconds. A dose of 1 mg/kg is recommended when rocuronium is used during modified rapid sequence induction, resulting in intubating conditions within 60 seconds in 93–96%. The increased speed of onset relates to the low potency of rocuronium. As a result of giving an increased dose (increased number of drug molecules), the concentration gradient at the neuromuscular junction is increased, leading to a faster diffusion of drug molecules and a reduction in drug onset time. The duration of action relates to the dose given, and, as a result, the usual recovery index of 8–17 minutes with a normal intubating dose is increased to nearly an hour when 1.0 mg/kg is used. The drug may also be infused at a rate of 300–600 micrograms/kg/hour. The drug is non-cumulative with repeated administration.

Effects

CVS Rocuronium has minimal cardiovascular effects; with large doses, a mild vagolytic effect leads to a slight (9%) increase in the heart rate and an increase in the mean arterial pressure of up to 16%.

RS Neuromuscular blockade leads to apnoea. Rocuronium causes an insignificant release of histamine; bronchospasm is extremely uncommon.

Toxicity/side effects There have been very rare reports of fatal anaphylactoid reactions with the administration of rocuronium. Cross-sensitivity may exist with other aminosteroid compounds (vecuronium, pancuronium). Pain on injection occurs in 16% of subjects when rocuronium is used in combination with propofol, compared with 0.5% of subjects when thiopental is used.

Kinetics

Distribution The drug is 30% protein-bound in the plasma; the V_D is 0.27 l/kg.

Metabolism No metabolites of rocuronium have been found in the plasma or urine.

Excretion Rocuronium is excreted primarily by hepatic uptake and hepato-biliary excretion. 30 to 40% of the dose is excreted unchanged in the bile, 13–31% in the urine. After administration of a bolus dose, the plasma concentration time course runs in three exponential phases. In adults, the mean elimination half-life is 73 (66–80) minutes, with a plasma clearance of 3.7 (3.5–3.9) ml/kg/min. The pharmacokinetics of rocuronium are not significantly altered in the presence of renal failure. The mean elimination half-life is prolonged by 30 minutes, and the mean plasma clearance is reduced by 1 ml/kg/min in the presence of hepatic dysfunction; the duration of action is correspondingly increased.

Special points The duration of action of rocuronium, in common with other non-depolarizing relaxants, may be prolonged by hypokalae-mia, hypocalcaemia, hypothermia, hypermagnesaemia, hypoproteinae-mia, dehydration, acidosis, and hypercapnia. The following drugs, when co-administered with non-depolarizing relaxants, increase the effect of the latter: volatile and induction agents, fentanyl, suxamethonium, diuretics, lithium, calcium antagonists, alpha- and beta-adrenergic antagonists, prota-mine, metronidazole, and the aminoglycoside antibiotics.

Rocuronium is physically incompatible with thiopental, methohexital, dexamethasone, erythromycin, trimethoprim, vancomycin, and diazepam. In animal studies, rocuronium does not appear to be a triggering factor for malignant hyperpyrexia.

Rocuronium causes significantly less rise in intraocular pressure, com-pared with suxamethonium.

Reversal of NMB activity by rocuronium may be achieved using neostig-mine (in combination with glycopyrrolate), but only after four twitches have returned to the train-of-four count. The alpha-cyclodextrin sugammadex may be used to reverse rocuronium-induced neuromuscular blockade by encapsulating rocuronium molecules within the plasma, thereby creating a concentration gradient favouring the movement of remaining rocuronium molecules from the neuromuscular junction back into the plasma.

The ideal body weight should be used to calculate drug dosage in mor-bidly obese individuals.

Ropivacaine

Uses Ropivacaine is used as a local anaesthetic.

Chemical An amino amide which is member of the pipecoloxylidide group of local anaesthetics.

Presentation As a clear, colourless solution containing racemic ropivacaine hydrochloride monohydrate (S- and R-enantiomers) in concentrations of 0.2/0.75/1.0% equivalent to 2.0, 7.5, and 10 mg/ml, respectively, of ropivacaine hydrochloride. A pure S-ropivacaine preparation is also available. It is not available in combination with a vasoconstrictor, as this does not alter its tissue uptake or the duration of action. The pKa of ropivacaine is 8.1, and it is 15% unionized at pH 7.4. The heptane:buffer partition coefficient is 2.9. The preparation also contains sodium hydroxide equivalent to 3.7 mg of sodium per ml.

Main action Local anaesthetic.

Mode of action Local anaesthetics diffuse in their uncharged base form through neural sheaths and the axonal membrane to the internal surface of cell membrane Na^+ channels; here they combine with hydrogen ions to form a cationic species which enters the internal opening of the Na^+ channel and combines with a receptor. This produces blockade of the Na^+ channel, thereby decreasing Na^+ conductance and preventing depolarization of the cell membrane.

S-ropivacaine is more potent and less cardiotoxic than R-ropivacaine.

Routes of administration/doses Ropivacaine may be administered topically, by infiltration, or epidurally; the drug is not currently intended for use in spinal anaesthesia. The maximum recommended dose of ropivacaine is 3 mg/kg. Sensory blockade is similar in time course to that produced by bupivacaine; motor blockade is slower in onset and shorter in duration than that after an equivalent dose of bupivacaine. Alkalinization of 0.75% ropivacaine significantly increases the duration of action of epidural blockade.

Effects

CVS Ropivacaine is less cardiotoxic than bupivacaine; in toxic concentrations, the drug decreases the peripheral vascular resistance and myocardial contractility, producing hypotension and possibly cardiovascular collapse. Ropivacaine has a biphasic vascular effect, causing vasoconstriction at low, but not at high, concentrations.

CNS The principal effect of ropivacaine is reversible neural blockade; this leads to a characteristically biphasic effect in the CNS. Initially, excitation (light-headedness, dizziness, visual and auditory disturbances, and seizure activity) occurs due to inhibition of inhibitory interneurone pathways in the cortex. With increasing doses, depression of both facilitatory and inhibitory pathways occurs, leading to CNS depression (drowsiness, disorientation, and coma). Local anaesthetic agents block neuromuscular transmission when administered intraneurally; it is thought that a complex of neuro-transmitter, receptor, and local anaesthetic is formed, which has negligible conductance.

GU Ropivacaine does not compromise uteroplacental circulation.

Toxicity/side effects Allergic reactions to the amide-type local anaes-thetic agents are extremely rare. The side effects are predominantly corre-lated with excessive plasma concentrations of the drug, as described above.

Kinetics

Absorption The absorption of local anaesthetic agents is related to:
1. the site of injection (intercostal > caudal > epidural > brachial plexus > subcutaneous)
2. the dose—a linear relationship exists between the total dose and the peak blood concentrations achieved and
3. the presence of vasoconstrictors which delay absorption.

Distribution Ropivacaine is 94% protein-bound in the plasma, predomi-nantly to alpha-1 acid glycoprotein; the V_D is 52–66 l. The drug demon-strates a biphasic absorption profile from the epidural space, with half-lives of 14 minutes and 4 hours in adults.

Metabolism Ropivacaine is metabolized in the liver by aromatic hydroxy-lation via cytochrome CYP1A2 to 3-hydroxy-ropivacaine, the major metabolite, 4-hydroxy-ropivacaine, and 4-hydroxy-dealkylated-ropivacaine. Co-administration of a CYP1A2 inhibitor (e.g. fluvoxamine, enoxacin) may reduce plasma clearance of the drug by up to 77% *in vitro*. The isoenzyme CYP3A4 is also involved in the metabolism of ropivacaine, as administra-tion of a CYP3A4 inhibitor (e.g. fluconazole) reduces the plasma clearance of the drug by 15% *in vitro*, although this is unlikely to cause a clinically significant effect. Ropivacaine has an intermediate hepatic extraction ratio of approximately 0.4. There is no evidence of *in vivo* racemization of ropivacaine.

Excretion The clearance is 0.44–0.82 l/min, and the terminal elimination half-life is 59–173 minutes. Eighty-six percent of the dose is excreted in the urine, 1% unchanged; 37% of 3-hydroxy-ropivacaine is excreted in the urine, predominantly conjugated. The elimination half-life is longer after epi-dural (4.2 hours) than after intravenous administration due to the biphasic absorption from the former, as described above.

Special points The onset and duration of conduction blockade are related to the pKa, lipid solubility, and the extent of protein binding. A low pKa and high lipid solubility are associated with a rapid onset time; a high degree of protein binding is associated with a long duration of action. Local anaesthetic agents significantly increase the duration of action of both depolarizing and non-depolarizing relaxants.

Salbutamol

Uses Salbutamol is used in the treatment of:
1. asthma
2. chronic obstructive airways disease and
3. uncomplicated preterm labour.

Chemical A synthetic sympathomimetic amine.

Presentation As 2/4/8 mg tablets, a syrup containing 0.4/2.5 mg/ml, an aerosol delivering 100 micrograms/puff, a dry powder for inhalation in capsules containing 200/400 micrograms, a solution for nebulization containing 2.5/5 mg/ml, and as a clear, colourless solution for injection containing 1 mg/ml of salbutamol sulfate.

Main actions Bronchodilatation and uterine relaxation.

Mode of action Salbutamol is a beta-adrenergic agonist (with a more pronounced effect at beta-2 than beta-1 receptors) that acts by stimulation of membrane-bound adenylate cyclase in the presence of magnesium ions to increase intracellular cAMP concentrations. It also directly inhibits antigen-induced release of histamine and slow-releasing substance of anaphylaxis from mast cells.

Routes of administration/doses The adult oral dose is 2–4 mg 6- to 8-hourly. One or two metered puffs of 200–400 micrograms of the powder may be inhaled 6- to 8-hourly; 2.5–5 mg of the nebulized solution may be inhaled similarly 6-hourly. The drug may also be administered subcutaneously or intramuscularly in a dose of 0.5 mg 4-hourly. Salbutamol should be administered intravenously as an infusion diluted in glucose or saline at a rate not exceeding 0.5 micrograms/kg/min. Bronchodilatation is observed 5–15 minutes after inhalation and 30 minutes after ingestion of the drug, and lasts for up to 4 hours.

Effects

CVS In high doses, the beta-1 actions of the drug lead to positive inotropic and chronotropic effects. At lower doses, the beta-2 effects predominate and cause a decrease in the peripheral vascular resistance, leading to a decrease in the diastolic blood pressure of 10–20 mmHg.

RS Bronchodilatation, leading to an increased peak expiratory flow rate (PEFR) and FEV_1, occurs after the administration of salbutamol. This is additive to the bronchodilatation produced by phosphodiesterase inhibitors. The drug interferes with the mechanism of hypoxic pulmonary vasoconstriction; an adequate inspired oxygen concentration should be ensured when the drug is used.

GU Salbutamol decreases the tone of the gravid uterus; 10% of an administered dose crosses the placenta and may lead to tachycardia in the fetus.

Metabolic/other Salbutamol may decrease the plasma potassium concentration by causing a shift of the ion into cells. It may also cause an increase in the plasma concentrations of free fatty acids and glucose; insulin release is therefore stimulated.

Toxicity/side effects Anxiety, insomnia, tremor (with no attendant change in motor strength), sweating, palpitations, ketosis, lactic acidosis, hypokalaemia, postural hypotension, and nausea and vomiting may occur, following the use of the drug.

Kinetics Data are incomplete.

Absorption 10% of the dose administered by inhalation reaches the bronchial tree, the remainder being swallowed.

Distribution Salbutamol is 8–64% protein-bound in the plasma; the V_D is 156 l.

Metabolism Salbutamol undergoes a significant first-pass metabolism in the liver; the major metabolite is salbutamol 4-O-sulfate.

Excretion 30% of the dose is excreted unchanged in the urine, the remainder in faeces, and as the sulfate derivative in the urine. The clearance is 28 l/hour, and the elimination half-life is 2.7–5 hours.

Special points Salbutamol appears to potentiate non-depolarizing muscle relaxants.

Sevoflurane

Uses Sevoflurane is used for the induction and maintenance of general anaesthesia.

Chemical A polyfluorinated isopropyl methyl ether.

Presentation As a clear, colourless liquid which is non-flammable; the commercial preparation contains no additives or stabilizers and is supplied in amber-coloured bottles. The molecular weight of sevoflurane is 200, the boiling point 58.6°C, and the saturated vapour pressure 22.7 kPa at 20°C. The MAC of sevoflurane is age-dependent and ranges from 1.4 in elderly patients to 3.3 in neonates (0.7–2.0 in the presence of 65% N_2O); the blood:gas partition coefficient is 0.63–0.69, and the fat:blood partition coefficient is 52. The oil:gas partition coefficient is 47–54. Degradation of sevoflurane may occur by two pathways in the presence of warm, dessicated alkaline CO_2 absorbants (potassium hydroxide > sodium hydroxide) at low fresh gas flows. The first pathway results in the loss of hydrogen fluoride, with the production of pentafluoroisopropenyl fluoromethyl ether (PIFE or 'Compound A') and trace amounts of pentafluoromethoxy isopropyl fluoromethyl ether (PMFE or 'Compound B'). The second pathway results in the production of HFIP and formaldehyde. The latter may further degrade into formate and methanol. Formate can contribute to carbon monoxide production, whilst methanol may react with Compound A to form Compound B. Compound B may undergo further loss of hydrogen fluoride to produce trace amounts of Compounds C, D, and E.

Main action General anaesthesia (reversible loss of both awareness and recall of noxious stimuli).

Mode of action The mechanism of general anaesthesia remains to be fully elucidated. General anaesthetics appear to disrupt synaptic transmission (especially in the area of the ventrobasal thalamus). This mechanism may include potentiation of the $GABA_A$ and glycine receptors and antagonism at NMDA receptors. Their mode of action at the molecular level appears to involve the expansion of hydrophobic regions in the neuronal membrane, either within the lipid phase or within hydrophobic sites in cell membranes.

Routes of administration/dose Sevoflurane is administered by inhalation; the agent has a pleasant, non-irritant odour. The concentration used for induction of anaesthesia is quoted as 5–8%. Maintenance of anaesthesia is usually achieved using between 0.5 and 3%.

Effects

CVS Sevoflurane causes a dose-related decrease in myocardial contractility and mean arterial pressure; the systolic pressure decreases to a greater degree than the diastolic pressure. The drug does not affect the heart rate, and myocardial sensitization to catecholamines does not occur. The drug does not appear to cause the 'coronary steal' phenomenon in man.

RS Sevoflurane is a respiratory depressant, causing dose-dependent decreases in the tidal volume and an increase in the respiratory rate. The drug depresses the ventilatory response to CO_2 and inhibits hypoxic pulmonary vasoconstriction. Sevoflurane appears to relax bronchial smooth muscle constricted by histamine or acetylcholine.

CNS The principal effect of sevoflurane is general anaesthesia. The drug causes cerebral vasodilation, leading to an increase in the cerebral blood flow; the cerebral metabolic rate is decreased. As with other volatile anaesthetic agents, sevoflurane may increase the intracranial pressure in a dose-related manner. Sevoflurane use is not associated with epileptiform activity.

GU Sevoflurane reduces renal blood flow and leads to an increase in fluoride ion concentrations (12 micrograms/l to 90 micrograms/l in anaesthesia lasting 1 to 6 hours, respectively). There is no evidence that sevoflurane causes gross changes in human renal function. The drug causes uterine relaxation.

Metabolic/other In animal models, the drug decreases liver synthesis of fibrinogen, transferrin, and albumin.

Toxicity/side effects Sevoflurane may cause PONV. It is a trigger agent for the development of malignant hyperthermia. There are no reports of renal toxicity occurring in patients who have received the drug. Rapid emergence in paediatric patients may lead to agitation in approximately 25% of cases. Paediatric patients with Down's syndrome receiving sevoflurane for inhalational induction may develop bradycardia in up to 52% of cases.

Kinetics

Absorption The major factors affecting the uptake of volatile anaesthetic agents are solubility, cardiac output, and the concentration gradient between the alveoli and venous blood. Due to the low blood:gas partition coefficient of sevoflurane, it is exceptionally insoluble in blood; the alveolar concentration therefore reaches inspired concentration very rapidly (fast washin rate), resulting in a rapid induction of (and emergence from) anaesthesia. An increase in the cardiac output increases the rate of alveolar uptake and slows the induction of anaesthesia. The concentration gradient between the alveoli and venous blood approaches zero at equilibrium; a large concentration gradient favours the onset of anaesthesia.

Distribution The drug is initially distributed to organs with a high blood flow (brain, heart, liver, kidney) and later to less well-perfused organs (muscle, fat, bone).

Metabolism Sevoflurane is metabolized by the process of defluorination via cytochrome P450 (CYP) 2EI, producing HFIP, inorganic fluoride, and CO_2. HFIP is rapidly conjugated with glucuronic acid and eliminated in the urine. Approximately 3–5% of an administered dose is metabolized. Cytochrome P450 2EI may be induced by chronic exposure to ethanol and isoniazid. It is not induced by exposure to barbiturates. Fluoride concentrations may increase significantly in the presence of increased CYP 2EI activity, although there are no reports from clinical trials regarding fluoride toxicity.

Excretion Excretion is via the lungs, predominantly unchanged. Elimination of sevoflurane is rapid, again due to its low solubility, resulting in a fast wash-out rate. HFIP peak excretion occurs within 12 hours; the elimination half-life is 55 hours. Fluoride ion concentrations peak within 2 hours at the end of anaesthesia; the half-life is 15–23 hours.

Special points Sevoflurane potentiates the action of co-administered depolarizing and non-depolarizing muscle relaxants to a greater extent than either halothane or enflurane.

As with other volatile anaesthetic agents, the co-administration of N_2O, benzodiazepines, or opioids lowers the MAC of sevoflurane.

Drug structure For the drug structure, please see Fig. 7.

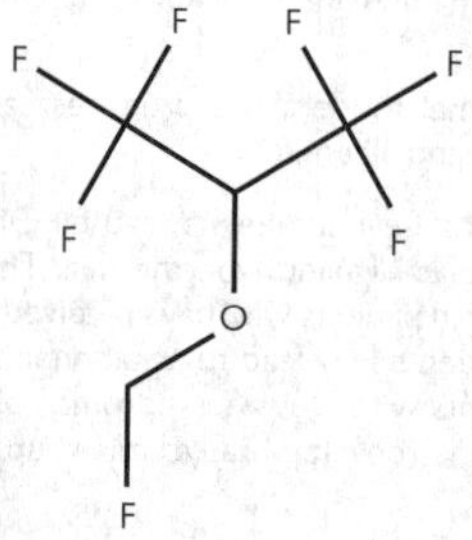

Fig. 7 Drug structure of sevoflurane.

Sodium bicarbonate

Uses Sodium bicarbonate is used:
1. for the correction of profound metabolic acidosis, especially that complicating cardiac arrest
2. for the alkalinization of urine and
3. as an antacid.

Chemical An inorganic salt.

Presentation As 300 mg tablets and as a clear, colourless, sterile solution containing 1.26/4.2/8.4% w/v sodium bicarbonate in an aqueous solution. The 8.4% solution contains 1 mmol/ml of sodium and bicarbonate ions and has a calculated osmolarity of 2000 mOsm/l.

Mode of action The compound freely dissociates to yield bicarbonate ions which represent the predominant extracellular buffer system. Each gram of sodium bicarbonate will neutralize 12 mEq of hydrogen ions.

Routes of administration/doses The adult oral dose for the relief of dyspepsia is 600–1800 mg as required. For the alkalinization of urine, an oral dose of 3 g is administered every 2 hours until the pH of the urine is 7.

When administered intravenously for the treatment of profound metabolic acidosis, the dose required to restore the pH to normal is usually calculated from the formula:

$$\text{Dose (mmol)} = [\text{base deficit (mEq/l)} \times \text{body weight (kg)}]/3$$

Half this amount is administered before the acid–base status is reassessed.

Effects

CVS Overenthusiastic correction of an acidosis will result in a metabolic alkalosis, which may result in myocardial dysfunction and peripheral tissue hypoxia due to a shift in the oxygen dissociation curve to the left.

RS Metabolic alkalosis diminishes pulmonary ventilation by an effect on the respiratory centre.

CNS The major clinical effect of metabolic alkalosis is excitability of the CNS, manifested as nervousness, convulsions, muscle weakness, and tetany.

AS Oral administration of the drug results in the release of CO_2 with subsequent belching.

Metabolic/other Hypernatraemia, hyperkalaemia, and hypocalcaemia may all result from the intravenous administration of sodium bicarbonate.

Toxicity/side effects Hypernatraemia and hyperosmolar syndromes may complicate the use of sodium bicarbonate. The compound is highly irritant to tissues when extravasated and may cause skin necrosis and sloughing.

Kinetics Data are incomplete.

Metabolism Bicarbonate ions react with hydrogen ions to yield CO_2 and water.

Excretion Occurs via renal excretion of bicarbonate and exhalation of CO_2.

Special points Sodium bicarbonate is physically incompatible with calcium salts (which it precipitates) and may cause inactivation of co-administered adrenaline, isoprenaline, and suxamethonium.

The use of sodium bicarbonate should be avoided in patients with renal, hepatic, or heart failure due to its high sodium content.

Hypertonic preparations of sodium bicarbonate appear to lower intracranial pressure in a manner similar to hypertonic saline.

Sodium chloride

Uses Sodium chloride is used:
1. to provide maintenance fluid and extracellular fluid replacement
2. to replace sodium and chloride ions under circumstances of reduced intake or excessive loss
3. in the management of hyperosmolar diabetic coma
4. as a priming fluid for haemodialysis and cardiopulmonary bypass machines
5. for rehydration of neonates and infants (0.45% solutions)
6. in the management of severe salt depletion (1.8% solutions)
7. for the dilution of drugs
8. for interspinous ligament injection in the treatment of chronic neck and back pain (10% solutions) and
9. in the management of raised intracranial pressure (5% solution).

Chemical An inorganic salt.

Presentation As clear, colourless, sterile 0.45/0.9/1.8/5% solutions in bags of various capacities. The 0.9% solution contains 154 mmol of both sodium and chloride ions per litre. The pH ranges from 4.5 to 7; they contain no preservative or antimicrobial agents.

Main action Volume expansion.

Routes of administration/doses Hypertonic saline solutions should be administered via a central venous line.

Effects

CVS The haemodynamic effects of sodium chloride are proportional to the prevailing circulating volume and are short-lived.

GU Renal perfusion is temporarily restored towards normal in hypovolaemic patients transfused with the crystalloid.

Toxicity/side effects The predominant hazard is that of overtransfusion, leading to hypernatraemia or pulmonary oedema. A hyperchloraemic metabolic acidosis may result from repeated administration of sodium chloride.

Kinetics

Absorption Sodium chloride is rapidly and completely absorbed when administered orally.

Distribution 0.9% solution is isotonic with extracellular fluid; it is initially distributed into the intravascular compartment where it remains for approximately 30 minutes before being distributed uniformly throughout the extracellular space.

Excretion In the urine.

Sodium nitroprusside

Uses Sodium nitroprusside is used in the management of:
1. hypertensive crises
2. aortic dissection prior to surgery
3. left ventricular failure and
4. to produce hypotension during surgery.

Chemical An inorganic complex.

Presentation As an intravenous solution of 10 mg/ml of sodium nitroprusside for dilution prior to infusion; it must be protected from light.

Main actions Vasodilation and hypotension.

Mode of action Sodium nitroprusside dilates both resistance and capacitance vessels by a direct action on vascular smooth muscle. It appears to act by interacting with sulfhydryl groups in the smooth muscle cell membrane, thereby stabilizing the membrane and preventing the Ca^{2+} influx necessary for the initiation of contraction.

Routes of administration/doses Sodium nitroprusside should be administered through a dedicated vein using a controlled infusion device at a rate of 0.5–6 micrograms/kg/min, titrated according to response. Invasive arterial pressure measurement during the use of the drug is considered mandatory. Onset of action is almost immediate; the desired response is usually achieved in 1–2 minutes.

Effects

CVS In hypertensive and normotensive patients, infusion of the drug causes a decrease in the systemic blood pressure and a compensatory tachycardia; the cardiac output is usually well maintained. In patients with heart failure, cardiac output increases due to a decrease in both venous return and systemic vascular resistance. The myocardial wall tension is decreased, and myocardial oxygen consumption falls; the heart rate tends to decrease due to improved haemodynamics with the use of the drug. The blood pressure is usually well maintained under these circumstances. Myocardial contractility is unaltered by the drug.

RS Sodium nitroprusside causes a reversible decrease in PaO_2 due to attenuation of hypoxic pulmonary vasoconstriction; an increased inspired oxygen concentration may be necessary.

CNS The drug causes cerebral vasodilation, leading to an increase in intracranial pressure in normocapnic patients; a 'steal' phenomenon may occur. The autoregulatory curve is shifted to the left.

AS Sodium nitroprusside decreases to lower oesophageal sphincter pressure and may cause a paralytic ileus.

GU The renal blood flow and glomerular filtration rate are well maintained during infusions of the drug.

Metabolic/other A compensatory increase in plasma catecholamine concentration and plasma renin activity occurs during the use of the drug. A metabolic acidosis may also occur.

Toxicity/side effects The major disadvantage of the drug is its liability to produce cyanide toxicity, the likelihood of which is increased by hypothermia, malnutrition, vitamin B12 deficiency, and severe renal or hepatic impairment. Cyanide ion toxicity is related to the rate of infusion of sodium nitroprusside, rather than to the total dose used; however, it is recommended that no more than 1.5 mg/kg of the drug is infused acutely and no more than 4 micrograms/kg/min is used chronically. The cyanide ion combines with cytochrome C and leads to impairment of aerobic metabolism; metabolic acidosis due to an increased serum lactic acid concentration may result. The signs of cyanide ion toxicity are tachycardia, dysrhythmias, hyperventilation, sweating, and the development of a metabolic acidosis; these occur at plasma cyanide ion concentrations in excess of 8 micrograms/ml. Treatment of cyanide ion toxicity involves curtailing the infusion of sodium nitroprusside, general supportive measures, and the administration of sodium thiosulfate or dicobalt edetate.

Additionally, profound hypotension produced by the drug may manifest itself as nausea and vomiting, abdominal pain, restlessness, headache, dizziness, palpitations, and retrosternal pain.

Kinetics Pharmacokinetic data are difficult to obtain due to the very short duration of action of the drug.

Absorption The drug is not absorbed orally.

Distribution Sodium nitroprusside in the blood is confined essentially to the plasma; scarcely any is present within red blood cells. The V_D is approximately the same as the extracellular space (15 l).

Metabolism Occurs by two separate pathways. In the presence of low plasma concentrations of sodium nitroprusside, the predominant route appears to be by reaction with the sulfhydryl groups of amino acids present in the plasma. In the presence of higher plasma concentrations of the drug, rapid non-enzymatic hydrolysis occurs within red blood cells. Five cyanide ions are produced by the degradation of each molecule of sodium nitroprusside; one reacts with methaemoglobin to form cyanomethaemoglobin. The remaining four cyanide ions enter the plasma; 80% of these react with thiosulfate in a reaction catalysed by hepatic rhodanese to form thiocyanate. The remainder of the cyanide ions reacts with hydroxycobalamin to form cyanocobalamin (vitamin B12).

Excretion Both thiocyanate and cyanocobalamin are excreted unchanged in the urine. The elimination half-life of the former is 2.7 days.

Special points Sodium nitroprusside is removed by haemodialysis.

Sodium valproate

Uses Sodium valproate is used in the treatment of:
1. primary generalized epilepsies, especially petit mal epilepsy, myoclonic seizures, infantile spasms, and tonic–clonic epilepsy
2. chronic pain of non-malignant origin.

Chemical Sodium valproate is the sodium salt of valproic acid, a fatty (carboxylic) acid.

Presentation As 100/200/500 mg tablets, a syrup containing 40 mg/ml, and in ampoules containing 400 mg of lyophilized sodium valproate for dilution in 4 ml of water.

Main action Anticonvulsant.

Mode of action The most likely mode of action is via GABA-ergic inhibition; sodium valproate increases brain GABA levels by inhibition of succinic semialdehyde dehydrogenase in the GABA shunt. Alternatively, it may:
1. mimic the action of GABA at post-synaptic receptors and
2. reduce excitatory inhibition (especially that due to aspartate).

Routes of administration/doses The adult oral dose is 600–2500 mg daily in two divided doses. The intravenous dose is 400–2500 mg daily in divided doses. The effective plasma range is 40–100 mg/l.

Effects

CNS The drug has anticonvulsant properties as described. Sodium valproate produces minimal sedation; an essential tremor may occasionally develop with the use of the drug.

Metabolic/other Hyperammonaemia occurs infrequently.

Toxicity/side effects Sodium valproate is generally well tolerated. Hepatic dysfunction, acute pancreatitis, gastrointestinal upsets, hair loss, oedema, and weight gain may occur, following administration of the drug. There are also reports of platelet disturbances (decreased platelet aggregation and thrombocytopenia) and coagulation disturbances (increased bleeding time, prothrombin time, and APTT) complicating the administration of sodium valproate.

Kinetics

Absorption Sodium valproate is rapidly and completely absorbed; the oral bioavailability is virtually 100%.

Distribution The drug is 90% protein-bound in the plasma, predominantly to albumin; the V_D is 0.1–0.41 l/kg. Brain concentrations are 7–28% of plasma levels.

Metabolism Sodium valproate is almost completely metabolized in the liver by oxidation and glucuronidation; some of the metabolites are active.

Excretion 1–3% is excreted unchanged in the urine. The clearance is 7–11 ml/kg/hour, and the elimination half-life is 8–20 hours.

Special points High concentrations of sodium valproate displace thiopental from its binding sites *in vitro* and similarly displace diazepam *in vivo*. Platelet function may need to be monitored prior to surgery or epidural or spinal anaesthesia.

The drug is contraindicated in patients with acute liver disease, and liver function should be monitored during chronic therapy. The sedative effects of the drug are additive with those of other CNS depressants.

Sodium valproate is not removed by dialysis.

Spironolactone

Uses Spironolactone is used in the treatment of:
1. congestive cardiac failure
2. hepatic cirrhosis with ascites and oedema
3. refractory oedema
4. hypertension
5. the nephrotic syndrome
6. in combination with loop or thiazide diuretics to conserve potassium and
7. in the diagnosis and treatment of Conn's syndrome.

Chemical A synthetic steroid.

Presentation As 25/50/100 mg tablets of spironolactone. Fixed-dose combinations with hydroflumethiazide or furosemide are also available.

Main actions Diuretic.

Mode of action Spironolactone acts as a competitive antagonist of aldosterone at the latter's receptor site in the distal convoluted tubule; consequently, Na^+ reabsorption is inhibited, and K^+ reabsorption is increased. The drug thus promotes saliuresis and also potentiates that produced by other diuretic agents.

Routes of administration/doses The adult oral dose of spironolactone is 100–400 mg daily; the corresponding dose of potassium canrenoate is 200–800 mg, administered by slow intravenous infusion. The drug has a slow onset of action; the diuretic effect takes 3–4 days to become established.

Effects

CVS The drug has an antihypertensive effect that may be mediated by alteration of the extracellular:intracellular Na^+ gradient or by antagonism of the effect of aldosterone on arteriolar smooth muscle.

CNS Spironolactone may produce both sedation and muscular weakness, presumably secondarily to electrolyte derangements.

GU The principal effect of the drug is diuresis with retention of K^+. The renal blood flow and glomerular filtration rate are unaffected, although the free water clearance may increase.

Metabolic/other Spironolactone has an anti-androgenic effect due to inhibition of ovarian androgen secretion and interference with the peripheral action of endogenous androgens. The drug increases renal Ca^{2+} excretion and may also lead to a reversible hyperchloraemic metabolic acidosis and an increased plasma urea concentration.

Toxicity/side effects The predominant side effect of spironolactone is hyperkalaemia, especially in the presence of renal impairment. The use of the drug is also associated with an appreciable incidence of nausea and vomiting and other gastrointestinal disturbances. Menstrual irregularities in the female and gynaecomastia in the male may result from the anti-androgenic effects of spironolactone.

Kinetics

Absorption Spironolactone is incompletely absorbed when administered orally and has a bioavailability by this route of 70%; the drug undergoes extensive first-pass hepatic metabolism.

Distribution The drug is 90% protein-bound in the plasma.

Metabolism Spironolactone is rapidly and extensively metabolized by deacetylation and dethiolation; some of the metabolites, including canrenone, are active.

Excretion The metabolites are principally excreted in the urine, with a small proportion undergoing biliary excretion. The elimination half-life of spironolactone is 1–2 hours.

Special points Spironolactone decreases the responsiveness to co-administered pressor agents and increases the effects of co-administered cardiovascular depressants, including anaesthetic agents. The drug increases the serum concentrations of co-administered digoxin and may interfere with digoxin assay techniques.

SSRIs

Uses Selective serotonin reuptake inhibitors (SSRIs) are used in the treatment of:
1. unipolar depression
2. obsessive–compulsive disorder
3. generalized anxiety disorder
4. social anxiety disorder
5. panic disorder
6. post-traumatic stress disorder and
7. bulimia nervosa.

Chemical SSRIs have a variety of chemical structures.

Presentation The following SSRIs are in common clinical use and are available in tablet or capsule form: fluvoxamine, fluoxetine, sertraline, paroxetine, citalopram, and escitalopram.

Main action Antidepressant and anxiolytic.

Mode of action SSRIs selectively inhibit the neuronal reuptake of serotonin by the pre-synaptic serotonin reuptake pump. *In vitro*, they exhibit very weak anticholinergic and histaminergic activity.

Routes of administration/doses SSRIs are usually administered orally as a single daily dose in the mornings. The specific dose of an SSRI administered is dependent on the clinical indication, age of the patient, and particular agent being used.

Effects

CVS SSRIs may cause an increase or decrease in the heart rate, together with a fall in the blood pressure which may be postural in nature.

CNS The effects of SSRIs are to improve mood and decrease feelings of anxiety.

Metabolic/other SSRIs may cause a decrease in plasma sodium concentration, possibly causing inappropriate ADH secretion. These drugs should be used with caution in patients concurrently receiving diuretics.

Toxicity/side effects SSRIs cause dose-related gastrointestinal effects (nausea, abdominal pain, diarrhoea). Hypersensitivity reactions of all types may occur. Urogenital side effects have been reported, including reduced libido, anorgasmia, impotence, and urinary frequency or retention.

Kinetics

Absorption SSRIs are well absorbed from the gastrointestinal tract. They undergo extensive first-pass metabolism, except for citalopram.

Distribution Due to the lipophilic nature of SSRIs, these drugs have large volumes of distribution and consequently take some time to reach a steady-state concentration.

Metabolism SSRIs undergo extensive hepatic metabolism via the cytochrome P450 system. In addition, the drugs are potent inhibitors of certain CYP isoenzymes, including CYP2D6. Fluoxetine is metabolized to the active metabolite norfluoxetine.

Excretion Metabolites undergo renal elimination.

Special points All SSRIs are associated with a withdrawal syndrome if treatment is discontinued abruptly. The commonest symptoms include: nausea, vomiting, headache, paraesthesiae, dizziness, sweating, sleep disturbances, and anxiety.

Concurrent administration of SSRIs to patients receiving MAOIs, lithium, L-tryptophan, sumatriptan, risperidone, or 3,4-methylenedioxy-methamphetamine (MDMA) may lead to serotonin syndrome. Serotonin syndrome is characterized by the acute onset of the following symptoms and signs: tachycardia, hypertension, hyperthermia, sweating, nausea, diarrhoea, agitation, pupillary dilatation, myoclonus, and hyperreflexia.

Statins

Uses Statins are used in the treatment of:
1. hypercholesterolaemia
2. primary prevention of cardiovascular events
3. secondary prevention of cardiovascular events.

Chemical Naturally occurring or synthetically derived inhibitors of 3-hydroxy-3-methyl-glutaryl-coenzyme A reductase (HMGCoA).

Presentation Six agents are available in the UK for oral administration. Atorvastatin and simvastatin comprise approximately 85% of statins prescribed in the UK.

Main action Reduction in total cholesterol.

Mode of action Inhibition of HMGCoA reductase, leading to early blockade of conversion of HMGCoA to mevalonate, thereby preventing subsequent conversion to cholesterol and isoprenoids.

Routes of administration/doses The specific dose of an agent administered is dependent on the clinical indication and particular agent being used. Statins are administered orally, usually at night.

Toxicity/side effects The most important side effect of statin therapy is muscle pains which may be associated with a myopathy, with subsequent development of rhabdomyolysis, and acute renal failure secondary to myoglobinuria. Sleep disturbance, memory loss, sexual dysfunction, depression, and rarely interstitial lung disease have all been reported, following use of these drugs. Hepatic serum transaminases may become elevated during treatment.

Kinetics

Absorption The bioavailability of statins is variable, depending on the specific agent. Atorvastatin has a bioavailability of 12% and simvastatin a bioavailability of 5%. Statins undergo extensive first-pass metabolism.

Distribution Statins are highly protein-bound in the plasma (90–98%), apart from pravastatin which has protein binding of 43–67%.

Metabolism The majority of statins are metabolized via the cytochrome P450 enzyme system. Atorvastatin and simvastatin are metabolized by CYP3A4. Atorvastatin is metabolized to orthohydroxylated and parahydroxylated metabolites during first-pass metabolism, which are pharmacologically active. Simvastatin is an inactive lactone that is metabolized during first-pass metabolism to the active metabolite beta-hydroxyacid.

Excretion The half-life of atorvastatin is 15 hours and that of simvastatin 1.9 hours. Up to 20% of a dose may be excreted renally. The majority of metabolites undergo biliary excretion. Minimal enterohepatic circulation occurs.

Special points There is growing evidence to suggest that statins act as inhibitors of the inflammatory process. Statins reduce leucocyte adhesion to endothelial cells during sepsis-driven leucocyte activation. The drugs also downregulate the production of the following pro-inflammatory cytokines: IL-6, IL-8, TNF-alpha, monocyte chemoattractant protein-1, and C-reactive protein (CRP). Statins also appear to reduce the procoagulant effects seen in sepsis and have anti-inflammatory effects mediated through upregulation of endothelial NO synthase activity, thereby enhancing NO production.

Co-administration of agents that act as CYP3A4 inhibitors may lead to increased drug levels of statins and a corresponding increased risk in the development of myopathy/rhabdomyolysis. The following agents require either discontinuation of statin therapy or dose reduction, depending on the specific drug(s) being used: itraconazole, ketoconazole, erythromycin, clarithromycin, HIV protease inhibitors, ciclosporin, diazole, amiodarone, verapamil, diltiazem, grapefruit juice.

Sucralfate

Uses Sucralfate is used:
1. in the treatment of peptic ulcer disease and
2. for the prevention of stress ulceration in the critically ill.

Chemical An aluminium salt of sulfated sucrose.

Presentation As tablets containing 1 g sucralfate and a white, viscous suspension containing 200 mg/ml of sucralfate.

Main actions Cytoprotection of the upper gastrointestinal tract.

Mode of action At acid pH, sucralfate forms a viscous paste which adheres preferentially to peptic ulcers via ionic binding. It acts by providing a physical barrier to the diffusion of acid, pepsin, and bile salts and also by forming complexes with proteins at the ulcer surface, which resist peptic hydrolysis.

Routes of administration/doses The adult dose for the prophylaxis of stress ulceration is 1 g 6-hourly.

Effects

AS Sucralfate has weak intrinsic antacid activity. It has no effect on gastric emptying time. The drug increases gastric blood flow and enhances gastric epithelial proliferation via stimulation of gastric mucosal epidermal growth factor and fibroblast growth factor.

Metabolic/other In uraemic patients, sucralfate increases aluminium absorption and therefore should be used with care. It acts as a phosphate binder which may induce hypophosphataemia.

Toxicity/side effects Sucralfate is essentially non-toxic. Constipation occurs in 2%.

Kinetics

Absorption Sucralfate is minimally (3–5%) absorbed after oral administration.

Distribution 85–95% of an oral dose remains in the gastrointestinal tract. The V_D and percentage of protein binding are unknown.

Metabolism No metabolism of the drug occurs in man.

Excretion Predominantly unchanged in the faeces. The fraction that is absorbed is excreted primarily in the urine.

Sufentanil

Uses Sufentanil is used for:
1. the induction and maintenance of general anaesthesia and has been used for
2. post-operative analgesia.

Chemical A phenylpiperidine which is the thienyl derivative of fentanyl.

Presentation As a clear solution containing 50 micrograms/ml of sufentanil citrate. The drug is not commercially available in the UK.

Main actions Analgesia and respiratory depression.

Mode of action Sufentanil is a highly selective mu-agonist; the MOP receptor appears to be specifically involved in the mediation of analgesia. Part of the analgesic effect of the drug may be attributable to stimulation of 5HT release. Opioids appear to exert their effects by increasing intracellular calcium concentration which, in turn, increases potassium conductance and hyperpolarization of excitable cell membranes. The decrease in membrane excitability that results may decrease both pre- and post-synaptic responses.

Routes of administration/doses The intravenous dose is 0.5–50 micrograms/kg, and the adult dose via the epidural route is 10–100 micrograms (the optimal post-operative dose being 30–50 micrograms). When administered intravenously, the drug acts in 1–6 minutes, and the duration of effect is 0.5–8 hours, dependent on the other components of the anaesthetic.

Effects

CVS Sufentanil causes little haemodynamic disturbance. Heart rate and blood pressure tend to decrease immediately post-induction. Venous pooling may lead to orthostatic hypotension.

RS The drug produces dose-dependent respiratory depression which may be delayed in onset. Chest wall rigidity (the 'wooden chest' phenomenon) may occur after the administration of sufentanil—this may be an effect of the drug on mu-receptors located on GABA-ergic interneurones.

CNS Sufentanil is 2000–4000 times as potent an analgesic as morphine. The EEG changes produced by the drug are similar to those produced by fentanyl—initial beta activity is decreased, and alpha activity is increased; subsequently, alpha activity disappears, and delta activity predominates. The drug has no intrinsic effect on intracranial pressure. Miosis is produced as a result of stimulation of the Edinger–Westphal nucleus.

AS Sufentanil appears to cause less nausea than fentanyl. The drug may cause spasm of the sphincter of Oddi.

Metabolic/other The drug tends to obtund the stress response to surgery, although it does not completely abolish it. Sufentanil may cause histamine release and may have less effect on immune function than fentanyl.

Toxicity/side effects Hypotension, tachycardia, bradycardia, nausea, and the 'wooden chest' phenomenon are the side effects most commonly reported with the use of sufentanil. Tonic/clonic movements of the limbs have also been reported.

Kinetics

Absorption The drug is normally administered intravenously; the drug is, however, 20% absorbed when administered transdermally.

Distribution Sufentanil is 92% protein-bound in the plasma, predominantly to alpha-1 acid glycoprotein. The drug is highly lipophilic; the V_D is 1.74–5.17 l/kg.

Metabolism The metabolic pathways are unknown in man, although two metabolites (norsufentanil and desmethylsufentanil) have been identified in the urine.

Excretion 60% of an administered dose appear in the urine and 10% in bile. The clearance is 11–21 ml/min/kg; the elimination half-life is 119–175 minutes.

Special points Sufentanil decreases the MAC of co-administered volatile agents by 60–70%. The drug should be used with caution in the presence of renal or hepatic failure, although the kinetics appears to be unaltered.

The drug increases the effect of non-depolarizing muscle relaxants to a similar extent to halothane.

Sugammadex

Uses Sugammadex is used to reverse neuromuscular blockade induced by rocuronium or vecuronium.

Chemical A modified gamma-cyclodextrin.

Presentation As a clear, colourless or pale yellow solution for injection, available in 2 ml and 5 ml glass vials, containing 100 mg/ml of sugammadex sodium (equivalent to sugammadex 100 mg/ml), needing to be stored below 30°C. It has a pH of between 7 and 8 and an osmolality of between 300 and 500 mOsm/kg. One ml of solution contains 9.7 mg of sodium. The solution may also contain 3.7% hydrochloric acid and/or sodium hydroxide for pH adjustment.

Main action Reversal of neuromuscular blockade induced by rocuronium or vecuronium.

Mode of action Sugammadex acts by encapsulating the steroid portion of aminosteroidal molecules within its hydrophobic interior. The negatively charged carboxyl groups bind to the positively charged nitrogen atom on the aminosteroidal molecule. This binding of the NMB drug decreases the amount of free drug within the central compartment, thereby establishing a concentration gradient and resulting in movement of the NMB drug away from the effector site towards the central compartment. The resultant reduction in competitive antagonism of acetylcholine at nicotinic (N2) receptors at the post-synaptic membrane of the neuromuscular junction leads to successful binding of acetylcholine and rapid re-establishment of neuromuscular function.

Routes of administration/doses The drug is administered intravenously as a single bolus injection in a variety of doses, depending on the extent of neuromuscular blockade present in a given patient. A dose of 4 mg/kg is recommended when recovery of neuromuscular function has reached at least 1–2 post-tetanic counts following administration of rocuronium or vecuronium (i.e. 'deep' neuromuscular block). The median time to recovery of the T4/T1 ratio to 0.9 is 3 minutes. A lower dose of 2 mg/kg is recommended when recovery of neuromuscular function has reached at least the reappearance of T2 (i.e. 'shallow' neuromuscular block), with a median time to recovery of the T4/T1 ratio to 0.9 of 2 minutes. The median recovery time is slightly faster in patients who have received rocuronium, compared to those receiving vecuronium. Sugammadex may also be administered immediately following the administration of rocuronium, as part of a modified rapid sequence induction (i.e. 'rescue reversal') when a 'can't intubate, can't ventilate' scenario has occurred. The recommended dose for 'rescue reversal' is 16 mg/kg. Following the administration of 1.2 mg/kg of rocuronium, if sugammadex is given 3 minutes later, the median time to recovery of the T4/T1 ratio to 0.9 is approximately 1.5 minutes. Sugammadex is not recommended for use in 'rescue reversal' following the administration of vecuronium. In the event of the re-establishment of neuromuscular block, a second dose of

4 mg/kg of sugammadex is recommended. The recommended dose for reversal in children aged between 2 and 17 years, when the recovery of neuromuscular function has reached at least the reappearance of T2, is 2 mg/kg. Use of the drug is not currently recommended in other reversal situations, including 'rescue reversal'. Sugammadex is not currently recommended for use in newborns and infants.

Effects

CVS Sugammadex has minimal cardiovascular side effects. There is no significant prolongation of the QT interval.

RS The drug has no respiratory effects.

CNS The drug has no effect on intracranial or intraocular pressure.

AS Administration of the drug may lead to a bitter or metallic taste.

Toxicity/side effects There has been one report of a patient developing symptoms of flushing, tachycardia, and palpitations, following the administration of 8.4 mg/kg of sugammadex. These symptoms were confirmed to be that of an allergic reaction and were self-limiting.

Kinetics

Distribution Sugammadex and the sugammadex–NMB complex do not bind to plasma proteins or erythrocytes. The V_D is 11–14 l, and the drug exhibits linear kinetics in the dosage range of 1–16 mg/kg.

Metabolism The drug does not undergo metabolism within the human body.

Excretion The clearance is 88–120 ml/min, and the elimination half-life is 1.8 hours. More than 90% of a given dose is excreted within 24 hours. Ninety-six percent of the dose is excreted in the urine, with up to 95% as unaltered drug. Excretion via faeces or expired air was <0.02% of the dose in clinical studies.

Special points In patients with mild and moderate renal impairment, no alteration in dosage is required. In patients with severe renal impairment, the excretion of sugammadex and the sugammadex–NMB complex is prolonged, and use of the drug is not recommended. The clearance of sugammadex by haemodialysis is variable.

No dose reduction is recommended in elderly patients, although the time to recovery of the T4/T1 ratio to 0.9 may be slightly prolonged.

No dose alteration is required for patients with mild and moderate hepatic impairment. No data are currently available in patients with severe hepatic impairment, and the use of sugammadex is not recommended.

Dose calculation in obese patients should be made, based on the actual body weight.

Reoccurrence of neuromuscular block following the administration of sugammadex has been reported as usually being due to suboptimal dosing of the drug. However, administration of drugs in the immediate postoperative period that potentiate the effects of neuromuscular block may theoretically lead to reoccurrence of block and should be used in caution in patients who have received sugammadex. In addition, displacement of bound neuromuscular block from sugammadex may theoretically occur, leading to reoccurrence of neuromuscular blockade if the following drugs are administered within 6 hours of a patient receiving sugammadex: toremifene, flucloxacillin, fusidic acid.

If neuromuscular blockade is required following reversal with sugammadex, then a non-steroidal agent (e.g. suxamethonium or a benzoisoquinolinium agent) should be used due to the risk of reduced efficacy of standard doses of rocuronium or vecuronium in the presence of residual sugammadex. A delay of 24 hours is recommended prior to repeat administration of rocuronium or vecuronium, following the use of sugammadex.

Due to the steroid-binding ability of sugammadex, the drug may interact with hormonal contraceptive agents. Administration of the drug may lead to a decrease in progesterone exposure (34% decrease) equivalent to missing one daily dose. It is recommended that patients taking oral hormonal contraceptive agents should consult the 'missed daily dose' advice contained in the product information leaflet. Patients receiving non-oral hormonal contraceptive agents should be advised to use an additional non-hormonal contraceptive method for the following 7 days after administration of sugammadex.

There is some evidence that sugammadex may interfere with the following laboratory tests: serum progesterone, APTT, prothrombin time. Data suggest that interference with these tests occurs following a dose of 16 mg/kg of sugammadex. The clinical relevance of this is uncertain.

Sulfonylureas

Uses Sulfonylureas are used in the treatment of non-insulin-dependent (type II) diabetes mellitus.

Chemical An S-phenylsulfonylurea structure with substitutions on the phenyl ring and urea terminus.

Presentation Three generations of sulfonylureas exist:
1. first-generation: tolbutamide
2. second-generation: gliclazide, glibenclamide
3. third-generation: glimepiride.

All are presented in tablet form. There is a modified-release preparation of gliclazide.

Main action Hypoglycaemia.

Mode of action Sulfonylureas act by liberating insulin from pancreatic beta-cells; they appear to act by binding to the plasma membrane of the beta-cell and producing prolonged depolarization, reducing the permeability of the membrane to potassium. This, in turn, leads to the opening of calcium channels; the resulting influx of calcium causes triggering of insulin release.

Routes of administration/doses These agents are only available for oral administration. The specific dose and frequency of an agent administered are dependent on the clinical indication and particular agent being used.

Effects
Metabolic/other Sulfonylureas cause a decrease in plasma triglyceride, cholesterol, and free fatty acid concentrations. Gliclazide decreases the incidence of microthrombosis by two methods, firstly by partial inhibition of platelet aggregation and adhesion and secondly by an action on the vascular endothelium fibrinolytic activity with an increase in tissue plasminogen activator activity. Glimepiride has extra-pancreatic effects. It increases the number of active glucose transport molecules, in addition to increasing the activity of the glycosyl phosphatidylinositol-specific lipase C, which may be correlated with drug-induced lipogenesis and glycogenesis in fat and muscle cells. The drug also inhibits hepatic gluconeogenesis by increasing the intracellular concentration of fructose-2,6-bisphosphate.

Toxicity/side effects Hypoglycaemia is a common complication of sulfonylurea therapy. Gastrointestinal disturbances, cholestatic jaundice, and alterations in liver function tests may complicate the use of sulfonylureas. Leucopenia and thrombocytopenia have also been reported. Sulfonylureas are potentially teratogenic.

Kinetics
Absorption Sulfonylureas are well absorbed from the gastrointestinal tract. Gliclazide and glimepiride have a 100% bioavailability.

Distribution The V_D of these agents is variable: gliclazide V_D 0.42 l/kg, glibenclamide V_D 0.15 l/kg, glimepiride V_D 0.12 l/kg. Protein binding is high, with 95–99% of agents bound to albumin.

Metabolism Sulfonylureas undergo extensive hepatic metabolism via CYP2C9 to inactive metabolites.

Excretion 30–50% of an administered dose is excreted in the urine, the remainder in the faeces. Clearance and elimination half-lives of the individual drugs vary—the half-life of gliclazide is 12–20 hours, and that of glibenclamide is 1–2 hours and of glimepiride is 5–8 hours. The elimination of these agents is impaired in the presence of severe renal impairment.

Special points The following drugs may potentiate the effect of sulfonylureas either by displacement from plasma proteins or by inhibition of their hepatic metabolism, resulting in hypoglycaemia: NSAIDs, salicylates, sulfonamides, oral anticoagulants, MAOIs, and beta-adrenergic antagonists. Conversely, the following drugs tend to counteract the effect of sulfonylureas and result in loss of diabetic control: thiazide and other diuretics, steroids, phenothiazines, phenytoin, sympathomimetic agents, and calcium antagonists.

The long-acting sulfonylureas should be stopped prior to anaesthesia for major surgery due to the risk of hypoglycaemia. Alternative methods of blood sugar control may need to be instituted.

Suxamethonium

Uses Suxamethonium is used:
1. wherever rapid and profound neuromuscular blockade is required, e.g. to facilitate tracheal intubation and
2. for the modification of fits after electroconvulsive therapy.

Chemical The dicholine ester of succinic acid (equivalent to two acetylcholine molecules joined back-to-back).

Presentation As a clear aqueous solution containing 50 mg/ml of suxamethonium chloride; the preparation should be stored at 4°C.

Main actions Neuromuscular blockade of brief duration in skeletal muscle.

Mode of action Suxamethonium causes prolonged depolarization of skeletal muscle fibres to a membrane potential above which an action potential can be triggered.

Routes of administration/doses The intravenous dose is 0.5–2.0 mg/kg; the onset of action occurs within 30 seconds, and the duration of action is 3–5 minutes. Infusion of a 0.1% solution at 2–15 mg/kg/hour will yield 90% twitch depression. The intramuscular dose is up to 2.5 mg/kg. Equal doses on a mg/kg basis have a shorter duration of action in infants. The drug may also be administered sublingually at a dose of 2 mg/kg.

Effects

CVS With repeated doses of suxamethonium, bradycardia and a slight increase in mean arterial pressure may occur.

RS Apnoea occurs subsequent to skeletal muscle paralysis.

CNS The administration of suxamethonium may initially cause fasciculations which are then followed by a phase I depolarizing block. The characteristics of this during partial paralysis are:
1. well-sustained tetanus during stimulation at 50–100 Hz
2. the absence of post-tetanic facilitation
3. train-of-four ratio >0.7 and
4. potentiation by anticholinesterases.

With repeated administration or a large total dose, a phase II block may develop. The characteristics of this during partial paralysis are:
1. poorly sustained tetanus
2. post-tetanic facilitation
3. train-of-four ratio <0.3
4. reversal by anticholinesterases and
5. tachyphylaxis.

Intracranial and intraocular pressures are both raised, following the administration of suxamethonium.

AS The intragastric pressure increases by 7–12 cmH$_2$O; the lower oesophageal sphincter tone simultaneously decreases with the use of suxamethonium. Salivation and gastric secretions are increased.

Metabolic/other Serum potassium concentration is briefly increased in normal individuals by 0.2–0.4 mmol/l.

Toxicity/side effects Bradycardia and other dysrhythmias may occur with single or repeated dosing. The hyperkalaemic response is markedly exaggerated in patients with burns or major denervation of muscle and acute or chronic renal failure; this may lead to cardiac arrest. Post-operative muscular pains are common, especially in women, the middle-aged, and those ambulant early in the post-operative period. Intraocular pressure is transiently raised, following the use of suxamethonium—the drug should be used with caution in patients with penetrating eye injuries. Suxamethonium is a potent trigger agent for the development of malignant hyperthermia and may cause generalized contractures in those patients exhibiting myotonia. Prolonged apnoea may occur in susceptible individuals. There have been many reports of fatal anaphylactoid reactions with the administration of suxamethonium. Cross-sensitivity exists with many of the non-depolarizing drugs, following administration of suxamethonium.

Kinetics

Distribution An initial rapid redistribution phase may contribute to the brief duration of action of the drug. Suxamethonium appears to be protein-bound to an unknown extent.

Metabolism The drug is hydrolysed by plasma cholinesterase (EC 3.1.1.8) to succinylomonocholine (which is weakly active) and choline; the former is further hydrolysed by plasma cholinesterase to succinic acid and choline. Eighty percent of an administered dose is hydrolysed before it reaches the neuromuscular junction.

Excretion 2–10% of an administered dose is excreted unchanged in the urine. The *in vivo* hydrolysis rate is 3–7 mg/l/min, and the half-life 2.7–4.6 minutes.

Special points The incidence of muscle pains after the administration of suxamethonium may be decreased by pre-treatment with:

1. low (0.2 mg/kg) dose of suxamethonium
2. small dose of a non-depolarizing relaxant
3. diazepam
4. dantrolene
5. aspirin or
6. vitamin C.

Plasma cholinesterase activity may be influenced by both genetic and acquired factors, leading to an altered pattern of response to suxamethonium. The normal gene encoding for plasma cholinesterase is E_i^u (usual); three abnormal genes also exist: E_i^a (atypical), E_i^s (silent), and E_i^f (fluoride-resistant).

Simple Mendelian genetics are involved; 94% of the population are heterozygous for the usual gene and are clinically normal in their response to suxamethonium. E_i^a homozygotes comprise 0.03%, E_i^s homozygotes 0.001%, and E_i^f homozygotes 0.0003% of the population, and all remain apnoeic for 1–2 hours after receiving the drug and develop a phase II block during this period (fresh frozen plasma may be used to provide a source of plasma cholinesterase under these circumstances). All possible combinations of heterozygotes exist—they constitute 3.8% of the population and remain apnoeic for approximately 10 minutes after receiving suxamethonium.

In addition, plasma cholinesterase concentrations may be reduced in pregnancy, liver disease, cardiac or renal failure, hypoproteinaemic states, carcinomatosis, thyrotoxicosis, tetanus, muscular dystrophy, and in patients with burns, and suxamethonium may have a prolonged action in these states. Drugs which decrease the activity of plasma cholinesterase include ecothiopate, tacrine, procaine, lidocaine, lithium and magnesium salts, ketamine, pancuronium, the oral contraceptive pill, and cytotoxic agents. Suxamethonium does not appear to be potentiated by volatile agents, although phase II block may appear more readily in their presence.

Suxamethonium is pharmaceutically incompatible with thiopental. The effects of digoxin may be enhanced by suxamethonium, leading to enhanced ventricular excitability.

Total body weight should be used to calculate drug dosage in morbidly obese individuals.

Drug structure For the drug structure, please see Fig. 8.

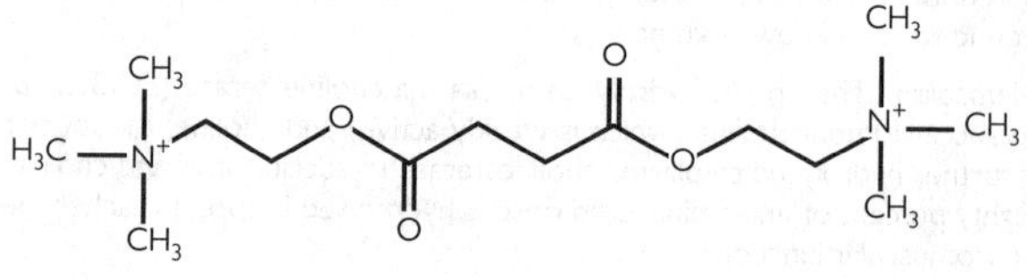

Fig. 8 Drug structure of suxamethonium.

Teicoplanin

Uses Teicoplanin is used in the parenteral treatment of severe infections:
1. complicated skin and soft tissue infections
2. bone and joint infections
3. hospital-acquired pneumonia
4. community-acquired pneumonia
5. urinary tract infections
6. infective endocarditis
7. peritonitis associated with continuous ambulatory peritoneal dialysis and
8. may be used orally as an alternative for *Clostridium difficile* infection-associated diarrhoea and colitis.

Commonly susceptible species are aerobic Gram-positive bacteria—*Corynebacterium jeikeium*, *Enterococcus faecalis*, *Staphylococcus aureus* (including MRSA), *Streptococcus agalactiae*, *Streptococcus dysgalactiae*, groups C and G streptococci, *Streptococcus pneumoniae*, *Streptococcus pyogenes*, streptococci in the *viridans* group; and aerobic Gram-positive bacteria *Clostridium difficile*, *Peptostreptococcus* spp. All Gram-negative organisms are resistant.

Chemical Teicoplanin is a glycopeptide antibiotic from cultures of *Actinoplanes teichomyceticus*, comprising five major components differentiated by a specific fatty acid.

Presentation As 200/400 mg powder for injection/infusion or oral solution with sodium chloride and sodium hydroxide (for pH adjustment). The solution is reconstituted by adding 3.14 ml of water for injection to the 200 mg and 400 mg powder vial. The water is slowly added to the vial which should be rotated until all the powder is dissolved to avoid foaming. If foam develops, stand for approximately 15 minutes. Only clear and yellowish solutions should be used. It then can be further diluted. Chemical and physical stability of the reconstituted solution prepared as recommended has been demonstrated for 24 hours at 2–8°C.

Main actions Teicoplanin has a limited spectrum of antibacterial activity (Gram-positive) and may not be suitable for use as a single agent for the treatment of some infections, unless the pathogen is already documented and known to be susceptible.

Mode of action Teicoplanin inhibits the growth of susceptible organisms by interfering with cell wall biosynthesis at a site different from that affected by beta-lactams. Peptidoglycan synthesis is blocked by specific binding to D-alanyl-D-alanine residues.

Teicoplanin antimicrobial activity depends essentially on the duration of time during which the substance level is higher than the MIC of the pathogen.

Routes of administration/doses Due to its long half-life, loading doses is required of 400/800 mg 12-hourly for 3–5 administrations, then a daily maintenance of 400/600 mg. The dose needs to be adjusted according to the infection, organism, and presence of renal failure.

Effects

CNS Teicoplanin does not readily penetrate into the CSF.

Metabolic/other It is unknown whether teicoplanin is excreted in human milk. Teicoplanin is not removed by haemodialysis and only slowly by peritoneal dialysis.

Toxicity/side effects Teicoplanin must be administered with caution in patients with known hypersensitivity to vancomycin, as cross-hypersensitivity reactions, including fatal anaphylactic shock, may occur. A previous history of 'red man syndrome' with vancomycin is not a contraindication to the use of teicoplanin. Life-threatening, or even fatal, cutaneous reactions have been reported. Increases in transaminase, alkaline phosphatase, and creatinine have all been recorded. Infusion-related reactions have been reported.

Kinetics

Absorption When administered by the oral route, teicoplanin is not absorbed from the gastrointestinal tract. Bioavailability after intramuscular injection is approximately 90%.

Distribution Teicoplanin is mainly bound to human serum albumin, and plasma protein binding ranges from 87.6 to 90.8%. The VD_{ss} varies from 0.7 to 1.4 ml/kg (>8 days). Teicoplanin is distributed mainly in the lungs, myocardium, and bone tissues, with tissue:serum ratios superior to 1.

Metabolism Minimal two metabolites are formed probably by hydroxylation and represent 2–3% of the administered dose.

Excretion Unchanged teicoplanin is mainly excreted by the urinary route (80% within 16 days), whilst 2.7% of the administered dose is recovered in faeces (via bile excretion) within 8 days after administration. The elimination half-life of teicoplanin varies from 100 to 170 hours. Teicoplanin has a low total clearance in the range of 10 to 14 ml/hour/kg, and a renal clearance in the range of 8 to 12 ml/hour/kg, indicating that teicoplanin is mainly excreted by renal mechanisms.

Special points The dose has to be decreased in renal failure.

During maintenance treatment, teicoplanin trough serum concentrations monitoring is recommended at least once a week to ensure concentrations are stable and appropriate.

Resistance to teicoplanin can be based on the following mechanisms:

1. modified target structure: this form of resistance has occurred particularly in *Enterococcus faecium*. The modification is based on exchange of the terminal D-alanine-D-alanine function of the amino acid chain in a murein precursor with D-Ala-D-lactate, thus reducing the affinity to vancomycin. The responsible enzymes are a newly synthesized D-lactate dehydrogenase or ligase

2. the reduced sensitivity of staphylococci to teicoplanin is due to the overproduction of murein precursors to which the antibiotic is bound.

Cross-resistance between teicoplanin and the glycoprotein vancomycin may occur, but a number of vancomycin-resistant enterococci are sensitive to teicoplanin (Van-B phenotype).

Temazepam

Uses Temazepam is used:
1. as a hypnotic and
2. for anaesthetic premedication.

Chemical A 3-hydroxy benzodiazepine which is a minor metabolite of diazepam.

Presentation As tablets containing 10/20 mg and an elixir containing 2 mg/ml of temazepam.

Main actions Temazepam has anxiolytic, hypnotic, anticonvulsant, and muscle relaxant properties.

Mode of action Benzodiazepines are thought to act via specific benzodiazepine receptors found at synapses throughout the CNS, but concentrated especially in the cortex and midbrain. Benzodiazepine receptors are closely linked with GABA receptors and appear to facilitate the activity of the latter. Activated GABA receptors open chloride ion channels which then either hyperpolarize or short-circuit the synaptic membrane.

Routes of administration/doses Temazepam is administered orally; the adult dose is 10–60 mg.

Effects

CVS Benzodiazepines have minimal effects on cardiovascular parameters; an insignificant decrease in blood pressure may occur. Benzodiazepines can dilate coronary blood vessels, whilst simultaneously reducing myocardial oxygen consumption.

RS High doses (40 mg) decrease the ventilatory response to hypercapnia.

CNS The drug causes muscular relaxation, sedation, hypnosis, and anxiolysis; it also has anticonvulsant properties.

Metabolic/other High doses (40 mg) cause a slight fall in temperature.

Toxicity/side effects Temazepam is normally well tolerated; gastrointestinal upsets, headaches, dreams, paraesthesiae, and a 'hangover effect' (in 10–15%) may occur. Tolerance and dependence may occur with prolonged use of benzodiazepines; acute withdrawal of benzodiazepines in these circumstances may produce insomnia, anxiety, confusion, psychosis, and perceptual disturbances.

Kinetics

Absorption Absorption of oral temazepam is virtually complete; antacids delay the absorption of benzodiazepines.

Distribution Temazepam is 76% protein-bound *in vivo*. The V_D is 0.8 l/kg.

Metabolism The drug is predominantly metabolized in the liver by direct conjugation to glucuronide; active metabolites are not formed to any great extent.

Excretion 80% of an administered dose appears in the urine as inactive conjugates; 12% is excreted in the faeces. The clearance is 6.6 l/hour, and the elimination half-life is 5–11 hours.

Special points The drug is not removed by haemodialysis. Temazepam is a drug of abuse and has controlled drug status.

Terbutaline

Uses Terbutaline is used in the treatment of:
1. asthma
2. chronic obstructive airways disease and
3. uncomplicated preterm labour.

Chemical An alcohol.

Presentation As 5 mg tablets, a syrup containing 0.3 mg/ml, a clear solution for injection containing 0.5 mg/ml, a respirator solution containing 2.5/10 mg/ml, and as an inhaler delivering 0.5 micrograms per actuation of terbutaline sulfate. It can be administered intravenously or subcutaneously 250–500 micrograms 6-hourly, and by infusion at a rate up to 5 micrograms/min in adults.

Main actions Bronchodilatation and uterine relaxation.

Mode of action Terbutaline is a beta-adrenergic agonist (with a more pronounced effect at beta-2 than beta-1 receptors) that acts by stimulation of membrane-bound adenylate cyclase in the presence of magnesium ions to increase intracellular cAMP concentrations.

Routes of administration/doses The adult oral dose is 2.5–5 mg 8-hourly; the subcutaneous, intramuscular, and intravenous dose is 0.25–0.5 mg once or twice a day. Terbutaline may be administered by intravenous infusion diluted in glucose or saline at the rate of 1.5–5 micrograms/min for 8–10 hours. The dose by inhalation is 0.25–0.5 micrograms 4-hourly or 2–5 mg 8- to 12-hourly if nebulized.

Effects

CVS When used in large doses, terbutaline has positive inotropic and chronotropic effects.

RS Bronchodilatation, leading to an increased PEFR and FEV_1, occurs after administration of the drug. This is additive to the bronchodilatation produced by phosphodiesterase inhibitors. The drug interferes with the mechanism of hypoxic pulmonary vasoconstriction; an adequate inspired oxygen concentration should be ensured when terbutaline is used.

GU Terbutaline relaxes uterine musculature. An increased tendency to bleeding has been reported in association with Caesarean sections.

Metabolic/other Hyperinsulinaemia, leading to hypoglycaemia and hypokalaemia, may follow administration of the drug. Antepartum administration of terbutaline stimulates release of surface-active material into the alveolar space of the fetus, improving the function of the neonatal lung.

Toxicity/side effects Tremor, palpitations, cramps, anxiety, and headache occur uncommonly after the administration of terbutaline.

Kinetics

Absorption The drug is incompletely absorbed after oral administration; the bioavailability is 7–26%. Less than 10% is absorbed after inhalation, the remainder being swallowed.

Distribution Terbutaline is 25% protein-bound in the plasma; the V_D is 1.6 l/kg.

Metabolism Terbutaline has an extensive first-pass metabolism; the drug is predominantly metabolized to a sulfate conjugate.

Excretion 60–70% is excreted unchanged in the urine, the remainder as the sulfated conjugate. The clearance is 1.75–2.75 ml/min/kg, and the elimination half-life is 11.5–23 hours.

Tetracycline

Uses Tetracycline is used in the treatment of infections of:
1. the respiratory, gastrointestinal, and urinary tracts
2. ear, nose, and throat
3. soft tissues and in the treatment of
4. venereal diseases, including non-specific urethritis
5. typhus fever
6. psittacosis
7. cholera
8. acne rosacea and for
9. the treatment of recurrent pleural effusions and
10. the prophylaxis of subacute bacterial endocarditis.

Chemical A napthacenecarboxamide derivative.

Presentation As 250 mg tablets, a syrup containing 25 mg/ml, in vials containing 100 mg (with procaine) for intramuscular injection, and 250/500 mg (with ascorbic acid) for intravenous injection of tetracycline hydrochloride. An ointment for topical use is also available.

Main actions Tetracycline is a broad-spectrum bacteriostatic antibiotic which is active against Gram-positive and Gram-negative bacteria, including *Clostridium*, *Streptococcus*, *Neisseria*, *Brucella*, and *Vibrio* spp., *Haemophilus influenzae*, *Yersinia pestis*, and *Rickettsiae*, *Mycoplasma*, *Chlamydia*, *Leptospira*, and *Treponema* spp.

Mode of action Tetracycline inhibits bacterial protein synthesis by binding to bacterial 30S ribosomes (in the same manner as do aminoglycosides) and preventing the access of aminoacyl transfer RNA (tRNA) to the mRNA–ribosome complex, thereby preventing further elongation of the polypeptide chain.

Routes of administration/doses The adult oral dose is 250–500 mg 6-hourly. The corresponding intramuscular dose is 100 mg 4- to 8-hourly, and the intravenous dose is 0.5–1 g 12-hourly. The intrapleural dose is 500 mg (of the intravenous preparation). Intramuscular injection of the drug is painful.

Effects

CVS Tetracycline may increase the intracranial pressure.

Metabolic/other The drug may cause an increase in the plasma urea concentration and decrease the plasma prothrombin activity.

Toxicity/side effects Occur in 1–5% of patients. The drug may cause renal and hepatic impairment, gastrointestinal and haematological disturbances, moniliasis, rashes, photosensitivity, and thrombophlebitis. Tetracycline may also cause tooth staining in infancy.

Kinetics

Absorption Tetracycline is incompletely absorbed when administered orally (it chelates with iron, calcium, and aluminium in the gut). The bioavailability is 77% by the oral route.

Distribution The drug is widely distributed and exhibits good tissue penetration. The drug is 62–68% protein-bound in the plasma; the V_D is 0.75–1.37 l/kg.

Metabolism 5% of the dose is metabolized to epitetracycline; the remainder is excreted unchanged.

Excretion 95% of the dose is excreted unchanged; 60% is excreted in the urine by glomerular filtration, the remainder in the faeces. The clearance is 1.43–1.91 ml/min/kg, and the half-life is 10–16 hours. A decreased dose should be used in the presence of renal failure.

Special points Tetracycline has been demonstrated to increase the action of non-depolarizing relaxants. It is pharmaceutically incompatible with a host of other drugs, including thiopental, sodium bicarbonate, and autologous blood.

Tigecycline is a glycylcycline antibacterial structurally related to the tetracyclines with similar side effects. It is used for complicated intra-abdominal and skin and soft tissue infections. It is active against MRSA and VRE.

Thiopental

Uses Thiopental is used:
1. for the induction of anaesthesia
2. in the management of status epilepticus and has been used
3. for brain protection.

Chemical A thiobarbiturate.

Presentation As a hygroscopic yellow powder, containing thiopental sodium and 6% sodium carbonate, stored under an atmosphere of nitrogen. The drug is reconstituted in water prior to use to yield a 2.5% solution with a pH of 10.8 and pKa of 7.6, which is stable in solution for 24–48 hours.

Main actions Hypnotic and anticonvulsant.

Mode of action Barbiturates are thought to act primarily at synapses by depressing post-synaptic sensitivity to neurotransmitters and by impairing pre-synaptic neurotransmitter release. Multi-synaptic pathways are depressed preferentially; the reticular activating system is particularly sensitive to the depressant effects of barbiturates. The action of barbiturates at the molecular level is unknown. They may act in a manner analogous to that of local anaesthetic agents by entering cell membranes in the unionized form, subsequently becoming ionized and exerting a membrane-stabilizing effect by decreasing Na^+ and K^+ conductance, decreasing the amplitude of the action potential, and slowing the rate of conduction in excitable tissue. In high concentrations, barbiturates depress the enzymes involved in glucose oxidation, inhibit the formation of ATP, and depress calcium-dependent action potentials. They also inhibit calcium-dependent neurotransmitter release and enhance chloride ion conductance in the absence of GABA.

Routes of administration/doses The dose by the intravenous route is 2–7 mg/kg; following bolus administration, thiopental acts in one arm–brain circulation time and lasts for 5–15 minutes; it is cumulative with repeated administration. The drug may also be administered rectally in a dose of 1 g/22 kg body weight when it acts within 15 minutes.

Effects

CVS Thiopental is a negative inotrope and decreases the cardiac output by approximately 20%; the blood pressure usually decreases as a result of both this effect and a decrease in systemic vascular resistance.

RS Thiopental is a potent respiratory depressant; following intravenous administration, a period of apnoea may occur, followed by a more prolonged period of respiratory depression with a decrease in the ventilatory response to hypercapnia. Laryngeal spasm is occasionally seen in association with the administration of thiopental; the drug may also produce a degree of bronchoconstriction.

CNS Thiopental produces a smooth, rapid induction of anaesthesia. Cerebral blood flow, intracranial pressure, and intraocular pressure are all decreased after the administration of the drug. As with all barbiturates, thiopental has anticonvulsant properties. The drug is antanalgesic when used in small doses. The characteristic EEG changes observed after thiopental administration are initially a fast activity which is subsequently replaced by synchronized low-frequency waves.

AS The drug causes some depression of intestinal activity and constriction of the splanchnic vasculature.

GU Thiopental decreases renal plasma flow and increases ADH secretion, leading to a decrease in the urine output. It has no effect on the tone of the gravid uterus.

Metabolic/other A slight transient decrease in the serum potassium concentration may occur, following the administration of thiopental.

Toxicity/side effects Severe anaphylactoid reactions may occur with the use of the drug, with a reported incidence of 1 in 20 000. Extravasation of the drug may lead to tissue necrosis; inadvertent intra-arterial injection may lead to arterial constriction and thrombosis. The treatment of the latter includes the administration of analgesia and alpha-adrenergic antagonists, sympathetic blockade of the limb, and anticoagulation.

Kinetics

Absorption Thiopental is absorbed when administered orally or rectally.

Distribution The drug is 65–86% protein-bound in the plasma, predominantly to albumin; 40% is sequestered in red blood cells; the V_D is 1.96 l/kg. The rapid onset of action of the drug is due to:
1. the high blood flow to the brain
2. the lipophilicity of the drug and
3. its low degree of ionization—only the non-ionized fraction crosses the blood–brain barrier (thiopental is 61% non-ionized at pH 7.4; hyperventilation increases the non-bound fraction and increases the anaesthetic effect).

The relatively brief duration of anaesthesia following a bolus of thiopental is due to redistribution to muscle and later to fat.

Metabolism Occurs in the liver by side-arm oxidation, oxidation to pentobarbital, and ring cleavage to form urea and 3-carbon fragments. Fifteen percent of the dose of the drug is metabolized per hour; 30% may remain in the body 24 hours after administration.

Excretion Occurs predominantly in the urine as inactive metabolites; 0.5% is excreted unchanged. The clearance is 2.7–4.1 ml/kg/min, and the elimination half-life is 3.4–22 hours.

Special points Volatile agents and surgery have no effect on the V_D or clearance of thiopental; morphine increases the hypnotic effect of the drug and increases its brain half-life. The drug may induce acute clinical and biochemical manifestations in patients with porphyria. Thiopental should be used with caution in patients with fixed cardiac output states, hepatic or renal dysfunction, myxoedema, dystrophia myotonica, myasthenia gravis, familial periodic paralysis, and in the elderly or in patients who are hypovolaemic.

Thiopental is not removed by dialysis.

Drug structure For the drug structure, please see Fig. 9.

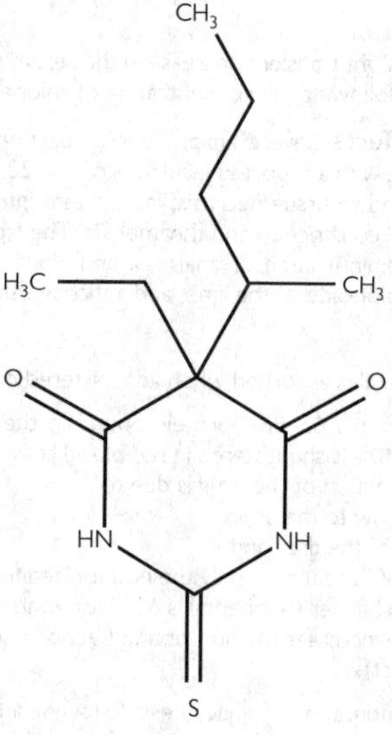

Fig. 9 Drug structure of thiopental.

Thrombolytics

Uses Thrombolytic agents are used:
1. in the treatment of acute myocardial infarction
2. in the treatment of acute ischaemic cerebrovascular events (alteplase only)
3. for the intravascular dissolution of thrombi and emboli (e.g. DVT and massive pulmonary embolism (alteplase only)) and
4. in the treatment of acute or subacute occlusion of peripheral arteries.

Chemical Thrombolytic agents are (glyco)protein structures that are either obtained from bacteria or genetically engineered. Streptokinase is a highly purified enzyme derived from beta-haemolytic streptococci of Lancefield Group C. Alteplase, reteplase, and tenecteplase are derived from Chinese hamster ovary cell lines using recombinant DNA technology.

Presentation Streptokinase, alteplase, reteplase, and tenecteplase are all presented in a powder form requiring subsequent dissolving prior to intravenous injection and/or infusion, depending on the specific agent.

Main action Fibrinolysis.

Mode of action Alteplase, reteplase, and tenecteplase are recombinant human tissue plasminogen activators (rtPA) that are fibrin-specific. These agents bind to fibrin within the thrombus, with subsequent conversion of thrombus-bound plasminogen to plasmin, leading to fibrin degradation. Streptokinase acts indirectly on plasmin; the first phase is the formation of a streptokinase–plasminogen activator complex, which then converts further plasminogen molecules to active plasmin. Plasmin then digests fibrin to produce lysis of thrombi.

Routes of administration/doses Thrombolytic agents are administered intravenously. This may be by bolus injection only, followed by further boluses and/or an intravenous infusion, depending on the type of agent being used and the regimen being followed. Streptokinase is administered by intravenous infusion. Alteplase is administered by a bolus, followed by infusion using either an 'accelerated' or a 'standard' regimen for acute myocardial infarction. For the treatment of pulmonary embolism, alteplase is administered as a 10 mg bolus over 1–2 minutes, followed by 90 mg over 2 hours. For the treatment of acute ischaemic stroke, alteplase is given over 1 hour at a dose of 0.9 mg/kg (maximum dose of 90 mg), with 10% of the dose given as a bolus. Tenecteplase is administered by a single weight-adjusted bolus, and reteplase is administered as two boluses 30 minutes apart.

Effects

CVS Transient hypotension and reperfusion arrhythmias may occur, following administration of thrombolytic agents.

Metabolic/other Fibrinolysis is produced by the action of the drug on plasmin. Following administration of streptokinase, anti-streptokinase antibodies are produced.

Toxicity/side effects Excessive haemorrhage may complicate the use of any thrombolytic agent; if serious, this should be treated by cessation of drug administration, resuscitation, and possible treatment with intravenous tranexamic acid. The risk of a haemorrhagic cerebrovascular event is 0.5–1%. Pyrexia occurs commonly, following administration of streptokinase. Allergic reactions are common with the use of streptokinase, which can be minimized with the administration of antihistamines and corticosteroids.

Kinetics Data are incomplete.

Distribution The V_D of thrombolytic agents are low: streptokinase 1.1 l, alteplase 2.8–4.6 l, reteplase 6 l, and tenecteplase 4.2–6.3 l.

Metabolism Thrombolytic agents undergo hepatic metabolism. Tenecteplase binds to specific hepatic receptors prior to conversion into small peptides.

Excretion The terminal elimination half-life of streptokinase is 83 minutes. Alteplase, reteplase, and tenecteplase undergo biphasic elimination. Alteplase is rapidly cleared from the plasma, with a plasma clearance of 550–680 ml/min. Reteplase and tenecteplase are cleared more slowly, with plasma clearance data of approximately 120 ml/min.

Special points Heparin is administered with all thrombolytic agents, apart from streptokinase. Due to the bolus-dose administration of reteplase and tenecteplase, these agents are used in pre-hospital thrombolysis, in addition to in-hospital use.

The current National Service Framework for thrombolysis for myocardial infarction states a 'call-to-needle' time of 60 minutes and a 'door-to-needle time' of 20 minutes. If the 'call-to-hospital' time is >30 minutes, then pre-hospital thrombolysis should be considered. Thrombolytic agents should not be administered to patients with contraindications to thrombolysis, as detailed in national guidelines and/or local policies.

Tramadol

Uses Tramadol is used in the management of moderate to severe pain.

Chemical A synthetic opioid of the aminocyclohexanol group. The drug is a racemic mixture of two enantiomers (+) and (−) tramadol.

Presentation As a clear aqueous solution for injection containing 50 mg/ml and tablets containing 50/100/150/200/300/400 mg of tramadol hydrochloride.

Main action Centrally mediated analgesia.

Mode of action Tramadol is a non-selective agonist at mu-, kappa-, and delta-opioid receptors (with a higher relative affinity for mu-receptors). It also inhibits neuronal reuptake of noradrenaline and enhances serotonin (5HT) release; inhibition of pain perception partly involves the activation of descending serotonergic and noradrenergic pathways.

Routes of administration/doses Tramadol may be administered orally, intramuscularly, or by slow intravenous injection or infusion. The adult dose is 50–100 mg 4- to 6-hourly for all routes of administration. The paediatric dose is 1–2 mg/kg 4- to 6-hourly.

Effects

CVS Tramadol has no clinically significant cardiovascular effects after intravenous administration.

RS The respiratory rate, minute volume, and $PaCO_2$ remain essentially unchanged, following intravenous administration of therapeutic doses of the drug.

CNS Tramadol has an analgesic potency equivalent to pethidine. The analgesic effect is only partially (30%) reversed by naloxone.

AS Tramadol has no demonstrable effect on bile duct sphincter activity. Constipation occurs uncommonly.

Toxicity/side effects The principal side effects of tramadol are nausea, dizziness, sedation, and diaphoresis. The potential for tolerance and dependence appears to be low.

Kinetics

Absorption The bioavailability following oral administration of the drug is 68–100%.

Distribution The drug is 20% protein-bound in the plasma; the V_D is 2.9–4.37 l/kg. Eighty percent of an administered dose crosses the placenta.

Metabolism 85% of an administered dose is metabolized by demethylation in the liver. One metabolite (O-desmethyltramadol) is active.

Excretion 90% of the dose is excreted in the urine, and 10% in the faeces. The clearance is 6.7–10.1 ml/kg/min, and the elimination half-life is 270–450 minutes. The elimination half-life is doubled in patients with impaired renal or hepatic function.

Special points The use of tramadol is not recommended in patients with end-stage renal failure; the dosage interval should be increased to 12 hours in patients with renal or hepatic impairment.

The drug is not licensed for intraoperative use, as it may enhance intraoperative recall during enflurane/N_2O anaesthesia.

Tramadol appears to be effective in the treatment of post-operative shivering.

The drug precipitates when mixed with diazepam or midazolam. The drug is only slowly removed by haemodialysis or haemofiltration.

Trichloroethylene

Uses Trichloroethylene is used:
1. for the induction and maintenance of general anaesthesia and has been used
2. for pain relief during labour.

Chemical A halogenated hydrocarbon.

Presentation As a blue liquid (that should be protected from light) that is coloured with waxoline blue to enable differentiation from chloroform. The commercial preparation contains 0.01% thymol, which prevents decomposition on exposure to light; it is non-flammable in normal anaesthetic concentrations. The molecular weight of trichloroethylene is 131.4, the boiling point 67°C, and the saturated vapour pressure 8 kPa at 20°C. The MAC of trichloroethylene is 0.17, the oil/water solubility coefficient 400, and the blood/gas solubility coefficient 9.

Main action General anaesthesia (reversible loss of both awareness and recall of noxious stimuli) and analgesia.

Mode of action The mechanism of general anaesthesia remains to be fully elucidated. General anaesthetics appear to disrupt synaptic transmission (especially in the area of the ventrobasal thalamus). This mechanism may include potentiation of the $GABA_A$ and glycine receptors and antagonism at NMDA receptors. Their mode of action at the molecular level appears to involve the expansion of hydrophobic regions in the neuronal membrane, either within the lipid phase or within hydrophobic sites in cell membranes.

Routes of administration/doses Trichloroethylene is administered by inhalation, conventionally via a calibrated vaporizer. The concentration used for the induction and maintenance of anaesthesia is 0.2–2%.

Effects

CVS Trichloroethylene is noted for its cardiovascular stability; the heart rate, blood pressure, and cardiac output are little altered by the administration of the drug. Trichloroethylene has a marked propensity to cause dysrhythmias and sensitizes the myocardium to the effects of circulating catecholamines.

RS The drug is moderately irritant to the respiratory tract and characteristically causes tachypnoea associated with a decreased tidal volume, which may lead to both hypoxia and hypercapnia.

CNS The principal effect of trichloroethylene is general anaesthesia; the drug also has a marked analgesic effect. The drug increases cerebral blood flow, leading to an increase in intracranial pressure. A slight decrease in skeletal muscle tone results from the use of trichloroethylene.

AS Nausea and vomiting occur commonly with the use of the drug.

GU Trichloroethylene reduces the tone of the pregnant uterus when used in concentrations of 0.5%.

Toxicity/side effects Trichloroethylene may provoke the appearance of myocardial dysrhythmias, particularly in the presence of hypoxia, hypercapnia, or excessive catecholamine concentrations.

Kinetics

Absorption The major factors affecting the uptake of volatile anaesthetic agents are solubility, cardiac output, and the concentration gradient between the alveoli and venous blood. Trichloroethylene is relatively soluble in blood; the alveolar concentration therefore reaches inspired concentration relatively slowly, resulting in a slow induction of anaesthesia. An increase in the cardiac output increases the rate of alveolar uptake and slows the induction of anaesthesia. The concentration gradient between the alveoli and venous blood approaches zero at equilibrium; a large concentration gradient favours the onset of anaesthesia.

Distribution The drug is initially distributed to organs with a high blood flow (brain, heart, liver, and kidney) and later to less well-perfused organs (muscles, fat, and bone).

Metabolism 20% of an administered dose is metabolized in the liver to yield trichloroacetic acid, monochloroacetic acid, and trichloroethanol (which is subsequently conjugated with glucuronide), and inorganic chloride.

Excretion 80% is exhaled unchanged; the metabolites are excreted in the urine over several days.

Special points Trichloroethylene should not be used in a closed circuit with soda lime, since it decomposes in the presence of heat and alkali to form hydrochloric acid, carbon monoxide, dichloroacetylene, and phosgene, all of which are toxic.

Vasopressin

Uses Vasopressin is used:

1. in the management of cranial diabetes insipidus
2. in the management of bleeding oesophageal varices
3. in the perioperative/trauma management of patients with haemophilia and von Willebrand's disease
4. in the management of polyuria and polydipsia post-hypophysectomy and
5. in the management of catecholamine-refractory septic shock.

Chemical Vasopressin is a naturally occurring nonapeptide prohormone synthesized in the paraventricular and supraoptic nuclei of the posterior hypothalamus. It is also available in three synthetic analogue forms: 8-arginine-vasopressin (argipressin) which is identical to endogenous human vasopressin; triglycyl-lysine-vasopressin (terlipressin/glypressin) which is a pro-drug requiring cleavage of three glycyl residues to form lysine-vasopressin which is found in pigs; and 1-deamino-8-O-arginine-vasopressin (desmopressin).

Presentation Argipressin is available as a clear, colourless solution in a glass ampoule containing 1 ml of argipressin for subcutaneous, intravenous, or intramuscular injection in a concentration of 20 IU/ml (= 0.4 mg argipressin). Terlipressin/glypressin is available as terlipressin acetate as a clear, colourless solution for intravenous administration in a concentration of either 0.12 mg/ml or 0.2 mg/ml. Terlipressin is also available as a white powder containing 1 mg of terlipressin acetate such that, when reconstituted in the provided 5 ml of solvent, 1 ml of solution contains 0.2 mg of the drug. Desmopressin is available as an oral lyophilizate containing 60, 120, and 240 micrograms of desmopressin acetate; as tablets containing 0.1 and 0.2 mg of desmopressin acetate; as a clear, colourless 1 ml solution containing 4 micrograms of desmopressin acetate; and as an aqueous solution for intranasal administration containing 0.01% w/v of the drug.

Main actions Antidiuresis, vasoconstriction.

Mode of action Endogenous vasopressin (or ADH) and its synthetic analogues act via G-protein vasopressin receptors V1, V2, and V3, and also has affinity for oxytocin-type receptors. V1 receptors are present in vascular smooth muscle, platelets, and myometrium. Activation of V1 receptors leads to increased intracellular calcium concentrations and vasoconstriction. V2 receptors are found in the distal renal tubule and collecting ducts, and activation leads to aquaporin-2 trafficking from intracellular vesicle membranes within renal epithelial cells into the apical cell membrane, allowing water reabsorption. V2 receptors are also present on endothelial cells, allowing von Willebrand factor (vWF) release that prevents the breakdown of factor VIII in plasma. V3 receptors are found in the pituitary and contribute to ACTH release. Oxytocin-type receptors are present on vascular smooth muscle and the myometrium, and activation results in increased NO synthase activity leading to vasodilation. Desmopressin has ten times the antidiuretic action of endogenous vasopressin, but 1500 times less vasoconstriction effect.

Routes of administration/doses Vasopressin can be administered subcutaneously, intramuscularly, intravenously, intranasally, orally, and via a sublingual route, depending on the synthetic vasopressin analogue being used. Argipressin is used in the treatment of cranial diabetes insipidus at a dose of 5–20 units subcutaneously or intramuscularly every 4 hours. In the management of bleeding varices, 20 units are administered by intravenous infusion over 15 minutes. It may also be used in the management of catecholamine-refractory septic shock by continuous infusion via a central venous catheter at a rate of 0.01–0.04 units/min. Terlipressin/glypressin is used in the management of bleeding varices, with a 2 mg dose being administered intravenously every 4 hours for a maximum of 48 hours. Desmopressin is used in the management of cranial diabetes insipidus and post-hypophysectomy polyuria/polydipsia. An initial dose of 60 micrograms sublingually, or 0.1 mg orally three times daily, is recommended. The dose should then be modified according to the clinical response. The drug may also be given intravenously, intramuscularly, or subcutaneously in the treatment of cranial diabetes insipidus at a dose of 1–4 micrograms once daily. Desmopressin may be given by intravenous infusion at a dose of 0.4 micrograms/kg in the perioperative or trauma management of patients with haemophilia or von Willebrand's disease.

Effects

CVS In the presence of shock, vasopressin causes an increase in the mean arterial pressure and systemic vascular resistance via its vasoconstrictor effect. At very low concentrations, vasopressin causes vasodilatation in certain vascular beds in animal models. It causes vasodilatation of the pulmonary artery in hypoxic and physiological conditions.

GU A reduction in the urine output and resolution of polydipsia are seen, following administration of the drug to patients with cranial diabetes insipidus.

Metabolic/other An increase in vWF and factor VIII can be detected, following administration of the drug.

Toxicity/side effects

Due to the vasoconstriction effect of vasopressin (and other catecholamines if concurrently administered), a significant reduction in cutaneous and splanchnic perfusion may occur.

Kinetics

Absorption Desmopressin is the only synthetic analogue that may be administered by an oral, sublingual, or nasal route. 0.25% of a sublingual dose is absorbed; oral administration results in 0.08–0.16% of a dose being absorbed; 10% of an administered intranasal dose is absorbed.

Distribution Argipressin is not protein-bound. It has a V_D of 0.14 l/kg. The V_D of terlipressin/glypressin is 0.5 l/kg and has a biphasic plasma level curve, suggesting a two-compartment pharmacokinetic model. The V_D of Desmopressin is 0.2–0.32 l/kg.

Metabolism Endogenous vasopressin is metabolized by vasopressinases and has a half-life of 10–35 minutes. Argipressin has a half-life of 10–20 minutes, and 35% of an administered dose undergoes enzymatic metabolism. Terlipressin/glypressin has a half-life of 50–70 minutes. Desmopressin undergoes minimal hepatic metabolism and has a half-life of 2–3 hours.

Excretion 65% of an administered dose of argipressin and desmopressin is excreted unchanged in the urine.

Vecuronium

Uses Vecuronium is used to facilitate intubation and controlled ventilation.

Chemical A bis-quaternary aminosteroid which is the mono-quaternary analogue of pancuronium.

Presentation As a lyophilized powder (containing citric acid monohydrate (20.75 mg), disodium hydrogen phosphate dihydrate (16.25 mg), mannitol (170 mg), sodium hydroxide or phosphoric acid) which is diluted in water prior to use to yield a clear, colourless, isotonic solution containing 2 mg/ml of vecuronium bromide. Mannitol is used to alter the tonicity, and the presence of either sodium hydroxide or phosphoric acid adjusts the pH to 4. The solution is stable for 24 hours.

Main action Competitive non-depolarizing neuromuscular blockade.

Mode of action Vecuronium acts by competitive antagonism of acetylcholine at nicotinic (N2) receptors at the post-synaptic membrane of the neuromuscular junction. The drug also has some pre-junctional action.

Routes of administration/doses The drug is administered intravenously. The ED90 of vecuronium is estimated to be 0.057 mg/kg. An initial dose of 0.08–0.1 mg/kg is recommended, providing muscle relaxation for between 25 and 40 minutes. Endotracheal intubation can be achieved within 90–120 seconds of an intravenous dose, with maximal resultant neuromuscular blockade achieved within 3–5 minutes following administration. Ninety-five percent recovery of the twitch height occurs within approximately 45 minutes. Maintenance of neuromuscular blockade may be achieved with bolus doses of 0.02–0.03 mg/kg. Vecuronium may be administered by intravenous infusion at a rate of 0.8–1.4 micrograms/kg/min. The drug is non-cumulative with repeated administration.

Effects

CVS Vecuronium has minimal cardiovascular effects; with large doses, a slight (9%) increase in the cardiac output and 12% decrease in the systemic vascular resistance may occur. Unlike pancuronium, the drug will not antagonize the haemodynamic changes or known side effects produced by other pharmaceutical agents or surgical factors.

RS Neuromuscular blockade leads to apnoea. Vecuronium has a very low potential for histamine release; bronchospasm is extremely uncommon.

CNS The drug has no effect on intracranial or intraocular pressure.

AS Lower oesophageal sphincter pressure remains unaltered after the administration of vecuronium.

Metabolic/other Vecuronium may decrease the partial thromboplastin time and prothrombin time.

Toxicity/side effects There have been rare reports of fatal anaphylactoid reactions with the administration of vecuronium. Cross-sensitivity may exist with rocuronium and pancuronium.

Kinetics

Distribution The drug is 60–90% protein-bound in the plasma. The V_D is 0.18–0.27 l/kg. The drug does not cross the blood–brain barrier. Very small amounts of vecuronium may cross the placenta, but not in clinically significant doses.

Metabolism Vecuronium is metabolized by deacetylation in the liver to the active metabolites 3- and 17-hydroxy and 3,17-dihydroxyvecuronium. These metabolites, which, in the case of 3-hydroxyvecuronium, may have up to 50% of the potency of vecuronium, are present in very low concentrations, although they may be of clinical significance after prolonged dosing.

Excretion 25–30% of the dose is excreted unchanged in the urine, and 20% unchanged in the bile. Metabolized drug is excreted in the bile. The clearance is 3–6.4 ml/kg/min, and the elimination half-life is 31–80 minutes. Renal failure leads to a prolongation of the elimination half-life, but to no clinically significant increase in the duration of action of vecuronium. Hepatic failure may cause a significant dose-dependent decrease in the clearance, and consequent increase in the duration of action, of the drug.

Special points The duration of action of vecuronium, in common with other non-depolarizing relaxants, is prolonged by hypokalaemia, hypocalcaemia, hypermagnesaemia, hypoproteinaemia, dehydration, acidosis, and hypercapnia. The following drugs, when co-administered with vecuronium, increase the effect of the latter: volatile anaesthetic agents, induction agents (including ketamine), fentanyl, suxamethonium, diuretics, calcium channel blockers, alpha- and beta-adrenergic antagonists, protamine, lidocaine, metronidazole, and the aminoglycoside antibiotics. Patients with burns may develop resistance to the effect of vecuronium. Onset of neuromuscular blockade is likely to be lengthened and the duration of action shortened in patients receiving chronic anticonvulsant therapy. The use of vecuronium appears to be safe in patients susceptible to malignant hyperpyrexia.

Reversal of neuromuscular-blocking activity by vecuronium may be achieved using neostigmine (in combination with glycopyrronium), but only after four twitches have returned on the train-of-four count. The gamma-cyclodextrin sugammadex may be used to reverse vecuronium-induced neuromuscular blockade by encapsulating vecuronium molecules within the plasma, thereby creating a concentration gradient favouring the movement of remaining vecuronium molecules from the neuromuscular junction back into the plasma.

Verapamil

Uses Verapamil is used in the treatment of:
1. hypertension of mild to moderate severity
2. angina and
3. paroxysmal supraventricular tachycardia, and atrial fibrillation and flutter.

Chemical A synthetic papaverine derivative.

Presentation As 40/80/120/160/180/240 mg tablets and as a clear solution for injection of a racemic mixture of verapamil hydrochloride containing 2.5 mg/ml.

Main actions Antihypertensive and antianginal.

Mode of action Verapamil causes competitive blockade of cell membrane slow Ca^{2+} channels, leading to a decreased influx of Ca^{2+} into vascular smooth muscle and myocardial cells. This results in electromechanical decoupling and inhibition of contraction and relaxation of cardiac and smooth muscle fibres, leading to coronary and systemic arterial vasodilation.

Routes of administration/doses The adult oral dose is 240–480 mg daily in 2–3 divided doses. The corresponding intravenous dose in 5–10 mg, administered over 30 seconds; the injection should cease as soon as the desired effect is achieved. The peak effect after intravenous administration occurs at 3–5 minutes, and the duration of action is 10–20 minutes.

Effects

CVS Verapamil is a class IV antiarrhythmic agent; it decreases automaticity and conduction velocity, and increases the refractory period. AV conduction is slowed; the drug appears to be taken up and bound specifically by AV nodal tissue. The drug causes a decrease in the systemic vascular resistance and is a potent coronary artery vasodilator. Verapamil has negative dromotropic and inotropic effects which are enhanced by acidosis.

CNS Cerebral vasodilation occurs after the administration of verapamil.

GU Verapamil decreases renovascular resistance.

Toxicity/side effects Oral administration of the drug may lead to dizziness, flushing, nausea, and first- or second-degree heart block. Intravenous administration may precipitate heart failure in patients with impaired left ventricular function and precipitate ventricular tachycardia or fibrillation in patients with Wolff–Parkinson–White syndrome.

Kinetics

Absorption Verapamil is completely absorbed when administered orally; the bioavailability is 10–22% due to a significant first-pass.

Distribution The drug is 90% protein-bound in the plasma; the V_D is 3.1–4.9 l/kg.

Metabolism Occurs by demethylation and dealkylation in the liver; the metabolites possess some activity.

Excretion 70% of the dose is excreted in the urine, and 16% in the faeces. The clearance is 6.8–16.8 ml/min/kg, and the elimination half-life is 3–7 hours. The dose should be reduced in patients with significant hepatic impairment.

Special points The effects of volatile agents and beta-adrenergic antagonists on myocardial contractility and conduction are synergistic with those of verapamil; caution should be exercised when these combinations are used. The drug increases the serum concentrations of co-administered digoxin.

Verapamil and dantrolene administered concurrently in animals cause hyperkalaemia, leading to ventricular fibrillation; these drugs are not recommended for use together in man. The drug decreases the MAC of halothane in animal models; chronic exposure to the drug may potentiate the actions of both depolarizing and non-depolarizing relaxants. Verapamil attenuates the pressor response to laryngoscopy and intubation.

Verapamil is not removed by haemodialysis.

Warfarin

Uses Warfarin is used:
1. in the prophylaxis of systemic embolization in patients with rheumatic heart disease and atrial fibrillation and in patients with prosthetic heart valves and
2. in the prophylaxis and treatment of DVT and pulmonary embolism.

Chemical A synthetic coumarin derivative.

Presentation As tablets containing 0.5/1/3/5 mg of a racemic mixture of warfarin sodium.

Main actions Anticoagulation.

Mode of action Warfarin prevents the synthesis of the vitamin K-dependent clotting factors (II, VII, IX, and X) in the liver. The formation of fully active clotting factors is dependent on the carboxylation of their precursor proteins; during this reaction, vitamin K is oxidized to vitamin K 2,3-epoxide; warfarin prevents the reduction of this epoxide back to vitamin K. This results in vitamin K depletion and a decrease in the rate of formation of complete clotting factors. The S-enantiomer is 2–5 times more potent than the R-enantiomer.

Routes of administration/doses The adult oral dose is usually 3–9 mg/day, according to response as measured by the prothrombin time. The maximum anticoagulant effect occurs 18–72 hours after the administration of a loading dose.

Effects Warfarin has no clinically significant effects other than its anticoagulant effect.

Toxicity/side effects Haemorrhage is the most frequent side effect. Hypersensitivity reactions and gastrointestinal upsets may occur. The drug appears to be teratogenic if taken during pregnancy.

Kinetics

Absorption The drug is rapidly and completely absorbed from the stomach and upper gastrointestinal tract, and has an oral bioavailability of 100%.

Distribution Warfarin is 99% protein-bound in the serum, predominantly to albumin. The V_D is 0.1–0.16 l/kg.

Metabolism Warfarin is virtually completely metabolized in the liver by oxidation (of the L-form) and reduction (of the D-form); these metabolites are then conjugated with glucuronide.

Excretion The metabolites are excreted in the faeces and urine. The clearance is 3.26–3.8 ml/min/kg, and the elimination half-life of warfarin ranges from 35 to 45 hours; this is decreased in patients with renal impairment.

Special points The response to warfarin treatment is monitored in the laboratory by the one-stage prothrombin time which is particularly sensitive to the activity of factors II, VII, and X. The INR should be maintained at 2–4.5 times the control value. Many factors may affect warfarin control; in particular, the drug may exhibit significant interactions with many other drugs. The activity of warfarin may be potentiated by alcohol, amiodarone, cimetidine, sulfonamides, salicylates and other NSAIDs, and many antibiotics, including co-trimoxazole, erythromycin, chloramphenicol, metronidazole, and tetracyclines. The activity of warfarin may be decreased by many drugs, including barbiturates, the oral contraceptive pill, and carbamazepine.

Control of anticoagulation in the perioperative period requires special attention. This is usually achieved by transferring the patient to heparin prior to, and immediately after, surgery; the INR should ideally be <2 for routine surgery. Acute reversal of the effects of warfarin can be achieved by the administration of prothrombin complex, especially in cases of life-threatening haemorrhage. Alternatively, 1 mg of vitamin K will reverse its effects within 12 hours, and 10 mg will prevent re-warfarinization due to the saturation of liver stores.

Spinal and epidural anaesthesia are contraindicated in patients anticoagulated with warfarin.

Xenon

Uses Xenon is used:
1. in the induction and maintenance of general anaesthesia and
2. for estimation of organ blood flow using a radioactive isotope.

Chemical An inert gas present in the atmosphere at a concentration of 0.0000087%.

Presentation As a colourless, odourless gas contained in 2, 5, and 10 l aluminium cylinders as a liquid. These correspond to a removable volume of 233, 555, and 1000 l, respectively, at 15°C and 1.013 bar. It has a molecular weight of 131, a specific gravity of 4.56, a critical temperature of 16.59°C, a critical pressure of 58.42 bar, and a boiling point of −108.1°C. The MAC of xenon is 60 ± 5, the oil:gas partition coefficient 1.9, and the blood:gas partition coefficient 0.115.

Main actions General anaesthesia and analgesia.

Mode of action The mechanism of general anaesthesia remains to be fully elucidated. Xenon non-competitively inhibits NMDA receptors by approximately 60%. Inhibition of glutamate-gated NMDA receptors by xenon provides a mechanism for its predominant analgesic profile. It also inhibits nicotinic acetylcholine receptors. In an animal model, it competitively inhibits $5HT_{3A}$ receptors. Xenon has no effect on $GABA_A$ receptors.

Routes of administration/doses Xenon is administered by inhalation, using a compatible anaesthetic machine. Maintenance of general anaesthesia is achieved at inhalational concentrations of between 51 and 69%.

Effects

CVS Xenon exhibits cardiovascular stability. No changes in the ventricular function occur during general anaesthesia, as measured by transoesophageal echocardiography. A reduction in the heart rate may be seen during use of the gas.

RS Xenon acts as a respiratory depressant, causing a reduction in the minute ventilation. The gas may improve the laminar flow and aeration of non-aerated alveoli, leading to recruitment and improved oxygenation.

CNS The principal effect of xenon is general anaesthesia, the mechanism of which remains to be fully elucidated. The analgesic effect of xenon may possibly be mediated by inhibition of NMDA receptors and effects on the spinal cord. Xenon may also confer an element of neuroprotection at sub-anaesthetic doses. However, the gas may also cause changes in cerebral blood flow, and its use can be associated with an increase in intracranial pressure in patients with traumatic brain injury.

Toxicity/side effects PONV may occur with the use of xenon.

Kinetics

Absorption As with other inhalational anaesthetic agents, the uptake of xenon is affected by its solubility, cardiac output, and the concentration gradient between the alveoli and venous blood. Due to the very low blood:gas partition coefficient of xenon, the alveolar concentration reaches inspired concentration rapidly (fast wash-in), resulting in a rapid induction (and emergence from) anaesthesia.

Distribution Xenon is initially distributed to organs with a high blood flow.

Metabolism Xenon does not undergo metabolism in man.

Excretion Xenon is excreted unchanged via the lungs.

Special points The use of xenon is safe in patients susceptible to malignant hyperpyrexia. The gas does not appear to have mutagenic, carcinogenic, or teratogenic properties. Xenon is environmentally safe to use. The gas does not potentiate the action of non-depolarizing muscle relaxants.

Appendix

Drug comparison tables

For drug comparison tables, please see Tables A1.1, A1.2, and A1.3.

Table A1.1 Physicochemical properties of inhalational anaesthetic agents

Agent	MW	BP (°C)	SVP (kPa)	MAC	Blood:gas partition coefficient	Oil:gas partition coefficient
Isoflurane	184.5	48.5	32	1.15	1.4	97
Enflurane	184.5	56.5	23.3	1.68	1.91	98
Sevoflurane	200	58.6	22.7	1.4–3.3	0.63–0.69	47–54
Desflurane	168	22.8	88.5	5.17–10.65	0.45	19
Halothane	197.4	50.2	32	0.75	2.5	224
Nitrous oxide	44	−88.5	5500	105	0.47	1.4
Xenon	131.293	−108.1	5800	60 ± 5	0.115	1.9

BP, boiling point; MAC, minimal alveolar concentration; MW, molecular weight; SVP, saturation vapour pressure.

Table A1.2 Comparison table of intravenous anaesthetic agents

Agent	pKa	pH	Protein binding (%)	Volume of distribution (l/kg)	Half-life
Propofol	11	7–8.5	98	4	9.3–69.3 minutes
Thiopental	7.6	10.8	65–86	1.96	3.4–22 hours
Ketamine	7.5	3.5–5.5	20–50	3	2.5 hours
Etomidate	4.2	8.1	76.5	4.5	1–4.7 hours

Table A1.3 Comparison table of local anaesthetic agents

Agent	pKa	% unionized at pH 7.4	Protein binding (%)	Toxic dose (mg/kg)	Onset (minutes)	Duration
Lidocaine	7.7	25%	64-70	3 (7 with adrenaline)	2-20	Variable
Bupivacaine	8.1	15%	95	2	10-20	5-16 hours
Prilocaine	7.7-7.9	33%	55	6	1-2	0.5-1 hours
Ropivacaine	8.1	15%	94	3	10-30	8-13 hours
Chloroprocaine	8.96	N/A	N/A	N/A	3-5	80-100 minutes

Index of drug derivation

Index of medical uses

Note: Tables are indicated by an italic *t* following the page number